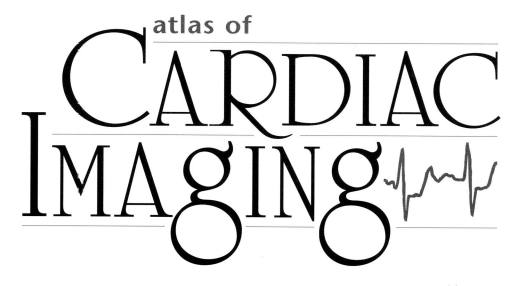

atlas of
CARDIAC IMAGING

Editors

RICHARD T. LEE, MD

Assistant Professor of Medicine
Department of Medicine
Division of Cardiology
Director
Echocardiography Laboratory
Brigham and Women's Hospital
Boston, Massachusetts

EUGENE BRAUNWALD, MD, MD (Hon), ScD (Hon)

Vice President for Academic Programs, Partners HealthCare System
Distinguished Hersey Professor of Medicine
Faculty Dean for Academic Programs at Brigham and Women's Hospital
and Massachusetts General Hospital
Harvard Medical School
Boston, Massachusetts

With 26 contributors

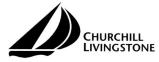
CHURCHILL
LIVINGSTONE

Developed by Current Medicine, Inc., Philadelphia

Current Medicine, Inc.

 400 Market Street
Suite 700
Philadelphia, PA 19106

Managing Editor:	Lori J. Bainbridge
Developmental Editor:	Danielle Shaw
Editorial Assistant:	Charlene French
Art Director:	Paul Fennessy
Design and Layout:	Jerilyn Bockorick
Illustration Director:	Ann Saydlowski
Illustrators:	Elizabeth Carrozza, Ann Saydlowski, and Debra Wertz
Production:	Lori Holland and Sally Nicholson
Indexing:	Alexandra Nickerson

Atlas of cardiac imaging / [edited by] Richard T. Lee, Eugene
    Braunwald.
        p. cm.
    Includes bibliographical references and index.
    ISBN 0-443-07567-0
    1. Heart–Imaging–Atlases. I. Lee, Richard T. II. Braunwald,
Eugene, 1929– .
    [DNLM: 1. Heart Diseases–diagnosis–atlases. 2. Diagnostic
Imaging–atlases.   WG 17 A8814 1998]
    RC683.5.I42A85 1998
    616.1'20754–dc21
    DNLM/DLC
    for Library of Congress

97-36794
CIP

Library of Congress Cataloging-in-Publication Data
ISBN 0-443-07567-0

Printed in the United States by Quebecor Printing
10 9 8 7 6 5 4 3 2 1

atlas of CARDIAC IMAGING

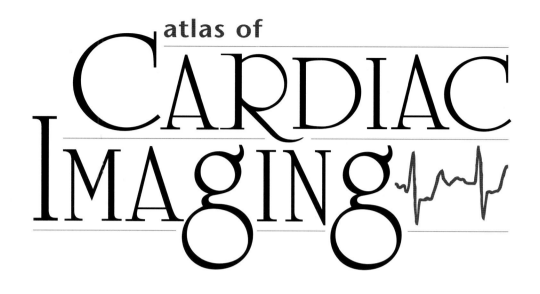

Preface

One can argue that advances in imaging have swept quickly in the era of modern cardiovascular medicine. For centuries, knowledge of the cardiovascular system often tiptoed forward very slowly through the use of postmortem examinations, such as those carried out by Leonardo da Vinci. When postmortem examination was insufficient to reveal the fundamentals of cardiovascular physiology, physicians such as William Harvey turned to animal experimentation. In contrast, in the 20th century, imaging technology allows us to make diagnoses and study pathophysiology rapidly and with great precision. It is interesting to ponder how rapidly cardiovascular medicine would have progressed if these brilliant investigators of the past had just one of the many imaging modalities available to us today.

The imaging revolution began in 1895, when roentgen rays were discovered. Only a year later, Francis Henry Williams described his work at the Massachusetts Institute of Technology showing the outline of the heart by fluoroscopy. In the past century, we have harnessed many other imaging techniques, providing patients with increased safety and improved diagnostic accuracy.

Frequently, physicians wonder which of the many available imaging techniques is best for a particular cardiovascular question. In this atlas, we present a visual overview of the rapidly changing world of cardiac imaging to try to help physicians answer this difficult question. Although imaging is entrenched in physics and engineering, no treatise on wave physics can substitute for the power of actual images of the human cardiovascular system. The widely used and invaluable techniques of ultrasound, nuclear cardiology, and angiography are presented. In addition, emerging modalities, such as magnetic resonance imaging and positron emission computed tomography scanning, are reviewed.

The imaging revolution is far from over. The costs of digital information storage and management are declining rapidly, and it is only a matter of time before all medical imaging will be digital. Faster, higher resolution, and more robust techniques will emerge as computer technology advances and costs decrease. Real-time three-dimensional ultrasound and other real-time three-dimensional techniques are on the horizon, providing the potential for three-dimensionally guided interventions. In addition, the capability of evaluating new drugs and other therapies with precise imaging will be of paramount importance in future clinical research.

Superficially, the imaging explosion is at odds with the growing constraints of health economics. How can we afford developing new technologies, and should we discourage use of these expensive tests? In fact, some imaging technologies may not find a place in cost-effective patient care and will be confined to research use or even to the graveyard of once-promising ideas. But other technologies will adapt to these economic constraints by becoming more cost-effective while continuing to improve. For example, today's ultrasound machines cost less than did machines only several years ago but provide dramatically superior images.

We are rapidly moving toward an era in which cardiovascular diagnosis will be almost exclusively noninvasive, and procedures with risk will be reserved only for carefully planned therapeutic interventions. We hope this atlas provides a glimpse of this exciting future.

– Richard T. Lee, MD
– Eugene Braunwald, MD, MD (Hon), ScD (Hon)

Contributors

JEAN M. ALESSI, RVT
Technical Director
Vascular Diagnostic Laboratory
Brigham and Women's Hospital
Boston, Massachusetts

JOSHUA A. BECKMAN, MD
Fellow
Department of Internal Medicine
Harvard Medical School
Brigham and Women's Hospital
Boston, Massachusetts

RICHARD C. BRUNKEN, MD
Staff
Director of Nuclear Cardiology
Department of Nuclear Medicine
The Cleveland Clinic Foundation
Cleveland, Ohio

ERIC Q. CHEN, PhD
Assistant Staff
Nuclear Instrumentation
The Cleveland Clinic Foundation
Cleveland, Ohio

STEFANO DE CASTRO, MD
Assistant Professor
Department of Clinical Medicine
University of Rome
Rome, Italy

ROBERT R. EDELMAN, MD
Associate Radiologist-in-Chief for Academic Affairs
Director, Magnetic Resonance Imaging
Professor of Radiology
Beth Israel Deaconess Medical Center
Boston, Massachusetts

MARIE GERHARD, MD
Instructor
Department of Internal Medicine
Harvard Medical School
Associate Physician
Brigham and Women's Hospital
Boston, Massachusetts

RAYMUNDO T. GO, MD
Chairman
Department of Nuclear Medicine
The Cleveland Clinic Foundation
Cleveland, Ohio

GEORGE G. HARTNELL, FRCR, FACC
Associate Professor of Radiology
Department of Radiology
Harvard Medical School
Director
Cardiovascular and Interventional Radiology
Beth Israel Deaconess Medical Center
Boston, Massachusetts

LISA K. HORNBERGER, MD
Assistant Professor
Department of Paediatrics
University of Toronto Faculty of Medicine
Staff Cardiologist
Director, Fetal Cardiac Program
The Hospital for Sick Children
Toronto, Ontario, Canada

TSUI-LIEH HSU, MD
Associate Professor
Department of Internal Medicine
Veterans General Hospital–Taipei
Taipei, Taiwan, Republic of China

KRISHNA KANDARPA, MD, PhD
Associate Professor
Department of Radiology
Harvard Medical School
Co-director
Cardiovascular and Interventional Radiology
Brigham and Women's Hospital
Boston, Massachusetts

SCOTT KINLAY, PhD, FRACP
Research Fellow
Department of Medicine
Harvard Medical School
Interventional Fellow
Brigham and Women's Hospital
Boston, Massachusetts

CHRISTOPHER M. KRAMER, MD
Assistant Professor
Department of Medicine
Allegheny University of the Health Sciences
Assistant Professor of Medicine
Allegheny General Hospital
Pittsburgh, Pennsylvania

RICHARD T. LEE, MD
Assistant Professor of Medicine
Department of Medicine
Division of Cardiology
Director
Echocardiography Laboratory
Brigham and Women's Hospital
Boston, Massachusetts

WARREN J. MANNING, MD
Associate Professor
Departments of Medicine and Radiology
Harvard Medical School
Co-director
Cardiac Magnetic Resonance Center
Beth Israel Deaconess Medical Center
Boston, Massachusetts

FINN MANNTING, MD, PhD
Associate Professor
Department of Radiology
Harvard Medical School
Director
Nuclear Medicine
Brigham and Women's Hospital
Boston, Massachusetts

MICHAEL V. McCONNELL, MD, MSEE
Instructor in Medicine
Department of Medicine
Cardiovascular Division
Harvard Medical School
Associate Physician
Brigham and Women's Hospital
Boston, Massachusetts

ADHIP MUKERJEE, MD
Instructor
Department of Radiology
Harvard Medical School
Radiologist
Brigham and Women's Hospital
Boston, Massachusetts

NATESA G. PANDIAN, MD
Associate Professor
Departments of Medicine and Radiology
Tufts University School of Medicine
Director
Cardiovascular Imaging and Hemodynamic
   Laboratory
New England Medical Center
Boston, Massachusetts

ROBERT N. PIANA, MD
Assistant Professor
Department of Medicine
Harvard Medical School
Associate Director of Interventional Cardiology
Brigham and Women's Hospital
Boston, Massachusetts

SHARON C. REIMOLD, MD
Assistant Professor of Medicine
Department of Medicine
Division of Cardiology
Harvard Medical School
Assistant Director
Echocardiography Laboratory
Brigham and Women's Hospital
Boston, Massachusetts

MARCY L. SCHWARTZ, MD
Instructor in Pediatrics
Department of Pediatrics
Harvard Medical School
Assistant in Cardiology
Children's Hospital
Boston, Massachusetts

JAMES D. THOMAS, MD, FACC
Professor of Medicine and Biomedical Engineering
Cleveland Clinic Health Sciences Center of The
   Ohio State University
Director of Cardiovascular Imaging
The Cleveland Clinic Foundation
Cleveland, Ohio

CHING-YEE OLIVER WONG, MD, PhD
Assistant Professor
Department of Radiology
Ohio State University College of Medicine
Assistant Staff
Director of Nuclear Neurologic Imaging
The Cleveland Clinic Foundation
Cleveland, Ohio

JIEFEN YAO, MD
Instructor in Medicine
Department of Medicine
Tufts University School of Medicine
Cardiology Research Fellow
New England Medical Center
Boston, Massachusetts

Contents

Chapter 5

DIGITAL ECHOCARDIOGRAPHY
James D. Thomas

Chapter 6

ADVANCED CORONARY IMAGING
Robert N. Piana and Scott Kinlay

Chapter 7

COMPUTED TOMOGRAPHY IMAGING OF THE HEART
George G. Hartnell

Chapter 8

MAGNETIC RESONANCE IMAGING OF CORONARY AND VASCULAR STRUCTURES
Michael V. McConnell, Warren J. Manning, and Robert R. Edelman

CHAPTER 1

Echocardiography in Acquired Heart Disease

Sharon C. Reimold ~ Richard T. Lee

Echocardiography is the most commonly used method of imaging the heart. Over the past two decades, advances in echocardiography have dramatically improved our clinical care of patients with valvular disease, myocardial disease, and pericardial disease. These advances include two-dimensional ultrasound imaging, color Doppler, and transesophageal imaging, with each major advance revealing new critical information. In addition to reliable evaluation of left ventricular function and regional wall motion, we can now study myocardial ischemia and viability with echocardiographic techniques. Echocardiography can also provide precise quantitative measurements of valve function, eliminating the need for catheterization in many patients. For some valvular diseases, Doppler echocardiography precision equals that of catheterization. The clinical diagnosis of cardiac tamponade is greatly aided by echocardiography, and the technical approach to relieving tamponade is often based on ultrasound images. Cardiac masses, even as small as a few millimeters in size, can be readily visualized.

Transesophageal echocardiography, considered experimental only a decade ago, is now a routine and important test with many clear indications. Transesophageal echocardiography is essential in the diagnosis of perivalvular abscesses, aortic dissection, left atrial thrombi, prosthetic valve disease, cardiac masses, and many other conditions.

Advances in imaging are offering higher frequency (and thus higher resolution) imaging with improved image quality. Improved image quality may even be found in more inexpensive and smaller new systems, as the use of digital ultrasound techniques becomes optimized. Because of the portability and relatively low cost of ultrasound technology, echocardiography will probably remain the foundation of cardiac imaging for the forseeable future.

The echocardiography revolution is not yet complete. Despite the advances of the past two decades, many important questions in echocardiography remain unanswered. How do we best evaluate mitral regurgitation, one of the most common and important adult cardiac diseases? How do we best use exercise and pharmacologic echocardiography? Will there be an ultrasonic myocardial perfusion agent that will enable echocardiographic perfusion imaging? How do we optimally use transesophageal echocardiography, a safe but more invasive test? In addition, the medical economic environment will create new questions on when to use echocardiography.

The expansion of echocardiography in clinical cardiology has been so explosive that many clinicians have lamented the substitution of echocardiography for bedside clinical skills. The first few decades of echocardiography's use have demonstrated that the technique does not substitute for bedside clinical cardiology skills but is a valuable adjunct in the hands of an experienced operator. With more advances on the way, we will continue to see echocardiography contribute to improved patient care.

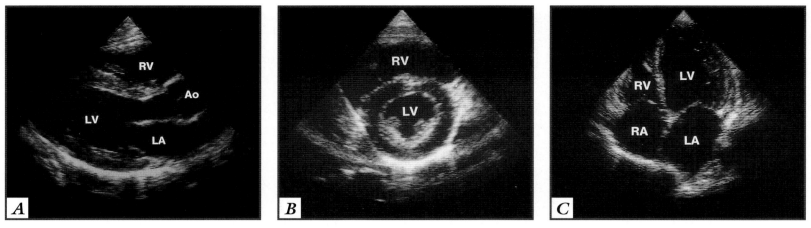

FIGURE 1-1. Echocardiographic features of a normal heart. The standard echocardiographic study includes parasternal long-axis, short-axis, apical, subcostal, and suprasternal imaging, including M-mode, two-dimensional, and Doppler information. Careful visualization of each valve and segment of myocardium is performed, often requiring optimization of images of one structure in a view, and then optimizing another portion of the image.

A, Parasternal long-axis view showing left ventricle (LV), aorta (Ao), left atrium (LA), and right ventricle (RV). **B,** Parasternal short-axis view at the midpapillary muscle level depicting the LV and the RV. **C,** Apical four-chamber view showing both ventricles, LA, and right atrium (RA). In addition to these views, subcostal and suprasternal images should be attempted as components of a complete two-dimensional imaging study. (*From* Kisslo [1]; with permission.)

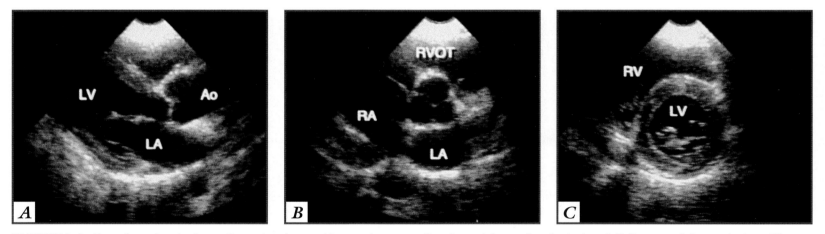

FIGURE 1-2. Two-dimensional echocardiography of normal heart valves. Direct imaging of the valves often reveals the nature of valvular pathology. Cardiac valvular structures may be visualized from parasternal, apical, and subcostal imaging windows in the adult subject. Two-dimensional echocardiography allows assessment of valvular morphology as well as function throughout the cardiac cycle. Shown here are parasternal long- and short-axis images of normal mitral and aortic valves. **A,** The mitral valve is open in

diastole, and the aortic valve is closed. **B,** Parasternal short-axis views. The normal aortic valve has three leaflets and forms a triangular-shaped opening in systole. This view demonstrates valve leaflet morphology, such as in aortic stenosis or bicuspid aortic valve. **C,** In parasternal short-axis views in diastole, the mitral leaflets open, forming a circular orifice. Ao—aorta; LA—left atrium; LV—left ventricle; RA—right atrium; RV—right ventricle; RVOT—right ventricular outflow tract. (*Courtesy of* Peter C. Nishan and Rick A. Nishimura.)

VALVULAR DISEASE: IDENTIFICATION AND QUANTIFICATION

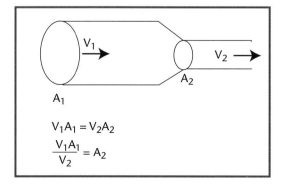

$$V_1 A_1 = V_2 A_2$$

$$\frac{V_1 A_1}{V_2} = A_2$$

FIGURE 1-3. Calculation of valve areas by the continuity equation. By the principle of conservation of mass, the flow passing through a cylindrical area is equal to the product of the area (A) and the velocity of blood (V) passing through that area. If blood passes through an area (A_1) and then must pass through a smaller area (A_2), flow through these two areas (Q_1 and Q_2) must be the same unless there are losses to the system. Therefore, $A_1 \bullet V_1 = A_2 \bullet V_2$. By rearranging this equation algebraically, one can solve for cross-sectional areas.

This principle may be applied when calculating valve areas in patients with valvular stenosis. The valve area in aortic stenosis may be calculated using the following variables: A_1 (the cross-sectional area of the left ventricular outflow tract), V_1 (the velocity of blood flow through the left ventricular outflow tract), and V_2 (the continuous-wave Doppler velocity of blood flow through the aortic valve). By integrating the velocity time integrals, the mean valve area during systole may be calculated. This method is also the basis of the Gorlin equation used in the catheterization laboratory. The Doppler echocardiographic correlation correlates well with catheterization laboratory–based calculations of aortic valve area when the measurements are made simultaneously [2].

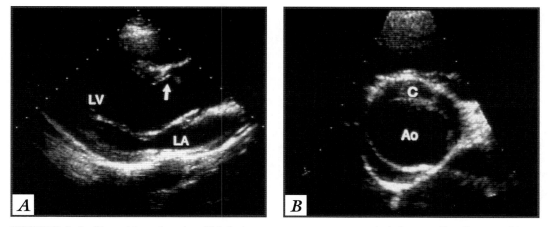

visualization of leaflet morphology is obtained from the parasternal short-axis view where the open orifice of a bicuspid valve has an ovoid shape. Bicuspid aortic valves may be associated with a raphe, a remnant of the third leaflet. The most common configuration for the bicuspid commissures is inadequate separation of the left and right coronary cusps. Bicuspid aortic valves may be associated with stenosis or regurgitation; even when there is no significant hemodynamic dysfunction, bicuspid valves are associated with increased risk of endocarditis or ascending aortic disease. As with other valvular abnormalities, determination of the degree of hemodynamic dysfunction is greatly aided by Doppler recordings. Ao—aorta; C—single cusp from "fused" right and left coronary cusps; LA—left atrium; LV—left atrium. (*Courtesy of Peter C. Nishan and Rick A. Nishimura.*)

FIGURE 1-4. Bicuspid aortic valve. This is the most common congenital abnormality diagnosed in adulthood. **A,** Bicuspid aortic valve may be suspected from the parasternal long-axis views if there is eccentric closure of the aortic leaflets or "doming" (*arrow*) of the aortic leaflets in systole. **B,** Direct

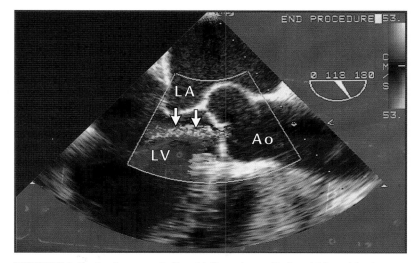

FIGURE 1-5. Aortic regurgitation. Unlike minor mitral and tricuspid valve regurgitation, aortic regurgitation is a normal finding in less than 1% of the population. Estimating the severity of aortic regurgitation is often based on a

composite assessment, which includes left ventricular (LV) systolic and diastolic dimensions as well as systolic function. LV size and function reflect the response of the ventricle to the regurgitant lesion. With the advent of color-flow Doppler, it became possible to assess disease severity by measuring the width of the diastolic color flow disturbance in the LV outflow tract. Jet widths of less than 25% of the outflow tract correlate with mild regurgitation, 25% to 40% of the outflow tract correlate with moderate regurgitation, and greater than 40% of the outflow tract correlates with severe regurgitation [3].

Color jet width may be directly measured by transesophageal echocardiography as well as transthoracic imaging. In this image from a transesophageal study, the outflow tract and diastolic flow disturbance is seen, in which 20% of the outflow tract is filled with the color jet abnormality (*arrows*), consistent with mild aortic regurgitation (AR). Use of jet width alone may lead to errors, however, because patients with nonuniform orifices may appear to have unusually narrow or wide jet widths by color-flow Doppler.

The assessment of AR severity should include pulsed-wave Doppler in the aortic arch. Patients with significant AR have diastolic flow velocity reversal that persists throughout diastole. As the amount of regurgitation increases, the absolute velocities of the flow reversal also increase. Velocities in excess of 18 cm/s indicate important AR. Ao—aorta; LA—left atrium; LV—left ventricle.

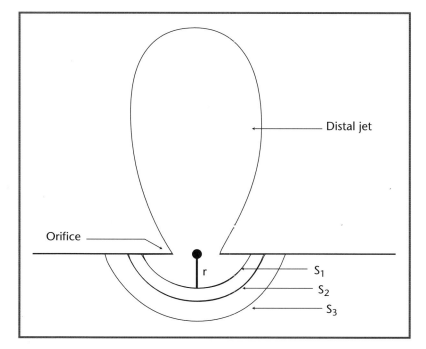

FIGURE 1-6. The proximal flow convergence method to calculate transvalvular flow rates. The size of a color Doppler regurgitant jet can be misleading as a parameter of regurgitant volume. Another method to evaluate regurgitation is based on blood flow in the proximal side of the regurgitant orifice, where blood flow is not turbulent. As blood flows toward a narrow orifice, flow accelerates. This pattern of flow acceleration may be visualized by color-flow Doppler. Color Doppler is based on repeated pulses of ultrasound, and any pulsed-wave technique will have an upper limit of velocity measurement, called the *Nyquist velocity*. This velocity is shown as a sudden change in color by the ultrasound device. For a uniform central orifice, acceleration of flow into the orifice is visualized as a series of hemispheric color rings that alternate colors as flow velocities exceed the Nyquist velocity. Flow rates through the orifice may be estimated by the PISA (proximal isovelocity surface area) method. The PISA may be approximated by $2\pi r^2$, where r is the radius of the isovelocity hemispheric shell. The flow rate may then be calculated by multiplying the PISA by the velocity of that shell as determined by the color velocity settings [4]. S_1—first isovelocity surface area; S_2—second isovelocity surface area; S_3—third isovelocity surface area.

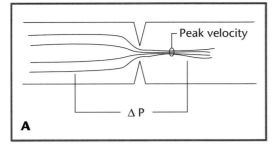

FIGURE 1-7. Calculating pressure gradients across stenotic valves. Estimates of gradients across the aortic valve (AV) may be made using continuous-wave Doppler of peak velocity through the AV by application of the modified Bernoulli equation. **A,** The peak velocity may be used to calculate the peak instantaneous gradient using the modified Bernoulli equation (pressure gradient [mmHg] = $4V^2$). This is a simplified equation but is very useful in clinical echocardiography. **B,** The instantaneous pressure gradient is almost always greater than is the catheterization laboratory–derived "peak to peak" gradient. This pressure tracing depicts simultaneous aortic and left ventricular pressure tracings from a patient with aortic stenosis. There is actually no true "peak to peak" gradient because the two peaks occur at different times, and the peak instantaneous gradient is the actual maximal gradient.

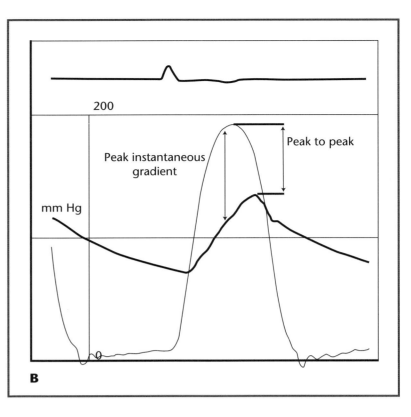

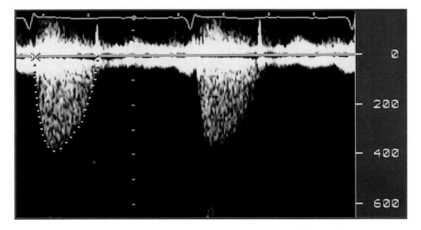

FIGURE 1-8. Aortic stenosis. The two most common etiologies associated with aortic stenosis (AS) are senile degeneration of a trileaflet valve and structural degeneration of a bicuspid aortic valve. Rheumatic AS is becoming less prevalent in the United States. Severe AS is often identified from two-dimensional images as an echogenic, nonmobile valve. In many cases of advanced disease, it is difficult to estimate severity of AS from images alone. However, by applying the modified Bernoulli equation, the pressure gradient in AS may be estimated by peak continuous-wave Doppler recordings of flow through the aortic valve. In addition, the valve area can be calculated using the continuity equation. Modern echocardiography devices have software packages to perform these calculations during the examination. In the example shown here, the peak instantaneous gradient is 59.6 mm Hg, and the calculated valve area is 0.73 cm^2, consistent with moderate to severe AS.

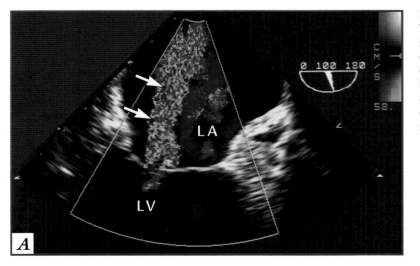

FIGURE 1-9. Eccentric versus noneccentric mitral regurgitant (MR) jets. The area of the systolic color flow disturbance in the left atrium reflects the severity of MR, but area alone can be deceiving. The area of the color-flow disturbance may be influenced by a number of parameters, including jet eccentricity. MR jets that are eccentric may appear smaller relative to the regurgitant volume due to the Coanda effect [5]. These jets may hug the atrial wall and wrap around the back of the atrium. In fact, the most severe cases of MR may have narrow eccentric jets. **A,** A central jet of MR (*arrows*) shown from a transesophageal echocardiographic image.

(Continued on next page)

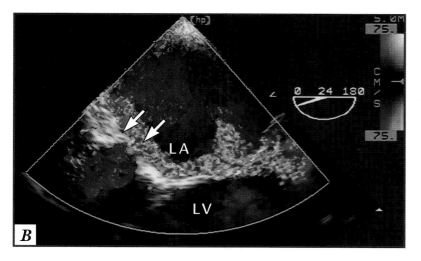

FIGURE 1-9. (*Continued*) **B,** An eccentric jet of MR (*arrows*) identified by transesophageal echocardiography. Although the jet sizes are relatively similar, the patient with the eccentric jet of regurgitation had much more severe MR as shown by left ventriculography. In patients with eccentric MR, it is crucial to carefully examine pulmonary venous flow by Doppler, because reversal of pulmonary venous flow in systole indicates important regurgitation. LA—left atrium; LV—left ventricle.

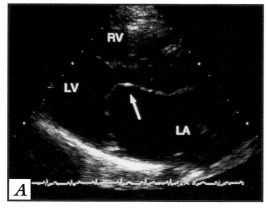

FIGURE 1-10. Mitral stenosis (MS). Rheumatic MS may be identified by transthoracic echocardiography, and the hemodynamic severity of the lesion is determined by Doppler echocardiography. **A,** The mitral valve (MV) anterior leaflet opens in a doming fashion due to fusion of the commissures. In this parasternal long-axis view, the anterior leaflet cannot open completely (*arrow*). **B,** From the parasternal short-axis view, the MV leaflets have the classic "fish-mouth" deformity. In addition, valve thickening, leaflet mobility, subvalvar calcification, leaflet fusion, and leaflet calcification should be noted because these features are useful in determining suitability for percutaneous balloon valvuloplasty in patients with severe MS [6]. Patients with extensive calcification as well as increased leaflet thickness and decreased pliability are less likely to have a successful outcome with percutaneous balloon valvuloplasty. LA—left atrium; LV—left ventricle; RV—right ventricle. (*Courtesy of* Peter C. Nishan and Rick A. Nishimura.)

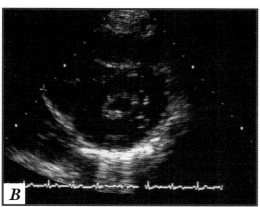

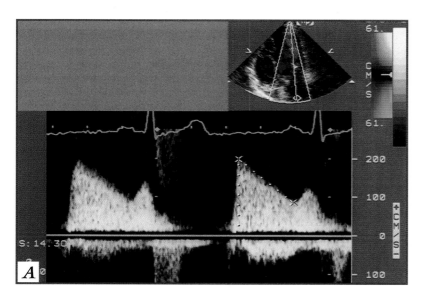

FIGURE 1-11. Quantitation of mitral stenosis (MS). Assessment of the severity of MS may be performed using various Doppler methods. The pressure half-time ($t_{1/2}$) method is based on an empiric relationship between mitral valve (MV) area and the deceleration time (DT) of the pressure decay. **A,** Continuous-wave Doppler is recorded through the tips of the mitral leaflets. Velocity is related to pressure by the relationship $4V^2 = P$, where V is velocity in m/sec and P is the pressure in mm Hg. The peak and mean pressure gradients across the MV may be calculated from continuous-wave Doppler recordings.

(Continued on next page)

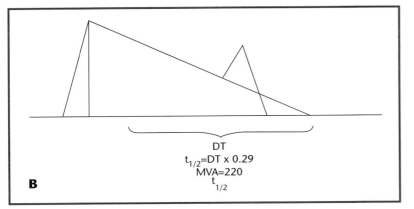

$$DT$$
$$t_{1/2}=DT \times 0.29$$
$$MVA=\frac{220}{t_{1/2}}$$

B

FIGURE 1-11. (*Continued*) **B,** The pressure half-time (the time it takes the pressure to drop by 50%) may be calculated as the time it takes velocity to fall to 70% of its original value. MV area (MVA; in cm^2) may be calculated as 220/pressure half-time [7]. Use of this equation to calculate the MVA is reliable in most cases; the presence of significant aortic regurgitation, recent valvuloplasty, or valve repair may lead to discrepancies.

An alternative method of determining MVA is to use planimetry. Using standard parasternal short-axis imaging, the smallest opening in the mitral leaflets is identified and traced in its most opened position. Although this technique generally correlates well with catheterization laboratory–based valve areas, increases in valve area associated with balloon valvuloplasty may be difficult to determine because the mechanism of increasing valve area with valvuloplasty is related to commissural fracture.

The third method for assessing MVA is the continuity equation. Left ventricular outflow tract diameter and velocity time integrals may be used as "knowns" in this calculation. Continuous-wave Doppler is recorded through the MV, and the valve area may be calculated. This is the most reliable method for determining MVA following balloon valvuloplasty and commissurotomy. Detection of mitral regurgitation, assessment of right heart function, and estimation of pulmonary arterial pressure are also important components of the assessment of a patient with MS.

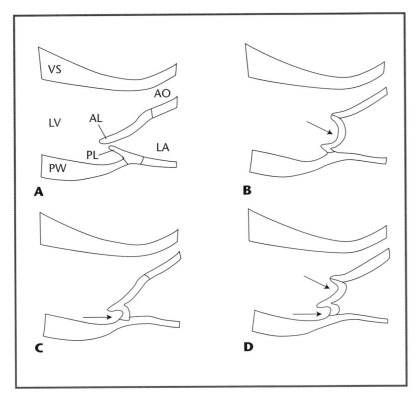

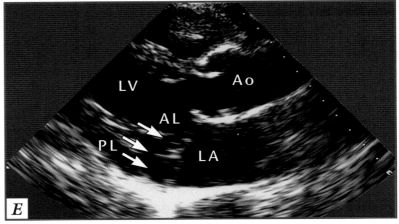

FIGURE 1-12. Mitral valve prolapse (MVP). MVP appears as systolic billowing of either or both mitral leaflets into the left atrium (LA). Determination of leaflet thickness and detection of valvular regurgitation are important in determining the management of these patients [8]. **A–D,** Patterns of mitral valve closure in the parasternal long-axis view. **A,** Normal mitral valve closure. **B,** Predominantly anterior leaflet prolapse (*arrow*). **C,** Predominantly posterior leaflet prolapse (*arrow*). **D,** Prolapse of both leaflets (*arrow*). **E,** Two-dimensional echocardiogram of prolapse of both mitral leaflets in systole (*arrows*). AL—anterior leaflet; Ao—aorta; LV—left ventricle; PL—posterior leaflet; PW—posterior wall; VS—ventricular septum. (*Courtesy of* Sumanth D. Pabhu and Robert A. O'Rourke.)

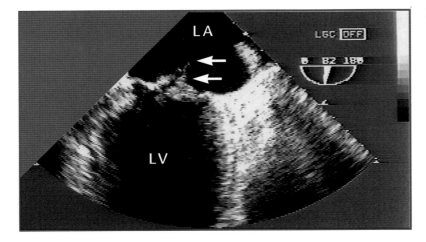

FIGURE 1-13. Myxomatous degeneration of the mitral valve (MV). Prolapse of MV leaflets should be given the most concern when accompanied by chordal rupture, leaflet thickening, or endocarditis. In this transesophageal echocardiogram, all three of these complications are present. Ruptured chords (*arrows*) are seen prolapsing into the left atrium (LA). In addition, the mitral leaflets are thick consistent with myxomatous degeneration. On the left ventricular (LV) side of the MV, a small additional structure is seen that proved to be a bacterial vegetation at surgery. It may be difficult to diagnose bacterial endocarditis in the presence of severe myxomatous degeneration of MV tissue due to the baseline distortion of the valve anatomy.

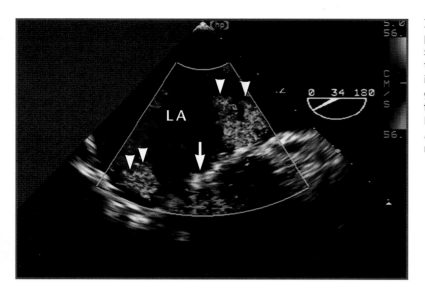

FIGURE 1-14. Perivalvular mitral regurgitation. The detection of mitral prosthetic regurgitation and perivalvular regurgitation may be difficult using standard transthoracic imaging due to shadowing of the left atrium (LA) by the nonbiologic materials of the prosthesis. For this reason, transesophageal imaging is much more sensitive to the detection of mitral prosthetic regurgitation. In this patient with hemolytic anemia and severe heart failure following mitral replacement with a St. Jude valve (*arrow*), color-flow Doppler imaging revealed two areas of abnormal regurgitation (*arrowheads*). These jets originate outside the sewing ring, indicating perivalvular regurgitation.

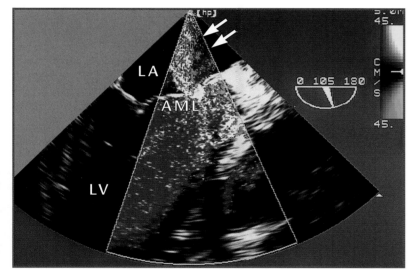

FIGURE 1-15. Mitral valve (MV) perforation. Perforation of valve leaflets is an uncommon complication of endocarditis. This complication may be suspected if a color jet of regurgitation arises from a site remote from commissures. In this patient undergoing transesophageal echocardiography for endocarditis, a turbulent jet of regurgitation (*arrow*) in the left atrium (LA) is seen arising from the anterior mitral leaflet (AML) away from the MV commissure. At the time of surgical repair, a 2-mm defect caused by bacterial erosion was found in the base of the AML. LV—left ventricle.

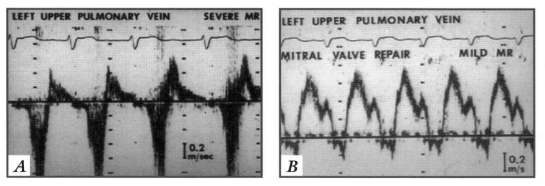

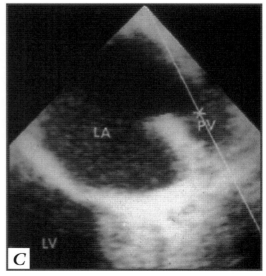

FIGURE 1-16. Pulmonary venous flow patterns. The evaluation of mitral regurgitant (MR) severity should include an assessment of pulmonary venous flow patterns. Pulmonary venous flow patterns normally show biphasic flow in systole and diastole. As MR severity increases, the systolic velocity of this flow becomes blunted, and systolic flow reversal is found in severe cases. **A,** Doppler recordings from the pulmonary veins (PVs) of a patient with severe MR are shown with prominent systolic flow reversal. **B,** Following mitral valve repair, not only has the systolic flow reversal resolved, the normal biphasic appearance of pulmonary venous flow has reappeared. **C,** With current imaging techniques, transthoracic determination of pulmonary venous flow patterns is possible in approximately 70% of patients. Determination of pulmonary venous flow patterns with transesophageal echocardiography, as shown here, is possible in nearly all patients. LA—left atrium; LV—left ventricle. (*Adapted from* Freeman and coworkers [9]; with permission.)

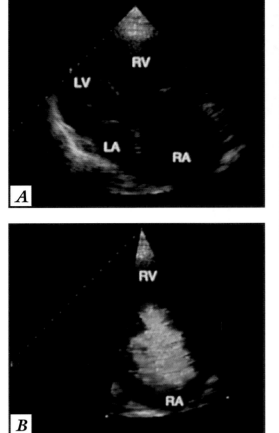

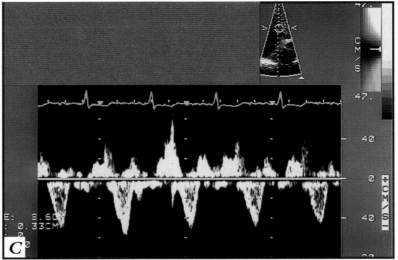

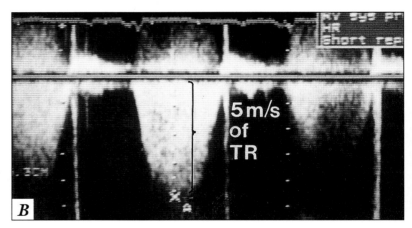

FIGURE 1-17. Tricuspid regurgitation. Doppler evidence of minor tricuspid regurgitation (TR) may be found in over 75% of normal subjects. Using two-dimensional and Doppler echocardiography, the degree of dysfunction is determined. **A,** The right atrium (RA) and right ventricle (RV) are dilated in this apical view from a patient with rheumatic TR. **B,** TR is detected as a systolic color-flow disturbance in the RA. The severity of TR may be estimated from the width and size of the jet within the RA. **C,** Severe TR is accompanied by pulsed-Doppler systolic flow reversal in the hepatic veins, the Doppler correlate of a "pulsatile liver" on physical examination. This pulsed-wave Doppler recording from the hepatic veins of a patient with severe TR shows retrograde flow in systole into the hepatic veins (flow above the baseline in systole). LA—left atrium; LV—left ventricle. (*Courtesy of* Peter C. Nishan and Rick A. Nishimura.)

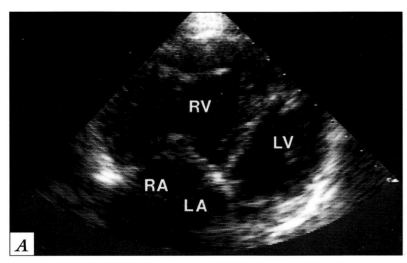

FIGURE 1-18. Pulmonary hypertension. Doppler echocardiography in primary and secondary causes of pulmonary hypertension may be used to estimate pulmonary pressures as well as right ventricular (RV) hypertrophy and function. **A,** In the apical four-chamber view of the heart, the RV is severely hypertrophied. Two-dimensional evaluation of motion allows assessment of RV function. **B,** Almost all patients with significant pulmonary hypertension will have at least mild tricuspid regurgitation (TR) that can be investigated with continuous-wave Doppler. The velocity of TR flow may be used to estimate the pulmonary artery systolic pressure. The RV systolic pressure may be estimated as $4V^2$ plus right atrial (RA) pressure. In patients

without significant RV outflow or pulmonic valve obstruction, RV systolic pressure will approximate pulmonic artery systolic pressure. In this example the peak velocity of the TR jet is 5 m/s, which is consistent with a pulmonary artery systolic pressures of 100 mm Hg greater than RA pressure.

In patients in whom an etiology for the pulmonary hypertension is unknown, it is important to exclude an atrial septal defect as cause for the disorder. Using a combination of pulsed and color Doppler echocardiographic methodologies as well as saline contrast echocardiography, it is usually possible to identify an intracardiac shunt if present. IVC—inferior vena cava; LV—left ventricle; TV—tricuspid valve. (*Courtesy of* Evan Loh.)

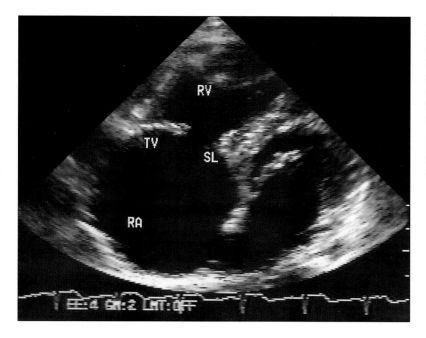

FIGURE 1-19. Carcinoid heart disease. Carcinoid tumors produce metabolites that injure cardiac valves [10]. Because 5-hydroxyindoleacetic acid and other metabolites are cleared by the pulmonary circulation, hepatic metastases from carcinoid tumors most commonly affect the tricuspid and pulmonic valves. Carcinoid valvular damage leads to diffuse leaflet thickening and shortening. This results in a decrease in valvular mobility that is frequently manifest as mixed regurgitation and stenosis of the valves. In this apical view, the right atrium (RA) is massively enlarged. The right ventricle (RV) is also enlarged due to the RV volume overload of tricuspid regurgitation, and the tricuspid leaflets are thickened and stenotic. SL—septal tricuspid leaflet; TV—anterior tricuspid valve leaflet. (*Courtesy of* Melvin D. Cheitlin and John S. MacGregor.)

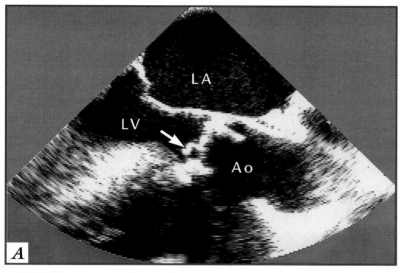

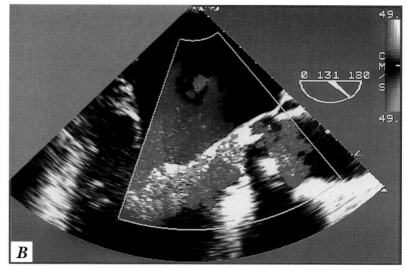

FIGURE 1-20. Aortic bioprosthetic endocarditis. Vegetations associated with bioprosthetic and mechanical valves often require transesophageal echocardiography for diagnosis. **A,** Transesophageal echocardiogram in a patient who presented with dyspnea and fatigue. A mobile lesion on the ventricular aspect of an aortic bioprosthesis is seen (*arrow*). This lesion is

approximately 8 mm long and was not visible by transthoracic echocardiography. **B,** Diastolic left ventricular (LV) outflow tract turbulence by color flow Doppler due to aortic regurgitation caused by this vegetation. Ao—aorta; LA—left atrium.

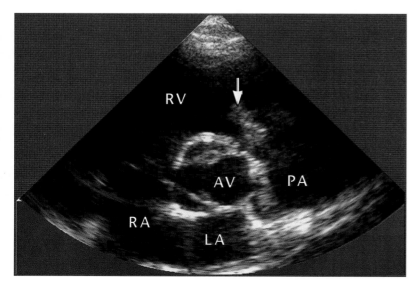

FIGURE 1-21. Pulmonic valve vegetation. Vegetations often appear as shaggy masses attached to the valve leaflets, but sometimes only as thickened leaflets. Transthoracic echocardiography can reliably identify vegetations that are 4 to 5 mm in diameter. Smaller lesions (1 to 2 mm) generally require diagnosis with transesophageal echocardiography. Transesophageal echocardiography is more sensitive in the detection of perivalvular abscesses, an important complication of endocarditis, and may more readily identify echocardiographic evidence of infection in patients with prosthetic valves.

Right-sided endocarditis involving the tricuspid or pulmonic valve is usually due to intravenous drug abuse. This short-axis transthoracic echocardiographic view shows a 2-cm-long mass engulfing the pulmonic valve (*arrow*). This vegetation caused severe pulmonic insufficiency as well as septic pulmonary embolization. Pulmonic valve vegetations are much less common than tricuspid valve lesions. AV—aortic valve; LA—left atrium; PA—pulmonary artery; RA—right atrium; RV—right ventricle.

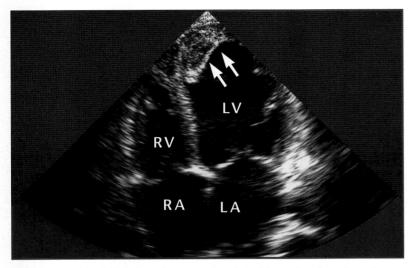

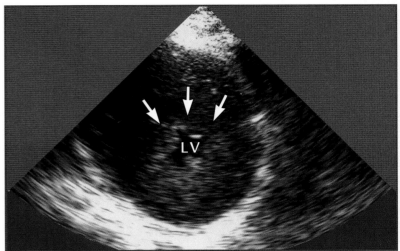

FIGURE 1-22. Dilated cardiomyopathy. Apical four-chamber view of dilated cardiomyopathy with apical thrombus. Dilated cardiomyopathy may have ischemic or nonischemic causes. In the nonischemic form, the left ventricle (LV) is dilated and has thin walls. Global systolic contractile function is depressed. Some mild regional dyssynergy may be apparent as well. Mitral regurgitation frequently accompanies dilated cardiomyopathy and is caused by mitral annular and LV dilatation. A complication of dilated cardiomyopathy is the formation of an LV thrombus due to stagnant blood flow. This apical four-chamber view demonstrates biatrial and LV enlargement. A laminated echodensity of 4.5 cm is seen in the LV apex consistent with an apical thrombus (*arrows*). The apical thrombus is more or less echogenic in its center, indicating liquefaction of the thrombus. LA—left atrium; RA—right atrium; RV—right ventricle.

FIGURE 1-23. Hypertrophic cardiomyopathy. Hypertrophic cardiomyopathy is an autosomal dominant disorder related to various mutations in the myosin heavy chain, tropomyosin, or other genes. This disorder is associated with atrial and ventricular arrhythmias and symptoms related to abnormal left ventricular (LV) filling and LV outflow tract obstruction. Some kindreds have a high incidence of sudden cardiac death.

The classic morphologic appearance of a patient with hypertrophic cardiomyopathy includes severe septal thickening (1.3 or greater times the posterior wall thickness [*arrows*]). As more cases have been examined, it is now clear that many patients exhibit concentric LV hypertrophy [11]. This short-axis view in a patient with familial hypertrophic cardiomyopathy demonstrates severe concentric hypertrophy, although the posterior wall of the LV is also severely hypertrophied. A complete echocardiogram would also include M-mode recordings evaluating systolic anterior motion of the mitral valve leaflets and Doppler recordings of the degree of LV outflow tract obstruction.

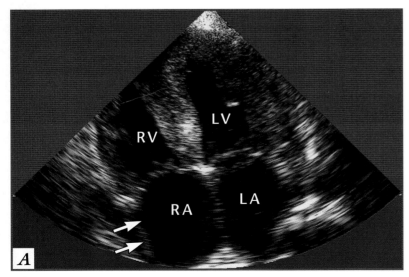

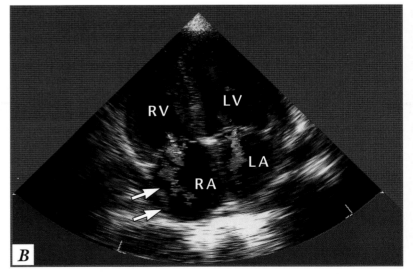

FIGURE 1-24. Amyloidosis. One of the most common infiltrative processes resulting in restrictive cardiomyopathy is amyloidosis due to amyloid protein deposition in the myocardium. Cardiac amyloid is more common in the "primary" light chain disease than the "secondary" amyloid of chronic inflammatory disorders. **A,** Apical four-chamber view demonstrating that left ventricular (LV) and right ventricular (RV) myocardium are thickened [12]. Often the myocardium may appear echogenic and has been called "sparkling." The absence of increased myocardial echogenicity, however, should not exclude the diagnosis of amyloidosis because this

finding is subjective and insensitive. The interatrial septum may become thickened and the atria dilate from the increased filling pressures. Small pericardial effusions are common (*arrows*). Systolic function is generally preserved until late in the disease, but diastolic filling abnormalities may be an early manifestation of this process. **B,** The amyloid protein may infiltrate the valves as well as the myocardium, resulting in thickened valve leaflets that are frequently at least mildly incompetent. *Arrows* indicate small pericardial effusions. LA—left atrium; RA—right atrium.

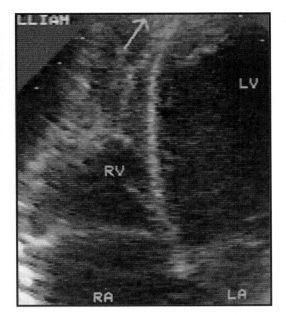

FIGURE 1-25. Chagas' disease. Chagasic myocarditis is one of the most common causes of cardiomyopathy in Central and South America. Chagas' disease causes severe left ventricular (LV) dilatation and dysfunction that may resemble typical idiopathic dilated cardiomyopathy. In 50% of patients, the LV apex or right ventricular (RV) apex will have an apical bulge or aneurysm (*arrow*). This abnormality may be small and appear as a finger-like projection. In this apical four-chamber view, a projection is seen extending off the apical segment of the RV. In addition to this focal abnormality, the LV is dilated and hypokinetic. LA—left atrium; RA—right atrium.

CARDIAC MASSES

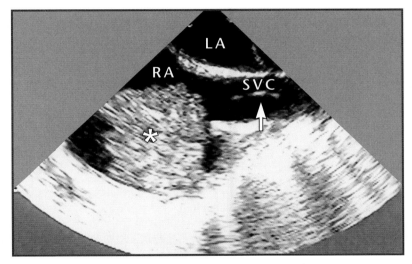

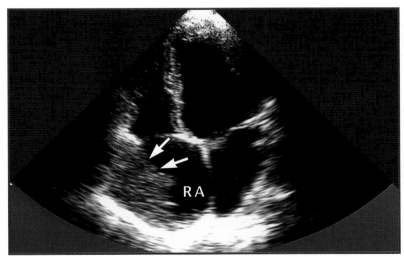

FIGURE 1-26. Atrial myxoma. Cardiac myxomas are the most common primary cardiac tumor. Usually located in the atrium, these masses tend to be mobile and typically attach to the interatrial septum. The tumors are more common in the left atrium (LA) than in the right atrium (RA), but may also be found in the ventricles. These tumors may be found incidentally but are more likely to be discovered after the development of symptoms of valve obstruction or embolization. Tumors may occur in multiple sites and in the ventricle as well, particularly in familial cases [13].

Visualization of the tumors is often possible with transthoracic echocardiography. In some cases, transesophageal echocardiography (TEE) may yield more definitive information. This TEE image demonstrates a large myxoma (*asterisk*) within the RA that was attached along the atrial free wall. Because of the patient's history of breast carcinoma and the site of attachment of the lesion, the patient underwent endovascular biopsy of the lesion with transesophageal guidance prior to surgical removal of the myxoma. *Arrow* indicates bioptome. SVC—superior vena cava.

FIGURE 1-27. Atrial sarcoma. The differential diagnosis for intracardiac masses includes thrombi, vegetations, primary cardiac tumors, and metastatic lesions to the heart [14]. This apical four-chamber view in a patient presenting with dyspnea shows an enlarged right atrium (RA). The lateral aspect of the RA is invaded by a homogenous mass (*arrows*). Note that the surface of the mass within the atrium appears irregular. Biopsy of lung and RA masses demonstrated angiosarcoma.

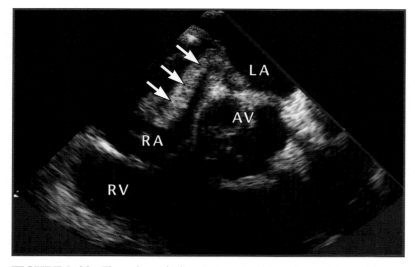

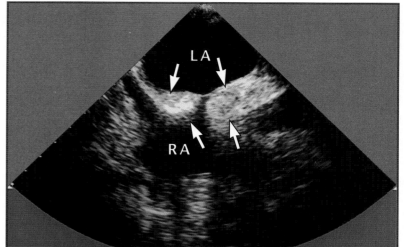

FIGURE 1-28. Thromboembolism in transit. Although most thrombi pass directly through the right heart and embolize to the lungs, some thrombi may become lodged in the right atrium (RA) or even become trapped in a patent foramen ovale (*arrows*). This transesophageal image was taken from a woman with a transient neurologic event. This thrombus is a linear deep venous thrombus lodged in the interatrial septum. Prompt surgical removal of thrombus as well as closure of the patent foramen is usually indicated in these cases. For mobile leg vein thrombi found in the RA, therapy with surgery and thrombolytic agents has been performed successfully. AV—aortic valve; LA—left atrium; RV—right ventricle.

FIGURE 1-29. Lipomatous hypertrophy of the interatrial septum. Fat may accumulate in the pericardial space, atrioventricular groove, and the interatrial septum. Because fat is echogenic, fat accumulation in the interatrial septum may create the appearance of a thick interatrial septum, which may exceed 1 cm in thickness and may be confused with a cardiac tumor. The appearance of the interatrial septum is distinctive in that fat rarely invades the fossa ovalis. In this transesophageal echocardiogram, the interatrial septum is quite thick (*arrows*) with a thin fossa ovalis. LA—left atrium; RA—right atrium.

AORTIC DISEASE

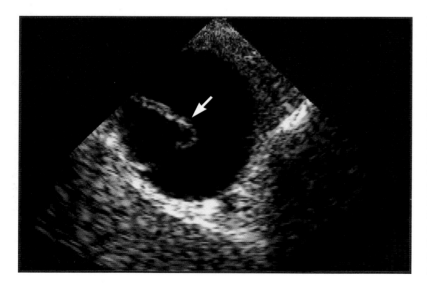

FIGURE 1-30. Aortic dissection. The descending aorta distal to the left subclavian artery may be visualized with transesophageal echocardiography (TEE). In this patient with a near circumferential aortic dissection, the intimal flap is visualized (*arrow*). The thickness of the intimal flap may vary. The sensitivity and specificity for detecting aortic dissections by TEE is similar to that of computed tomography and only slightly less than that of magnetic resonance imaging. The aortic arch is a blind-spot for transesophageal imaging due to the interposition of the trachea. The sensitivity of transthoracic imaging is far less than that of transesophageal imaging. In addition to localization and identification of the dissection flap, the echocardiographer should note the presence or absence of a pericardial effusion and aortic valve dysfunction as well as the location of the flap relative to the coronary artery ostia. Because mortality from aortic dissections is very high (1% to 2% per hour), a primary advantage of TEE is that the diagnosis can be established in the emergency room in minutes. Intramural hematoma occurs when the dissection is contained within the aortic media. This may occur in the ascending or descending aorta and is identified on imaging studies as a regionally thickened aortic wall (> 7 mm), which may be crescentic or circular [15,16].

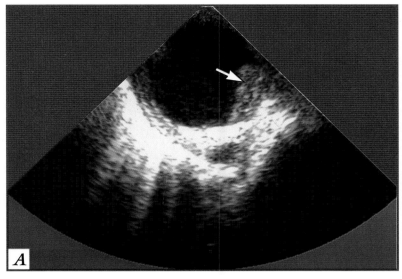

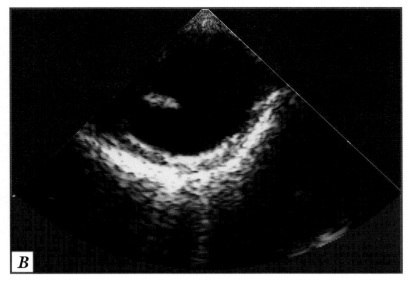

FIGURE 1-31. Aortic atheroma. In addition to the detection of dissections, aortic atheroma may be detected by transesophageal imaging. Atheroma appears as increased thickening of the aortic wall or as a complex of lesions with protruding masses or mobile thrombi [17]. **A,** This image shows an eccentric lesion found at the three o'clock position (*arrow*).

B, Increased aortic wall thickness with a mobile protruding mass consistent with an attached thrombus. Multiple studies have found a correlation between the complexity of aortic atheromata and the subsequent development of cerebrovascular accidents. Atheroma may be seen in both the ascending and the descending aorta.

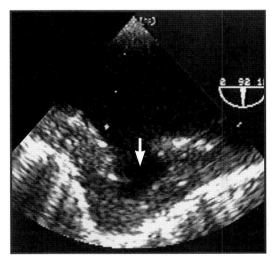

FIGURE 1-32. Aortic pseudoaneurysm. Rupture of the aorta is usually fatal. On occasion the rupture is "contained" and forms a pseudoaneursym, similar to a left ventricular pseudoaneursym, which may form after a myocardial infarction. This image is a longitudinal view of the descending aorta with a finger-like projection off the aorta (*arrow*). The walls of this projection were made of inflammatory material at the time of surgery with adjacent adherent lung tissue. *Haemophilus* species were cultured from the periaortic fluid but not from the aortic wall, which is consistent with an inflammatory pseudoaneurysm.

CORONARY ARTERY DISEASE

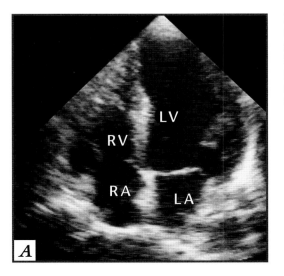

FIGURE 1-33. Coronary artery disease and wall motion abnormalities. Wall motion abnormalities may provide objective evidence of the presence of coronary artery disease. In patients suffering myocardial infarction, the involved myocardium becomes dysfunctional. This myocardium may thicken in systole less than normal (hypokinesis), fail to thicken (akinesis), or bulge outward in systole (dyskinesis). Wall motion abnormalities are often localized by identifying hinge points, an area of the myocardium that abruptly changes from normal to abnormal. **A,** In this four-chamber apical view, the myocardium appears normal at end-diastole.

(*Continued on next page*)

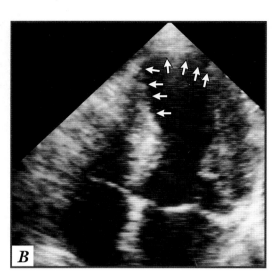

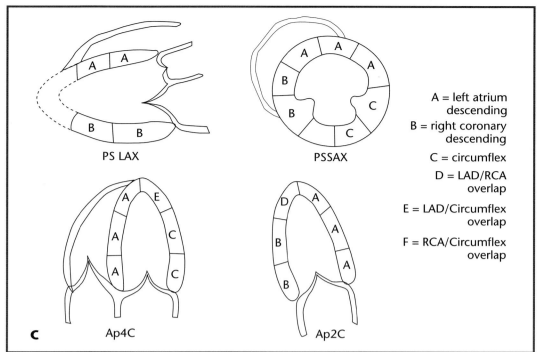

A = left atrium
descending

B = right coronary
descending

C = circumflex

D = LAD/RCA
overlap

E = LAD/Circumflex
overlap

F = RCA/Circumflex
overlap

PS LAX

PSSAX

Ap4C

Ap2C

FIGURE 1-33. (*Continued*) **B,** At end-systole, the base of the heart thickens. The apex of the heart (*arrows*) does not thicken and is akinetic. **C,** Correspondence between coronary artery distribution and the underlying myocardial segments in typical echocardiographic views. Understanding the correspondence between coronary artery anatomy and underlying myocardium may be useful in predicting the diseased vessel on stress echocardiographic images. A—left anterior descending artery; Ap2C—apical two chamber; Ap4C—apical four chamber; B—right coronary artery; C—circumflex; D—left anterior descending/right coronary artery overlap; E—left anterior descending/circumflex artery overlap; F—right coronary artery/circumflex overlap; LA—left atrium; LV—left ventricle; PS LAX—parasternal long axis; PS SAX—parasternal short axis at the midventricular level; RA—right atrium; RV—right ventricle. (*Courtesy of* Michael H. Picard and Arthur E. Weyman.)

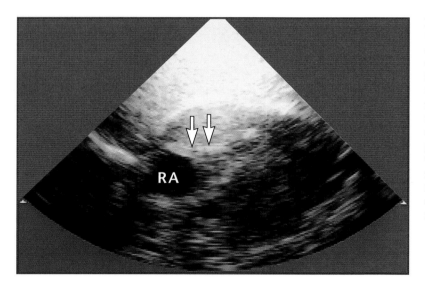

FIGURE 1-34. Myocardial rupture. Myocardial rupture is an uncommon but frequently lethal complication of myocardial infarction (MI). This complication generally occurs 3 to 5 days following an MI and is more common in single-vessel than in multivessel disease. It may be heralded by a brief episode of chest pain, but frequently presents as cardiac arrest. Echocardiographic evidence of myocardial rupture generally involves identification of echodense material (*arrows*) in the pericardial space. This material may appear gelatinous or homogeneous, and is caused by blood in the pericardial space. Identification of this abnormality constitutes a surgical emergency; rarely this finding is noted antemortem. If identified following cardiovascular collapse, surgical survival is very poor. This subcostal view shows normal-sized right and left ventricular chambers. There is 3 to 4 cm of dense material inferior to the right ventricle consistent with thrombus in the pericardial space. In this case the rupture was caused by an anterior MI. RA—right atrium.

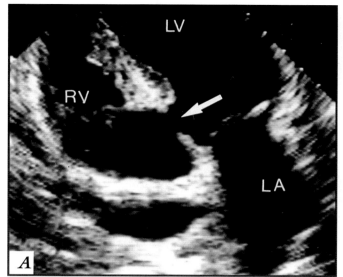

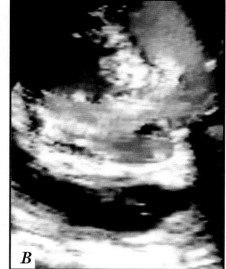

FIGURE 1-35. Ventricular septal rupture. Rupture of the interventricular septum is an uncommon complication of myocardial infarction (MI). The clinical presentation of a patient with a ventricular septal defect (VSD) following MI may include symptoms of acute heart failure and the detection of a new systolic murmur. The primary differential diagnosis of a new systolic murmur following MI is mitral regurgitation and VSD.

Imaging patients with suspected VSDs involves careful attention to all views for echo-dropout of the interventricular septum and color Doppler evidence of interventricular flow.

For example, inferior septal rupture may be difficult to identify except with subcostal imaging. **A,** In this image, a VSD is noted by transthoracic imaging (*arrow*). **B,** Color-flow Doppler confirms the presence of left-to-right flow across the septum. In addition to identifying the site and magnitude of shunting across the defect, careful attention should be paid to right ventricular systolic function, because this affects the outcome of surgery in patients with this complication. LA—left atrium; LV—left ventricle; RV—right ventricle. (*Courtesy of* Michael H. Picard and Arthur E. Weyman.)

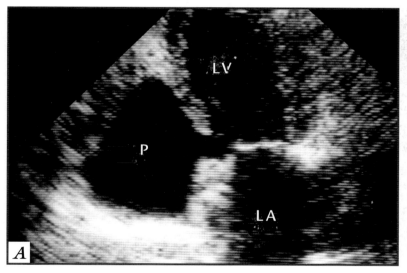

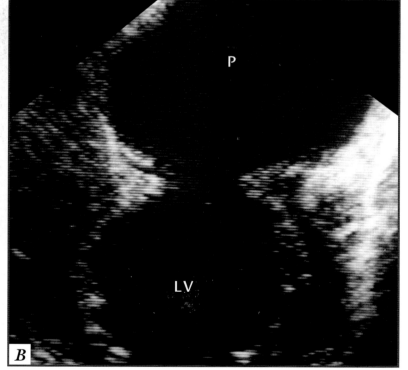

FIGURE 1-36. Left ventricular pseudoaneurysm (P). Myocardial rupture frequently results in marked hemodynamic instability and cardiac arrest. Occasionally, blood from the myocardial rupture is contained by the pericardium, and a pseudoaneurysm forms. The walls of the pseudoaneurysm are composed of organized thrombus instead of myocardium. Blood flows between the left ventricle (LV) and the pseudoaneurysm cavity with a "to and fro" pattern. Flow velocities into the pseudoaneurysm may be extremely low, and thrombus may form within this area. In general, pseudoaneurysms have a narrow neck relative to the size of the chamber. Surgical repair of pseudoaneurysms is generally recommended due to the increased risk of late rupture. **A,** Inferior wall pseudoaneurysm. The neck is narrow relative to the size of the pseudoaneurysm. **B,** Transesophageal echocardiogram in the same patient. LA—left atrium. (*Courtesy of* Michael H. Picard and Arthur E. Weyman.)

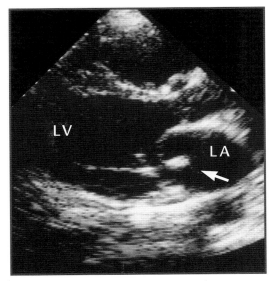

FIGURE 1-37. Papillary muscle rupture. Parasternal long-axis view showing a portion of a papillary muscle prolapsing into the left atrium (LA). In this example, the anterolateral papillary muscle was ruptured—a very unusual complication. Papillary muscle rupture may cause acute mitral regurgitation (MR) following myocardial infarction. Acute rupture results in severe MR. The ruptured muscle and its attached chordae and leaflet prolapse into the LA (*arrow*). This complication most frequently occurs in the posteromedial papillary muscle because it derives its blood supply from one coronary artery (posterior descending artery). The anterolateral papillary muscle has a dual blood supply that tends to protect the muscle. This structural abnormality may be accompanied by color-flow Doppler evidence of severe MR. In many cases, jet eccentricity, elevated LA pressure, and tachycardia may lead to an underestimation of the severity of MR based on color Doppler area. LV—left ventricle. (*Courtesy of* Michael H. Picard and Arthur E. Weyman.)

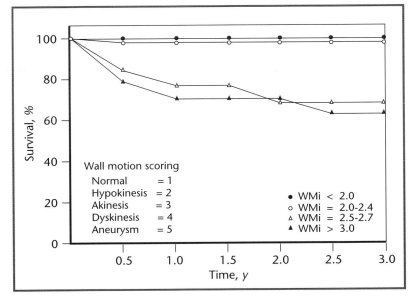

FIGURE 1-38. Prognosis depending on wall motion index (WMi). Survival following myocardial infarction is strongly related to residual left ventricular (LV) function, which is influenced by infarct size as well as by the presence or absence of ischemia. The extent and severity of wall motion abnormalities on transthoracic echocardiograms correlate with clinical status and likelihood of complications. This figure displays the survival of 50 patients with chronic coronary artery disease stratified by WMi. Survival is inversely related to an increase in the WMi (worsening of LV function). (*Adapted from* Shiina and coworkers [18]; with permission.)

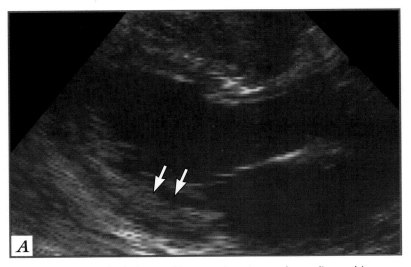
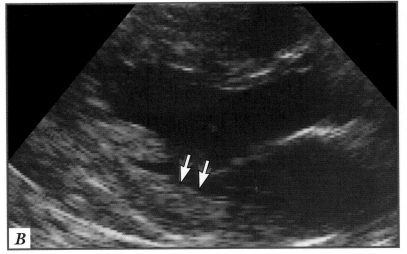

FIGURE 1-39. Displaying and interpreting stress echocardiographic images. Echocardiography may be used as an imaging tool to assess regional wall motion abnormalities that occur in response to stress [19]. Many different modalities may be combined with echocardiography, including those that increase myocardial oxygen demand (*eg*, exercise or dobutamine) and those that alter coronary artery blood flow distribution (*eg*, dipyridamole and adenosine).

Most stress echocardiographic studies are acquired and displayed using a digital technique that allows selection and storage of a cardiac cycle from each plane. For exercise echocardiography, images from rest, peak exercise, and recovery may be selected and displayed in a format for side-by-side comparison. For dobutamine echocardiography, images from rest, low dose, peak dose, and recovery are selected and displayed. Each segment may be compared for each stage of the protocol and compared with the distribution of coronary arteries. This figure shows the quad screen format of parasternal long-axis images from a patient undergoing a dobutamine stress echocardiogram following an inferoposterior myocardial infarction.

A, Stage 1 displays rest images; the posterior base is severely hypokinetic (*arrows*). **B,** Stage 2 is at low dose (5 μg/kg/min) with improvement of motion in the posterior base (*arrows*).

(*Continued on next page*)

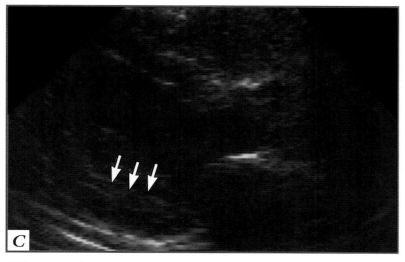

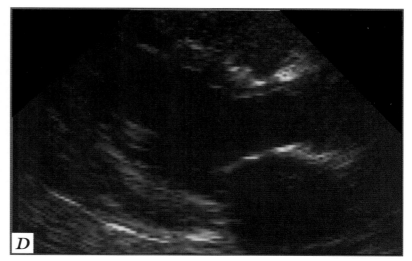

FIGURE 1-39. (*Continued*) **C,** Stage 3 is at peak dose (40 µg/kg/min); the posterobase has become akinetic (*arrows*). **D,** Stage 4 image is obtained at recovery and demonstrates hypokinesis of the posterior base.

These results may be interpreted as follows: the posterior base has viable myocardium because it is hypokinetic at baseline and augments with low-dose dobutamine infusion. The posterior base is also ischemic because it becomes akinetic with high-dose dobutamine infusion. This patient was found to have 75% stenoses in the left circumflex and posterior descending coronary arteries. (*Courtesy of* Michael H. Picard and Arthur E. Weyman.)

Sensitivity and Specificity of Exercise Echocardiography Compared with Thallium-201 SPECT

	Echocardiography, n/n(%)	Thallium-201 SPECT, n/n(%)
Sensitivity		
One vessel	24/41(58)	25/41(61)
Two vessel	25/29(86)	25/29(86)
Three vessel	15/16(94)	15/16(94)
Specificity	23/26(88)	21/26(81)

FIGURE 1-40. Sensitivity and specificity of exercise echocardiography compared with thallium-201 single photon emission computed tomography (SPECT). In this study of 112 patients, significant coronary artery disease was defined by a greater than 50% narrowing on angiography. Sensitivity was almost identical between stress echocardiography and thallium, but a small difference was noted in the specificities between these two techniques in this study [20].

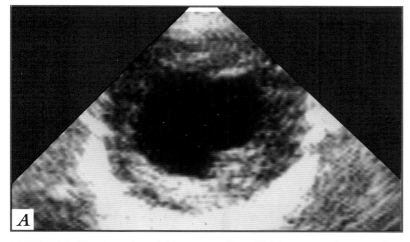

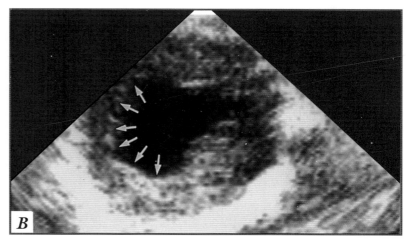

FIGURE 1-41. Assessing viable myocardium. Viable myocardium may be identified by dobutamine echocardiography [21]. These parasternal short-axis images are from an animal model of viable but ischemic myocardium.

This model is performed by flow reduction in the mid–left anterior descending artery. **A,** At baseline, the left ventricle has normal shape at end-diastole. **B,** Akinetic area in the anterior wall (*arrows*) at end-systole.

(Continued on next page)

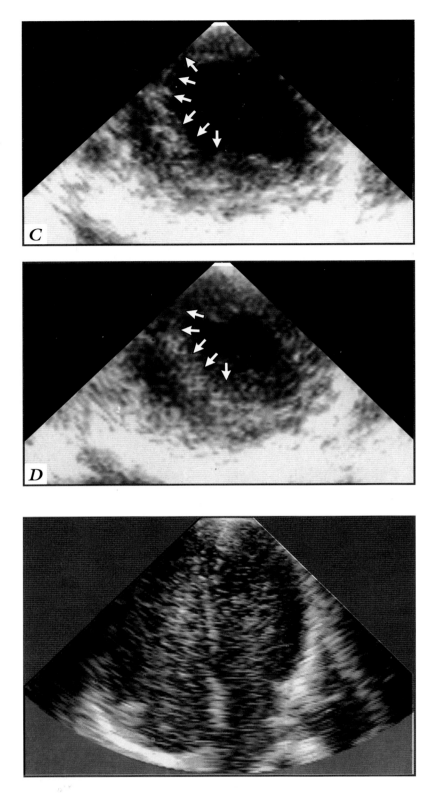

FIGURE 1-41. (*Continued*) Following a 10 µg/kg/min infusion of dobutamine, an improvement in wall motion is seen in end-diastole (**C**) and end-systole (**D**). (*Courtesy of* Michael H. Picard and Arthur E. Weyman.)

FIGURE 1-42. Contrast echocardiography. Agitated saline may be used to produce ultrasonic contrast in the heart. In normal individuals, the agitated saline is injected into an intravenous line and passes into and through the right heart, where the microbubbles are visible. The microbubbles in the injection are cleared by the pulmonary circulation and never reach the left heart. Contrast may reach the left heart via an intracardiac or extracardiac communication. In patients with atrial septal defects or patent foramen ovale, contrast may be shunted from the right to left atrium when the right atrial pressure is elevated relative to left atrial pressure.

Extracardiac shunting may occur when contrast passes into the pulmonary vasculature containing one or more pulmonary arteriovenous malformations. The air is not cleared by the malformations and is returned to the left heart via the pulmonary veins. This example is from a patient with dyspnea and systemic oxygen desaturation. The underlying disorder is cirrhosis. Six cardiac cycles after the contrast is seen in the right heart, dense saline contrast is seen in the left heart consistent with the diagnosis of pulmonary arteriovenous malformations. The time delay between appearance of contrast in the right and left heart is crucial because contrast from intracardiac shunting is generally seen in the left heart after 1 to 2 cardiac cycles. New contrast agents that can pass through the pulmonary vasculature are being evaluated. These new agents may prove useful for evaluating myocardial perfusion and enhancing endocardial definition by echocardiography [22].

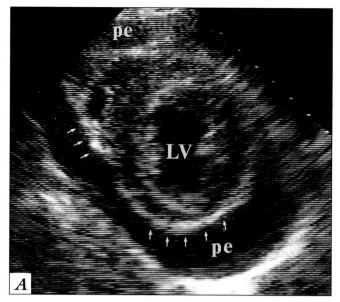 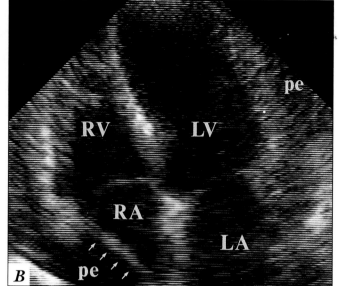

FIGURE 1-43. Pericardial effusion (pe). Echocardiography has the ability to identify pericardial fluid and evaluate the hemodynamic effects of a pericardial effusion. Effusions may be localized or circumferential. These figures show a moderate-sized effusion in a patient with scleroderma. **A,** In the parasternal short-axis view the effusion is located predominantly posteriorly. Posteroinferior visceral pericardial thickening (*arrows*) can also be seen.

B, The right atrium (RA) appears compressed (*arrows*) on the apical view. Hemodynamic abnormalities associated with pericardial tamponade include RA collapse, right ventricular diastolic indentation, respirophasic flow velocity changes, and a nonpulsatile, dilated inferior vena cava. LA—left atrium; LV—left ventricle; RV—right ventricle. (*Courtesy of* Carlos A. Roldan.)

REFERENCES

1. Kisslo J: *Echocardiography: A Slide Atlas.* New York: Medi Cine Productions; 1988.

2. Oh JK, Taliercio CP, Holmes DR Jr, *et al.*: Prediction of the severity of aortic stenosis by Doppler aortic valve area determination: prospective Doppler-catheterization correlation in 100 patients. *J Am Coll Cardiol* 1988, 11:1227–1234.

3. Perry GJ, Helmcke F, Nanda NC, *et al.*: Evaluation of aortic insufficiency by Doppler color flow mapping. *J Am Coll Cardiol* 1987, 9:952–959.

4. Bargiggia G, Tronconi L, Sahn D, *et al.*: A new method for quantification of mitral regurgitation based on color-flow Doppler imaging of flow convergence proximal to regurgitant orifice. *Circulation* 1991, 84:1481–1489.

5. Cape E, Yoganathan P, Weyman A, *et al.*: Adjacent solid boundaries alter the size of regurgitant jets on Doppler color-flow maps. *J Am Coll Cardiol* 1991, 17:1094–1102.

6. Reid CL, Chandratna PA, Kawanishi DT, *et al.*: Influence of mitral valve morphology in double balloon catheter balloon valvuloplasty in patients with mitral stenosis. *Circulation* 1989, 80:515–524.

7. Hatle LK, Angelson B, Romsdal T, *et al.*: Noninvasive assessment of the atrioventricular halftime by Doppler ultrasound. *Circulation* 1979, 60:1096–1104.

8. Devereux RB, Kramer-Fox R, Kligfield P: Mitral valve prolapse: causes, clinical manifestations, and management. *Ann Intern Med* 1989, 111:305–317.

9. Freeman WK, Schaff HV, Khandheria BK, *et al.*: Intraoperative evaluation of mitral valve regurgitation and repair by transesophageal echocardiography: incidence and significance of systolic anterior motion. *J Am Coll Cardiol* 1992, 20:599–609.

10. Pellikka PA, Tajik AJ, Khandheria BK, *et al.*: Carcinoid heart disease: clinical and echocardiographic spectrum in 74 patients. *Circulation* 1993, 87:1188–1196.

11. Solomon SD, Wolff S, Watkins H, *et al.*: Left ventricular hypertrophy and morphology in familial hypertrophic cardiomyopathy associated with mutations of the beta-myosin heavy chain gene. *J Am Coll Cardiol* 1993, 22:498–505.

12. Klein MD, Hatle LK, Burstow DJ, *et al.*: Characterization of left ventricular diastolic function in amyloidosis. *J Am Coll Cardiol* 1989, 13:1017–1026.

13. Carney JA: Differences between nonfamilial and familial cardiac myxoma. *Am J Surg Pathol* 1985, 9:53–55.

14. Colucci WS, Braunwald E: Primary tumors of the heart. In *Heart Disease: A Textbook of Cardiovascular Medicine* Edited by Braunwald E. Philadelphia: WB Saunders Co; 1992:1451–1464.

15. Nienaber CA, von Kodolitsch Y, Nocolas V, *et al.*: The diagnosis of thoracic aortic dissection by noninvasive imaging procedures. *N Engl J Med* 1993, 328:1–9.

16. Nienaber CA, Kodolitsch Y, Petersen B, *et al.*: Intramural hemorrhage of the thoracic aorta: diagnostic and therapeutic implications. *Circulation* 1995, 92:1465–1472.

17. Amarenco P, Cohen A, Rzourio C, *et al.*: Atherosclerotic disease of the aortic arch and the risk of ischemic stroke. *N Engl J Med* 1994, 331:1474–1479.

18. Shiina A, Tajik AJ, Smith HC, *et al.*: Prognostic significance of regional wall motion abnormality in patients with prior myocardial infarction: a prospective correlative study of two-dimensional echocardiography and angiography. *Mayo Clin Proc* 1986, 61:254–262.

19. Sawada SG, Segar DS, Ryan T, *et al.*: Echocardiographic detection of coronary artery disease during dobutamine infusion. *Circulation* 1992, 82:1605–1614.

20. Quinones MA, Verani MS, Haichin RM, *et al.*: Exercise echocardiography versus 201Tl single-photon emission computed tomography in evaluation of coronary artery disease. *Circulation* 1992, 85:1026–1031.

21. Perrone-Filardi P, Pace L, Prastano M, *et al.*: Assessment of myocardial viability in patients with chronic coronary artery disease. Rest-4-hour-24 hour 201Tl tomography versus dobutamine echocardiography. *Circulation* 1996, 94:2712–2719.

22. Sabia PJ, Pewers ER, Ragosta M, *et al.*: An association between collateral blood flow and myocardial viability in patients with recent myocardial infarction. *N Engl J Med* 1992, 327:1825–1831.

CHAPTER 2

Echocardiography in Congenital Heart Disease

Lisa K. Hornberger ~ Marcy L. Schwartz

Echocardiographic imaging of congenital heart disease requires a clear understanding of cardiovascular anatomy. Knowledge of the features that distinguish chambers or great arteries and the spatial relationships of the cardiovascular structures within the thorax and their relationships to each other are necessary for an accurate and complete assessment of the cardiac pathology. The physiology and hemodynamics of a particular defect must also be fully appreciated for a thorough assessment.

Sequential analysis of the cardiac segments and connections enables the echocardiographer to quickly assess the pathology in an organized manner [1–4]. To make an accurate and complete diagnosis, the following should be determined: 1) situs of the viscera; 2) cardiac position within the chest; 3) atrial morphology and situs, including the systemic and pulmonary venous connections; 4) ventricular morphology and looping; 5) atrioventricular (AV) connection and alignment; 6) ventricular-arterial connection and alignment; 7) conal (infundibular) anatomy; and the 8) relationship of the great arteries. Additional major or minor cardiac abnormalities must also be identified, including the presence of interatrial or interventricular communications, valve anomalies, and branch pulmonary artery or distal arch pathology.

Most diagnoses are made using transthoracic echocardiographic imaging. All cardiac imaging views are necessary to fully assess complex congenital heart disease. In contrast to adult imaging, pediatric echocardiography relies heavily on the subxyphoid view for segmental analysis as well as some details of anatomy. Pulsed- and continuous-wave Doppler are important in the hemodynamic assessment of congenital heart disease. With an improvement in our understanding of the structural and hemodynamic information provided by two-dimensional and Doppler echocardiography, the number of diagnostic catheterizations needed in patients with congenital heart disease has been significantly reduced [5]. This has resulted in the echocardiographer assuming much of the responsibility in the preoperative assessment of patients and in guiding medical and surgical management.

Assessment of the patient following surgical palliation or correction of congenital heart disease requires knowledge of the preoperative spectrum of the lesion encountered and the specific procedure performed. The echocardiographic examination should be directed to the areas of potential residual disease. For example, following AV septal defect repair, the left or right AV valve regurgitation and stenosis, left ventricular outflow tract obstruction and residual atrial or ventricular septal defect, and left ventricle to right atrial shunt should be excluded [6].

Several specialized echocardiographic techniques have been developed over the past decade. Two of the most important ones are transesophageal echocardiography and fetal echocardiography. Transesophageal echocardiography plays an extremely important role in the assessment of the patient with congenital heart disease in whom transthoracic acoustic windows are poor, such as in an affected adult or postoperative patient [7]. It is also useful in real-time evaluation during interventional catheterization procedures and in the immediate postcardiopulmonary bypass assessment of patients in the operating room [8,9].

Finally, high-resolution, high-frequency imaging has made it possible to evaluate cardiovascular anatomy, function, and rhythm in the developing human fetus by 16 to 17 weeks [10–12], and even as early as 12 to 14 weeks of gestation using transvaginal fetal echocardiography [13]. This technology has provided insight into the normal human fetal circulation [14], and serial study of affected pregnancies has provided information about the pathogenesis of the spectrum of postnatally encountered disease [15,16].

SEQUENTIAL AND SEGMENTAL ANALYSIS OF THE HEART

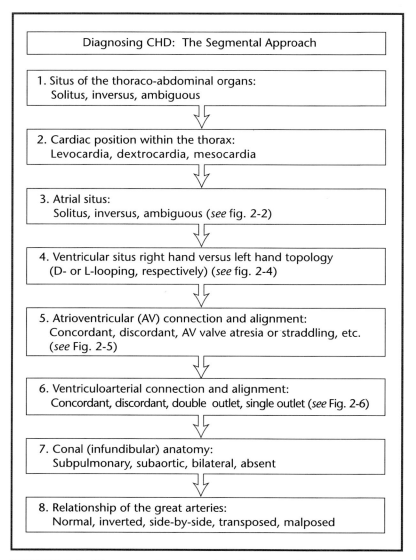

FIGURE 2-1. The segmental approach to the diagnosis of congenital heart disease (CHD). Use of the segmental approach allows the echocardiographer to accurately and thoroughly assess the cardiac anatomy. Each segment is assessed based on specific morphologic features unique to that segment [17]. Associated major and minor anomalies can then be identified. AV—atrioventricular. (*Adapted from* Geva [17].)

Features that Distinguish the Right Atrium from the Left Atrium

	Right Atrium	Left Atrium
Veins	Receives the major horn of the sinus venosus: IVC*, SVC†, CS‡	Normally receives all pulmonary veins§
Appendage	Broad-based, triangular, anterior	Narrow, fingerlike, posterior
Septum	Septum secundum (limbus of the fossa ovale)	Septum primum (valve of the foramen ovale)
Musculature	Crista terminalis, tinea sagittalis	Thin, few trabeculations¶

*In cases with interrupted IVC, the RA receives all hepatic veins and CS.
†The SVC is not a reliable marker of the RA because a persistent left SVC may drain directly into the LA when the CS is unroofed.
‡When the CS is unroofed and the IVC is interrupted, the shape, size, and location of the atrial appendages may be used for identification of atrial situs.
§The pulmonary veins are not a reliable marker of the LA due to their potential for variable connections.
¶When a persistent left SVC drains directly into the LA a muscle bar similar to a crista terminalis may be present in the left SVC-LA junction.

FIGURE 2-2. Morphologic features that distinguish the right atrium (RA) from the left atrium (LA) CS—coronary sinus; IVC—inferior vena cava; SVC—superior vena cava. (*Adapted from* Geva [17].)

Morphologic Features that Distinguish the Right Ventricle from the Left Ventricle

Morphologic Feature	Right Ventricle	Left Ventricle
Trabeculae carneae	Coarse, few	Fine, numerous
Papillary muscles	Numerous, small	Two, large
	Attachments to the septum	Smooth septal surface
AV valve leaflets	Three	Two
Infundibulum	Well developed	Absent
Semilunar-AV fibrous continuity	Absent	Present
Coronaries	Single	Two
Conduction system	Single radiation	Two radiations

FIGURE 2-3. Morphologic features that distinguish the right ventricle from the left ventricle [18]. AV—atrioventricular.

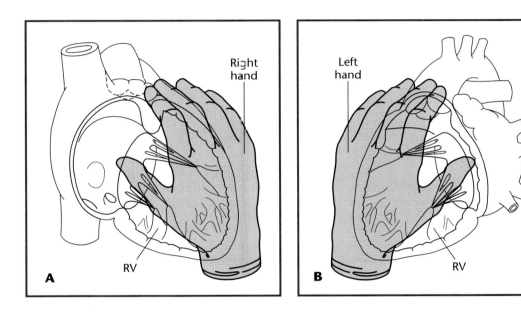

FIGURE 2-4. Determination of ventricular situs. After the right ventricle (RV) and left ventricle (LV) are identified, the ventricular looping or topology can be determined by chirality. **A,** In D-looped ventricles (right hand topology) the palm of the right hand can be placed over the RV septal surface with the thumb in the tricuspid valve and the fingers through the outflow. **B,** In L-looping (left hand topology), the palm of the left hand can be placed on the RV aspect of the septum with the thumb in the inflow and the fingers of the left hand in the RV outflow tract. (*Adapted from* Geva [17].)

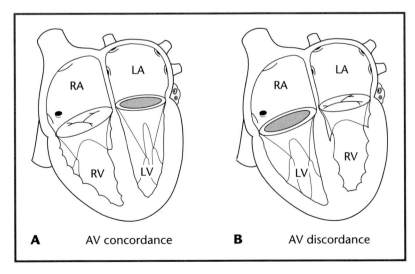

FIGURE 2-5. Atrioventricular (AV) alignments and connections. When both ventricular inflows are present, the AV connection may be concordant (**A**; *see* Fig. 2-6*A*), with the morphologic right atrium (RA) connecting to the morphologic right ventricle (RV), or discordant (**B**; *see* Fig. 2-6*B*), with the morphologic RA connecting to the morphologic left ventricle (LV). There may also be double inlet of the AV valves in which both AV valves communicate predominantly with one ventricle, or atresia straddling or overriding an AV valve. (*Adapted from* Geva [17].)

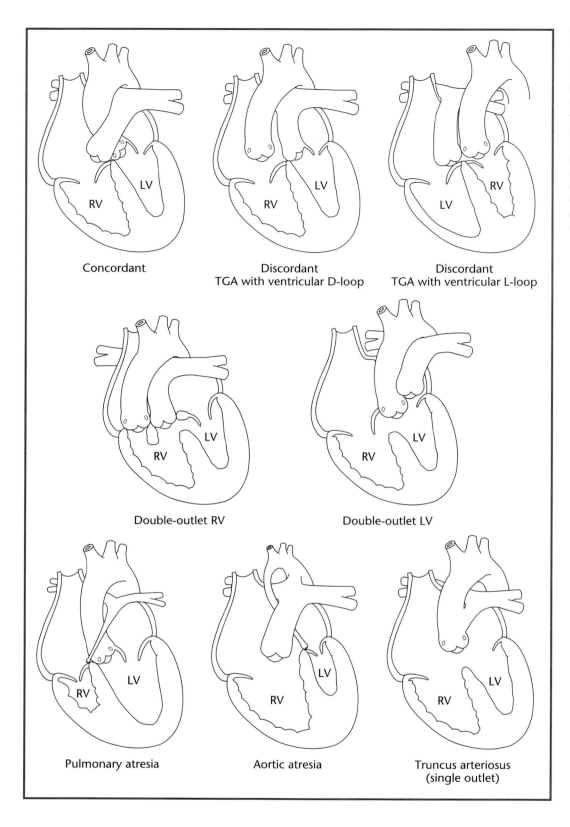

FIGURE 2-6. Ventriculoarterial relationships. These relationships are determined by looking at which great artery arises entirely or predominantly from which ventricle. The most common types of ventriculoarterial connections are 1) concordant, with the pulmonary artery arising from the morphologic right ventricle (RV) and the aorta arising from the morphologic left ventricle (LV), and 2) discordant, with the vessels arising in a transposed arrangement, as shown. Other types of ventriculoarterial connections include a double-outlet ventricle (*eg,* double-outlet RV), or single cardiac outlet (*eg,* truncus arteriosus or aortic or pulmonary atresia). TGA—transposition of the great arteries. (*Adapted from* Geva [17].)

Concordant

Discordant
TGA with ventricular D-loop

Discordant
TGA with ventricular L-loop

Double-outlet RV

Double-outlet LV

Pulmonary atresia

Aortic atresia

Truncus arteriosus
(single outlet)

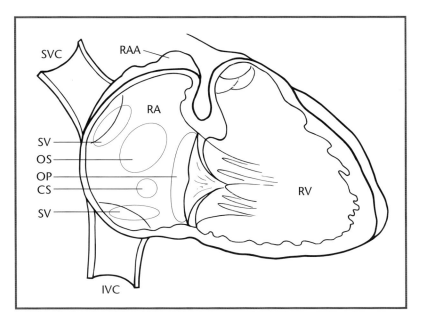

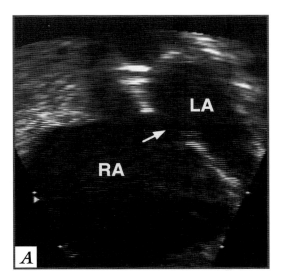

FIGURE 2-7. Atrial septal defects (ASDs). **A,** The types of ASDs that may be encountered as seen from the right atrium (RA). The classic site of an ostium secundum (OS) defect is within the confines of the fossa ovalis, the most common site for ASDs. Ostium primum (OP) defects lie adjacently to the atrioventricular valves. Sinus venosus (SV) defects are located at the junction of the superior vena cava (SVC) or inferior vena cava (IVC) and are typically associated with partially anomalous pulmonary venous drainage. Finally, interatrial communications may also occur through the coronary sinus (CS) related to a deficiency of the roof of the CS. RAA—right atrial appendage; RV—right ventricle; SV—sinus venous. (*Courtesy of* Norman H. Silverman.)

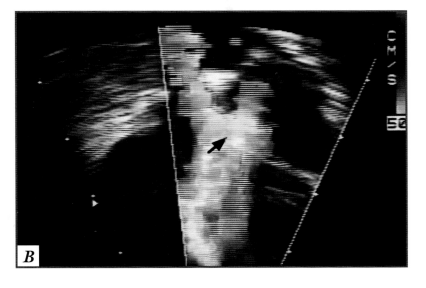

FIGURE 2-8. Atrial septal defects (ASDs). Long-axis subxiphoid view demonstrating a large secundum ASD by imaging (**A,**; *arrow*) and color-flow mapping (**B**; *arrow*) with left atrium (LA) to right atrium (RA) flow. ASDs of any type are most clearly identified using the subxiphoid long- and short-axis views [19]. The ostium secundum ASD is the most common type of ASD. A rim of septum beneath the superior vena cava and posteriorly distinguishes this type of ASD from the sinus venosus ASD, the latter of which is usually associated with anomalous pulmonary venous drainage [20]. When an ASD is identified, the pulmonary and systemic venous anatomy should be assessed. The degree of hemodynamic significance, including the presence of right ventricular volume overload and the pulmonary artery pressure, should be determined.

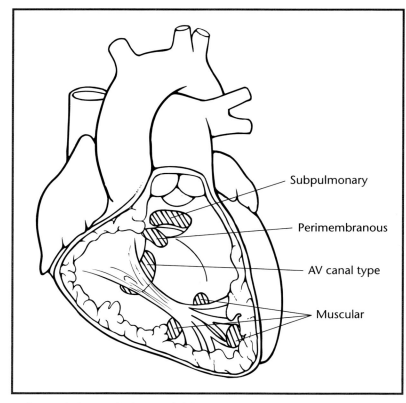

FIGURE 2-9. Ventricular septal defects (VSDs). As is the case for atrial septal defects, there are several types of VSDs classified according to their position within the ventricular septum, as shown in the diagram. These include perimembranous, subpulmonary, muscular, atrioventricular (AV) canal type, and malalignment, as in tetralogy of Fallot (the latter not shown). VSDs should be identified in long-axis or short-axis imaging of the heart. (*Adapted from* Fyler [22].)

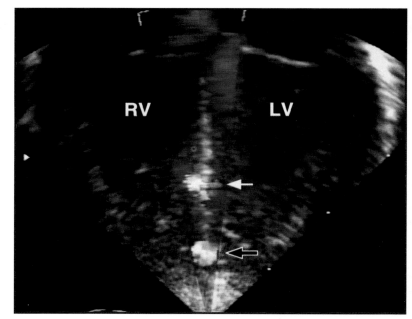

FIGURE 2-10. Ventricular septal defects (VSDs). Apical four-chamber view demonstrating multiple midmuscular VSDs. Color-flow mapping, as shown, is particularly useful in the detection of smaller muscular and perimembranous VSDs [23]. Muscular VSDs may involve four areas of the ventricular septum: 1) posterior muscular septum; 2) mid-muscular within the vicinity of the moderator band (*white arrow*); 3) apical, below the moderator band (*black arrow*); and 4) anterior muscular septum, near the base of the heart. In the presence of elevated right ventricular (RV) pressures, the use of color-flow mapping with a low-velocity scale and high frame rate should improve the detection of one or more small VSDs. LV—left ventricle.

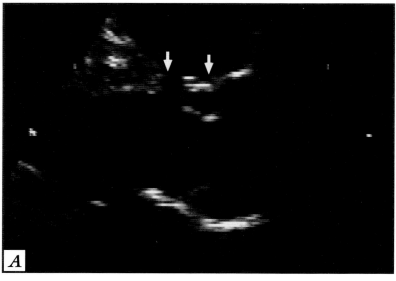

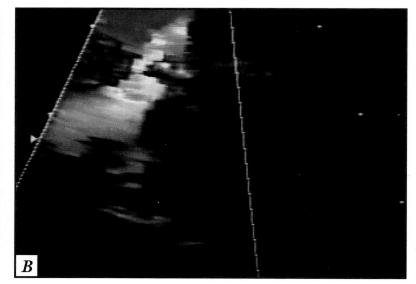

FIGURE 2-11. Ventricular septal defect (VSD). **A,** Parasternal long-axis view demonstrating a perimembranous VSD with subpulmonary extension. The right coronary cusp prolapses into the defect [21]. The *arrows* indicate the true margins of the defect. **B,** The prolapse of the right coronary cusp into the defect results in a much smaller residual defect orifice, as shown by color Doppler. This prolapse may distort the valve, resulting in aortic insufficiency. Associated cardiac lesions to be excluded in the presence of a perimembranous VSD include aortic valve prolapse, a discrete subaortic ridge or membrane, and muscle bundles in the right ventricular outflow, which cause obstruction (also referred to as *double-chamber right ventricle*).

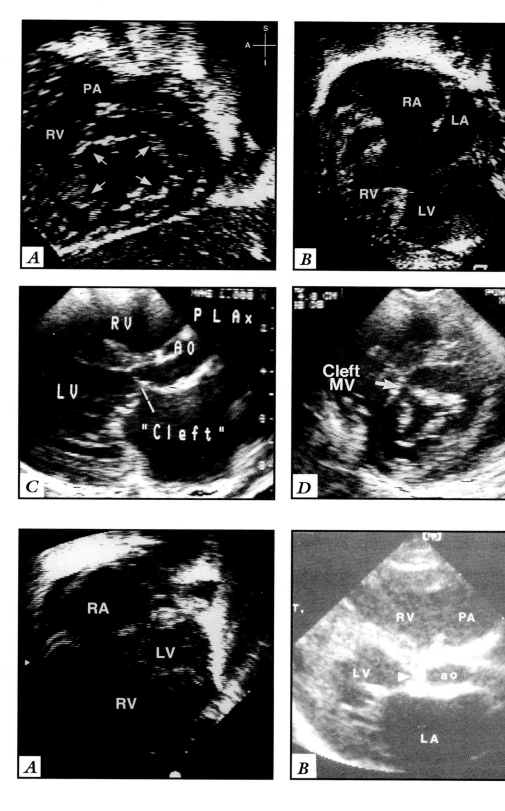

FIGURE 2-12. Atrioventricular septal defects (AVSDs). **A,** The subxiphoid short-axis view is very useful in the assessment of AVSDs. In this subxiphoid short-axis view, the large common atrioventricular (AV) valve with its right ventricular (RV) and left ventricular (LV) components is indicated by the *arrows*. This view permits assessment of the valve morphology and attachments. The LV and RV components of the valve can be assessed to determine whether the valve is "balanced," or "not balanced," over the ventricles, with one ventricle receiving a greater proportion of the AV valve tissue.

B, Apical four-chamber view of a common AVSD. Absence of the crux of the heart or endocardial cushion area, characteristic of an AVSD, is best seen in this view. An AVSD may also be partial, with only a ventricular or atrial component (AVSD-type VSD or a primum atrial septal defect, respectively), or complete, with both atrial and ventricular septal components. When there are AV valve attachments to the crest of the ventricular septum that result in a small ventricular septal defect component are referred to as *transitional AVSD.*

C, Parasternal long-axis view showing cleft mitral valve (MV) attachments to the anterior LV outflow tract (LVOT), which may result in LVOT obstruction.

D, Parasternal short-axis (PLAx) view demonstrating a cleft in the MV in a patient with a primum atrial septal defect. Additional information in the assessment of the AVSD should include further evaluation of the morphology of the left AV valve and its chordal attachments to the papillary muscles (eg, parachute, double orifice, and so on), and the degree of AV valve regurgitation. AO—aorta; LA—left atrium; PA—pulmonary artery; RA—right atrium. (Parts C and D *courtesy of* Norman H. Silverman.)

FIGURE 2-13. Left heart obstructive lesions. A broad spectrum of cardiovascular lesions involving the mitral valve and supramitral area, the left ventricle (LV), the LV outflow tract (LVOT), the aortic valve, and the aortic arch are encompassed in left heart obstructive lesions. Minor lesions, such as a bicommissural aortic valve, to severe lesions, such as those associated with Shone syndrome [24] or hypoplastic left heart syndrome, are included in this group of lesions.

A, Apical four-chamber view in a patient with hypoplastic left heart syndrome. There is obvious LV hypertrophy, and the LV is severely hypoplastic in its short- and long-axis dimensions. The degree of LV hypoplasia, which may determine the prognosis and management of the patient, is variable in significant neonatal aortic stenosis (AS).
B, Parasternal long-axis view demonstrating a thickened, poorly mobile aortic valve (*arrow*) and a hypoplastic ascending aorta (ao).

(Continued on next page)

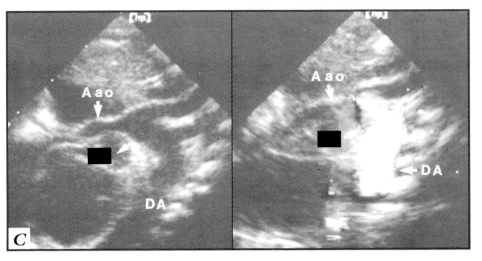

FIGURE 2-13. (*Continued*) **C,** Suprasternal notch view demonstrating the aortic arch in critical AS. The largest diameter of the arch in critical AS may be found near the distal aortic arch and descending aorta (DA). Retrograde flow through the distal and transverse aortic arch, as shown by color-flow mapping, as well as right to left flow in the patent ductus arteriosus (not shown), are typical of severe LVOT obstruction in the newborn. AAo—ascending aorta; LA—left atrium; PA—pulmonary artery; RA—right atrium; RV—right ventricle. (Parts B and C *courtesy of* Christine Boutin.)

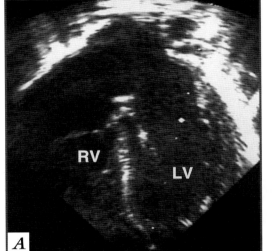

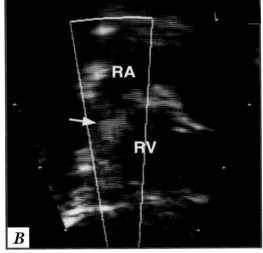

FIGURE 2-14. Pulmonary atresia with intact ventricular septum. **A,** Four-chamber view in pulmonary atresia with intact ventricular septum. Pulmonary atresia with intact ventricular septum is associated with a variable-sized right ventricle (RV). In this case, there is significant tricuspid valve and RV hypoplasia. These intracardiac features may also be observed in the presence of critical pulmonary stenosis. **B,** In pulmonary atresia or critical pulmonary valvar stenosis with intact ventricular septum, there may be fistulous connections between the RV and the right or left coronary artery, as shown in this four-chamber view magnified on the RV free wall. As seen in this image of the RV to coronary fistula (*arrow*), high RV systolic pressures may result in flow reversal during ventricular systole [25]. Proximal coronary stenoses with distal fistula may preclude surgical decompression of the RV [26,27]. LV—left ventricle; RA—right atrium.

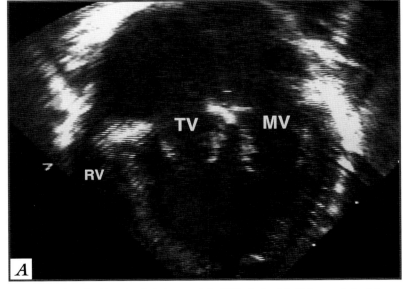

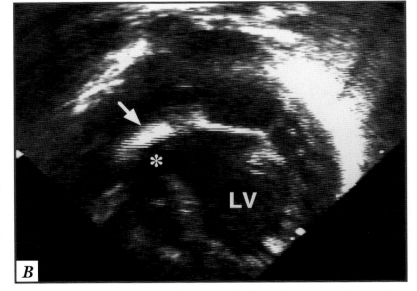

FIGURE 2-15. The single left ventricle (LV). **A,** In this D-looped double-inlet LV, both atrioventricular valves empty into a single, morphologic LV. **B,** In tricuspid atresia, there is usually a thick band of tissue in the tricuspid valve (TV) position (*arrow*) with a normal LV and mitral valve (MV). In both conditions, a ventricular septal defect (VSD) allows flow to enter the smaller right ventricular (RV) chamber and provide flow to the pulmonary artery when they are normally related or to the aorta when the great arteries are transposed. *Asterisk* indicates VSD.

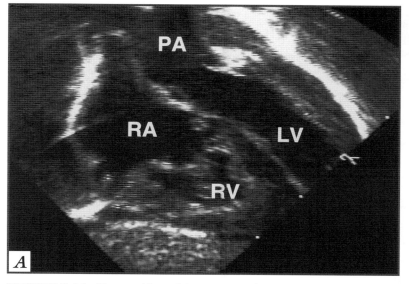
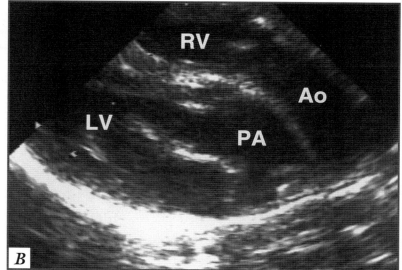

FIGURE 2-16. Transposition of the great arteries. Imaging of the heart in the presence of conotruncal abnormalities such as transposition of the great arteries requires detailed assessment of the ventricular outflow tracts and great arteries. **A,** Subxiphoid long-axis view demonstrating the abnormal left ventricle (LV) to pulmonary artery (PA) connection (ventriculoarterial discordance). The PA bifurcation can be seen from this view. **B,** Parasternal long-axis view showing both ventricular to arterial connections, with the aorta (Ao) more anterior relative to the PA and arising from the right ventricle (RV). The Ao and PA arise in a parallel fashion characteristic of transposition of the great arteries. From this view, the mitral valve to pulmonary valve continuity can be seen. In the assessment of transposition of the great arteries, a ventricular septal defect may be present in as many as 50% of affected infants, and LV and RV outflow tract obstruction should be excluded. The coronary artery anatomy (not shown) should also be evaluated because of the potential for coronary artery abnormalities and their implications for the arterial switch operation [28]. RA—right atrium.

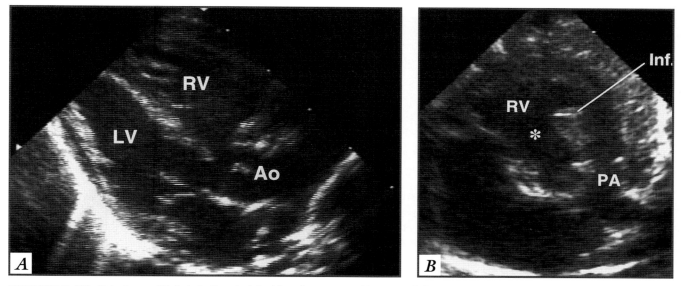

FIGURE 2-17. Tetralogy of Fallot. Both subxiphoid and parasternal long- and short-axis images demonstrate the most important aspects of tetralogy of Fallot. **A,** Parasternal long-axis view demonstrating the large anterior malalignment ventricular septal defect (VSD) with aortic overriding of the crest of the ventricular septum. **B,** Parasternal short-axis view of the right ventricular outflow tract (RVOT) demonstrating anterior malalignment of infundibular septum (Inf). The large subaortic, malalignment VSD can be seen (*asterisk*). Other lesions to be excluded in tetralogy of Fallot include additional VSDs, branch pulmonary artery (PA) stenoses, mitral valve abnormalities, and coronary abnormalities, particularly the left anterior descending from the right coronary artery (which crosses over the RVOT) or a single right coronary artery. A prominent conal branch from the right coronary that partially crosses the infundibulum is common in tetralogy of Fallot. Ao—aorta; LV—left ventricle; RV—right ventricle.

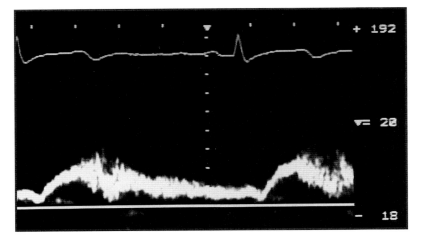

FIGURE 2-18. The descending aortic Doppler flow pattern may give a clue or support for a hemodynamically significant lesion. In this example, the presence of significant aortic coarctation is suggested. The systolic flow velocity peaks late and is of low magnitude, and there is continued antegrade flow throughout ventricular diastole. When there is flow reversal in diastole, a run-off lesion such as a patent ductus arteriosus, an aortopulmonary window, or aortic regurgitation, is likely to be present.

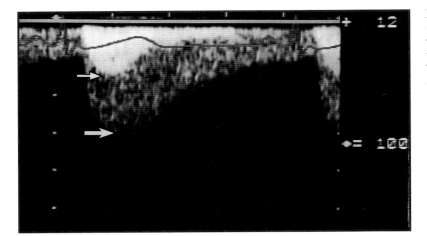

FIGURE 2-19. Gradient assessment. Doppler gradient estimation requires use of the simplified Bernoulli equation, $\Delta P \sim 4v_2{}^2 - 4v_1{}^2$, where v_1 is the velocity of flow proximal to an obstruction and pressure difference between the vessel proximal to the obstruction, and v_2 is that distal to the obstruction. To obtain a true gradient, the proximal pressure must be subtracted from the distal pressure [29]. In most cases, the proximal velocity is negligible; however, there are times when the proximal velocity must be considered, including across a valve that is both stenotic and regurgitant, when an intracardiac shunt and stenosis are present, when multiple levels of obstruction in series are present, and when valve gradients are assessed during exercise or a high-output state [29]. There is also often flow acceleration around the aortic arch proximal to a potential coarctation due to the curvature of the vessel [30]. This figure shows the continuous-wave Doppler signal obtained through the distal arch of a patient with coarctation of the aorta. The *small arrow* indicates the velocity proximal to the coarctation and the *large arrow* indicates the total maximum instantaneous velocity through the arch.

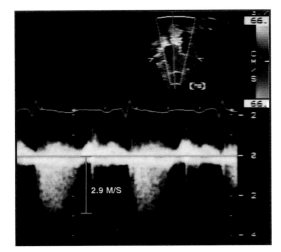

FIGURE 2-20. The simplified Bernoulli equation may also be applied to estimate right ventricular (RV) pressure. Using the jet of tricuspid insufficiency [31], the gradient calculated is equivalent to the right atrial (RA) pressure subtracted from the RV systolic pressure. In this example, the RV pressure is approximately 30 to 35 mm Hg plus the RA pressure (v-wave). Similarly, a ventricular septal defect (VSD) or patent ductus arteriosus gradient permits assessment of RV pressure relative to the LV pressure. In the absence of LV outflow tract obstruction, the LV systolic pressure is approximately equal to the systolic systemic blood pressure. The VSD Doppler spectra is only a peak instantaneous gradient between the two ventricles and may provide an inaccurate assessment of the difference in the RV and LV peak systolic pressures if the timing of ventricular contraction is different between the ventricles [32].

Postoperative Assessment of Congenital Heart Disease

Surgical Procedure	Potential Residual Cardiovascular Lesions
Tetralogy of Fallot repair	Residual VSD, residual RVOT obstruction, RV function and systolic pressure, TR, branch PA stenosis, LVOT obstruction
AVSD repair	Left and right AV valve regurgitation and stenosis, LVOT obstruction, residual ASD, VSD, or LV-RA shunt
Arterial switch operation	Obstruction at the Ao and PA anastomoses, branch PA stenosis, neoaortic or pulmonary regurgitation, regional wall motion abnormalities
Mustard/Senning operation	Systemic or pulmonary venous pathway obstruction, LVOT obstruction, TR, RV dysfunction
Ross procedure	Global or regional LV dysfunction, neoaortic regurgitation, LVOT obstruction, MR, RVOT obstruction, VSD (particularly with Konno procedure)
Rastelli operation (RV-PA conduit, VSD closure)	LVOT obstruction, RVOT obstruction, residual VSD, LV or RV dysfunction, branch PA stenosis
Coarctation of the aorta repair	Residual distal arch obstruction, LV dysfunction, development of MS or LVOT obstruction
Subaortic stenosis resection	Residual subaortic stenosis, AR, MR, LV dysfunction
Fontan procedure (lateral tunnel)	IVC or SVC anastomosis obstruction, cavopulmonary obstruction, patch leak with right to left atrial shunting, branch PA stenosis, ventricular dysfunction, AV valve regurgitation, pulmonary vein stenosis

FIGURE 2-21. Postoperative assessment of congenital heart disease (CHD). Cardiac anatomy should be evaluated following common surgical reparative or palliative procedures for CHD. A directed approach to imaging the postoperative patient with CHD is crucial for a complete assessment. This table lists several common palliative and reparative surgical techniques used in CHD. Ao—aorta; AR—aortic regurgitation; ASD—atrial septal defect; AV—atrioventricular; AVSD—atrioventricular septal defect; IVC—inferior vena cava; LV—left ventricle; LVOT—left ventricular outflow tract; MR—mitral regurgitation; MS—mitral stenosis; PA—pulmonary artery; RA—right atrium; RV—right ventricle; RVOT—right ventricular outflow tract; SVC—superior vena cava; TR—tricuspid regurgitation; VSD—ventricular septal defect.

TRANSESOPHAGEAL ECHOCARDIOGRAPHY

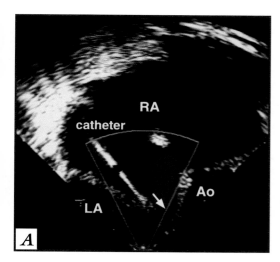

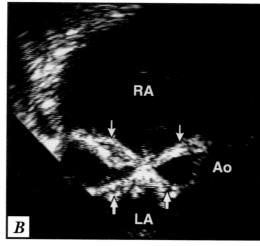

FIGURE 2-22. Transesophageal echocardiography (TEE) imaging. TEE is useful in patients with poor transthoracic acoustic windows, particularly adults with congenital heart disease. It is also important for real-time imaging during interventional cardiac catheterization procedures, such as device placement in atrial septal defects (ASDs) and ventricular septal defects. **A**, TEE image of an ASD with left to right flow. The catheter is seen crossing through the defect (*arrow*). **B**, This image was obtained following device closure of this ASD. After device placement, the position of the individual arms of the device (including the potential for impingement of the device and its arms on other cardiac structures) and the presence of a residual ASD can be evaluated. In this case, the device is in stable position. The *thin arrows* point to the arms on the right atrium (RA) side of the septum, and the *thick arrows* point to those on the left atrium (LA) side of the septum. Ao—aorta; LA—left atrium.

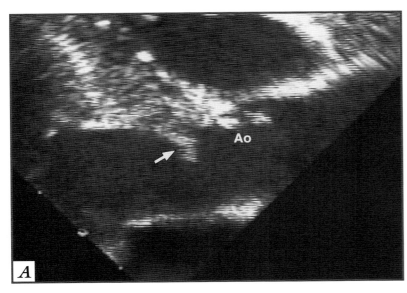

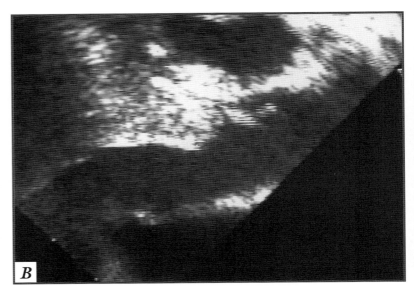

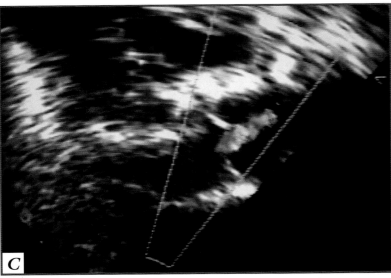

FIGURE 2-23. Intraoperative assessment of a discrete subaortic membrane. **A,** Image demonstrating the preoperative anatomy with significant left ventricular outflow tract (LVOT) obstruction due to a fibromuscular ridge (*arrow*). **B** and **C,** In the postoperative images, the LVOT is widely patent, with mild aortic regurgitation. Ao—aorta.

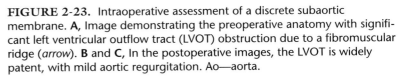

FETAL ECHOCARDIOGRAPHY

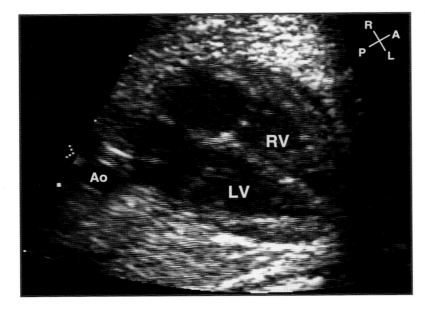

FIGURE 2-24. Four-chamber view of a normal fetal heart at 24 weeks of gestation. The fetal heart can be reliably evaluated by transabdominal imaging beginning at 17 to 18 weeks of gestation. As is true in the postnatal evaluation of congenital heart disease, sequential and segmental assessment of the fetal heart are also important, and the same criteria for delineating structures should be used. This four-chamber view demonstrates symmetry between the left and right chambers of the heart. Symmetry between the great arteries is also important. A—anterior; Ao—aorta; L—left; LV—left ventricle; P—posterior; R—right; RV—right ventricle.

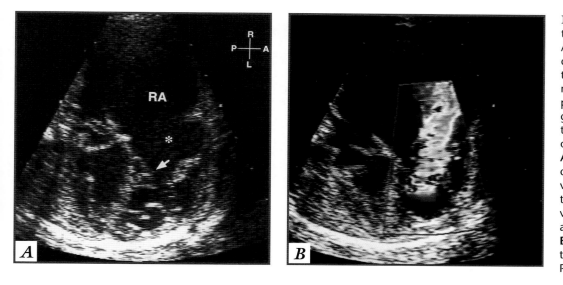

FIGURE 2-25. Ebstein's anomaly of the tricuspid valve in a 32-week gestational-age fetus. As demonstrated in these two images, fetal heart disease typically represents a more severe spectrum of disease than is encountered in the postnatal population. This is due to the referral patterns established as defects, which are more grossly abnormal in the four-chamber view and thus are most likely to be detected at the time of a routine obstetrical ultrasound examination. **A,** In this image, the right atrium (RA) is massively dilated as are both left ventricle (LV) and right ventricle (RV), and the heart consumes most of the fetal chest. Displacement of the tricuspid valve leaflet into the RV apex (*arrow*) and the amount of atrialized RV (*asterisk*) can be seen. **B,** Color-flow mapping demonstrating the severe tricuspid regurgitation. A—anterior; L—left; P—posterior; R—right.

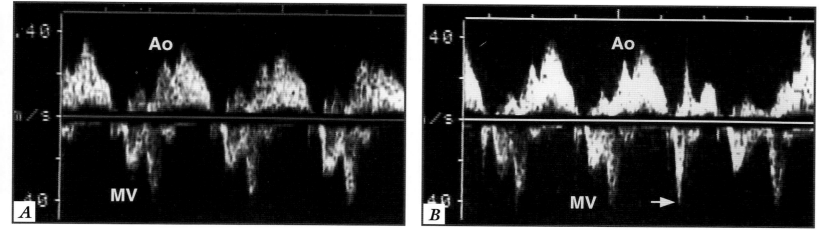

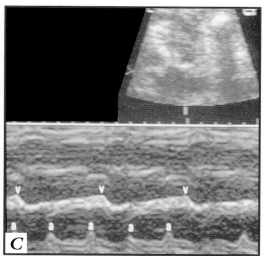

FIGURE 2-26. Fetal rhythm evaluation. **A,** Spectral Doppler tracing demonstrating normal left ventricular (LV) flow and outflow spectra. The Doppler sample volume is increased, and the cursor is placed between the LV inflow and outflow to obtain signals that are in opposite directions to each other. **B,** Atrial premature beat. The third Doppler spectral tracing through the mitral valve (MV) demonstrates an atrial premature beat seen only as an "A" wave during atrial systole (*arrow*) rather than the normal biphasic flow pattern as seen in the two beats before. **C,** M-mode in complete atrioventricular (AV) block. M-mode imaging with the cursor angled through one of the atria (preferably the right atrial appendage) and the ventricle can also be useful in the delineation of fetal dysrhythmias as well as in the assessment of ventricular function. This is an example of fetal complete AV block in which the atrial systoles (a) are completely independent of the ventricular systoles (v; ventricular contraction). The fetal rate is approximately 60 bpm. AO—aorta.

REFERENCES

1. Van Praagh R: The segmental approach to diagnosis of congenital heart disease. *Birth Defects: Original Article Series* 1972, 8:4–23.

2. Anderson RH, Becker AE, Freedom RM, *et al.*: Sequential segmental analysis of congenital heart disease. *Pediatr Cardiol* 1984, 5:281–287.

3. Shinebourne EA, Macartney FJ, Anderson RH: Sequential chamber localization: logical approach to diagnosis in congenital heart disease. *Br Heart J* 1976, 38:327–340.

4. Rao PS: Systematic approach to differential diagnosis. *Am Heart J* 1981, 102:389–403.

5. Gomez R, Maitre MJ, Leon JP, *et al.*: Surgery for congenital cardiopathies without previous catheterization: preoperative evaluation and surgical indication using bidimensional echocardiography and Doppler. *Esp Cardiol* 1989, 42:653–660.

6. Chin AJ, Keane JF, Norwood WI, *et al.*: Repair of complete common atrioventricular canal in infancy. *J Thorac Cardiovasc Surg* 1982, 84:437–445.

7. Fleischer DE, Goldstein SA: Transesophageal echocardiography: what the gastroenterologist thinks the cardiologist should know about endoscopy. *J Am Soc Echocardiogr* 1990, 3:428–435.

8. Muhiudeen IA, Roberson DA, Silverman NH, *et al.*: Intraoperative echocardiography for evaluation of congenital heart disease in infants and children. *Anesthesiology* 1992, 76:165–172.

9. Ritter SB: Transesophageal real-time echocardiography in infants and children with congenital heart disease. *J Am Coll Cardiol* 1991, 18:569–580.

10. Allan LD, Tynan M, Campbell S, *et al.*: Identification of congenital cardiac malformations by echocardiography in the midtrimester fetus. *Br Heart J* 1981, 46:358–362.

11. Benacerraf BR, Pober BR, Sanders SP: Accuracy of fetal echocardiography. *Radiology* 1987, 165:847–849.

12. Kleinman CS, Hobbins JC, Jaffe C, *et al.*: Echocardiographic studies in the human fetus: prenatal diagnosis of congenital heart disease and cardiac dysrhythmias. *Pediatrics* 1980, 65:1059–1067.

13. Bronshtein M, Zimmer EZ, Milo S, *et al.*: Fetal cardiac abnormalities detected by transvaginal fetal sonography at 12-16 weeks gestation. *Obstetr Gynecol* 1991, 78:374–378.

14. Kenny JF, Plappert T, Doubilet P, *et al.*: Changes in intracardiac blood flow velocities and right and left ventricular stroke volumes with gestational age in the normal human fetus: a prospective Doppler echocardiographic study. *Circulation* 1986, 74:1208–1216.

15. Hornberger LK, Sanders SP, Sahn DJ: In utero pulmonary artery and aortic growth and the potential for progression of pulmonary outflow tract obstruction in tetralogy of Fallot. *J Am Coll. Cardiol* 1995, 25:739–745.

16. Hornberger LK, Sanders SP, Rein AJJT: Left heart obstructive lesions and left ventricular growth in the midtrimester fetus: longitudinal study. *Circulation* 1995, 92:1531–1538.

17. Geva T: Segmental approach to the diagnosis of congenital heart disease. In *Atlas of Heart Diseases: Congenital Heart Disease*, vol 12. Edited by Braunwald, E, Freedom RM. Philadelphia: Current Medicine; 1996.

18. Van Praagh R, VanPraagh S: Morphologic anatomy. In *Nadas' Pediatric Cardiology* Edited by Fyler DC. Philadelphia: Hanley & Belfus; 1992:17–26.

19. Shub C, Dimopoulos IN, Seward JB, *et al.*: Sensitivity of two-dimensional echocardiography in the direct visualization of atrial septal defects utilizing a subcostal approach: experience with 154 patients. *J Am Coll Cardiol* 1983, 4:127–135.

20. Ettedgui JA, Siewers RD, Anderson RH, *et al.*: Diagnostic echocardiographic features of the sinus venosus defect. *Br Heart J* 1991, 64:329–331.

21. Rhodes LA, Keane JF, Keane JP, *et al.*: Long term follow-up (to 43 years) of ventricular septal defect with audible aortic regurgitation. *Am J Cardiology* 1990, 66:340–345.

22. Fyler DC: Ventricular septal defect. In *Nadas' Pediatric Cardiology* Edited by Fyler DC. Philadelphia: Hanley & Belfus; 1992:437.

23. Ortiz E, Robinson PJ, Deanfield JE, *et al.*: Localisation of ventricular septal defects by simultaneous display of superimposed colour Doppler and cross-sectional echocardiographic images. *Br Heart J* 1985, 54:53–60.

24. Shone JD, Sellers RD, Anderson RC *et al.*: The developmental complex of "parachute mitral valve" supramitral ring of the left atrium, subaortic stenosis and coarctation of the aorta. *Am J Cardiol* 1963, 11:714–716.

25. Leung MP, Mok C-K, Hui P-W: Echocardiographic assessment of neonates with pulmonary atresia with intact ventricular septum. *J Am Coll Cardiol* 1988, 12:718–725.

26. Giglia TM, Mandell VS, Connor AR, *et al.*: Diagnosis and management of right ventricle dependent coronary circulation in pulmonary atresia with intact ventricular septum. *Circulation* 1992, 86:1516–1528.

27. Akagi T, Benson LE, Williams WG, *et al.*: Ventriculo-coronary arterial connection in pulmonary atresia with intact ventricular septum and their influence on ventricular performance and clinical course. *Am J Cardiol* 1993, 72:586–590.

28. Wernovsky G, Sanders SP: Coronary artery anatomy and transposition of the great arteries. *Coron Art Dis* 1993, 4:148–154.

29. Snider AR, Serwer GA, Ritter SB: Methods for obtaining quantitative information form the echocardiographic examination. In *Echocardiography in Pediatric Heart Disease*. St Louis: Mosby; 1997:133–234.

30. Sarin V. Flow of an elastico-viscous liquid in a curved pipe of slowly varying curvature. *Int J Biomed Computing* 1993;32:135–149.

31. Berger M, Haimowitz A, Van Josh A, *et al.*: Quantitative assessment of pulmonary hypertension in patients with tricuspid regurgitation using continuous wave Doppler ultrasound. *J Am Coll Cardiol* 1985, 6:359–365.

32. Murphy DJ Jr, Ludomirsky A, Huhta JC: Continuous wave Doppler in children with ventricular septal defect. noninvasive estimation of interventricular pressure gradient. *Am J Cardiol* 1986, 57:428–432.

Vascular Ultrasound

Joshua A. Beckman ~ Jean M. Alessi ~ Marie Gerhard

Vascular diseases are among the most common causes of death and disability in the United States and the world. The occurrence of atherosclerosis, thrombosis, embolization, and vasospasm result in clinical manifestations such as myocardial infarction, peripheral atherosclerotic disease, stroke, and deep venous thrombosis. These clinical manifestations are commonly observed in daily interactions with patients. Peripheral atherosclerotic disease affects at least 20% of those over the age of 75 [1], approximately 300,000 patients are hospitalized each year for deep venous thrombosis [2], and stroke is the third leading cause of death in the United States [3]. Vascular diseases frequently complicate the management of other illnesses, and the impact ranges from mild disability to death.

Ultrasonography is an extremely useful, noninvasive modality to detect and document vascular disease. This documentation includes localization of its anatomic site, characterization of obstruction and its functional significance, confirmation of appropriate indications for angiography in questionable cases, and evaluation of results of treatment. From venous thromboses to carotid stenoses, ultrasonography can aid in disease detection and assessment, both quickly and accurately. This chapter discusses the application of ultrasound to detect changes in blood flow and abnormalities in vascular structures in the upper and lower extremities and neck.

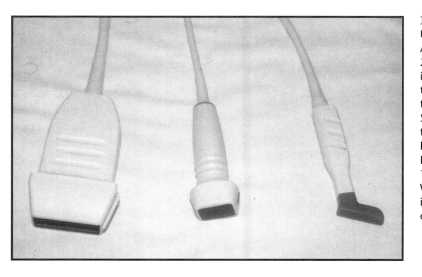

FIGURE 3-1. Various probes used to image different vascular beds. Ultrasound imaging relies on the transmission and reception of sound waves. A piezoelectric, usually ceramic, crystal transmits a beam with a frequency of 2 to 10 MHz or million cycles per second. Either the same or another crystal in the probe receives the sound waves as they are reflected from the imaged tissues. An image can be constructed by taking into account the velocity of the returning wave, the time of the return, and the direction of the wave [4]. Several different types of ultrasound imaging are used in the assessment of the vasculature, including B-mode, Doppler ultrasonography, and color-flow Doppler. From left to right, the probes pictured are a 7- to 4-MHz Broadband Linear Array probe, a 3- to 2-MHz Broadband Phased Array probe, and a 10- to 5-MHz Intraoperative Scanhead (all probes are made by ATL, Bothell, WA). Linear array probes, rather than sector, are typically used for optimal imaging of the linear blood vessel structures in the extremities and the intraoperative field.

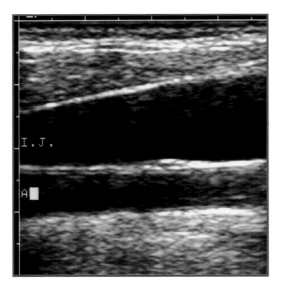

FIGURE 3-2. Neck ultrasound. The earliest ultrasound tools used a single beam to determine the position of a tissue. Oscillations on paper from the horizontal indicated the reflectivity of the tissue. B-mode (brightness modulation) imaging uses many beams from a single source or in parallel to determine the qualities of many points below the probe. By transmitting and receiving many beams 10 to 60 times per second in seemingly real time, a two-dimensional image is produced. This black and white image is constructed by interpreting the intensity of the reflected beams. Highly reflective tissues, like the vessel wall, appear more white and those with poor reflection, more dark. If blood is moving perpendicularly from the transmitted sound waves, the erythrocytes disperse the beams and appear black, whereas the relatively static walls appear lighter. At higher frequencies, the resolution of tissue structures increases, but the depth of penetration of the ultrasound decreases. Vascular ultrasonography is generally performed with probes that use 3.5- to 5-MHz linear array sound waves [5]. IJ—internal jugular vein.

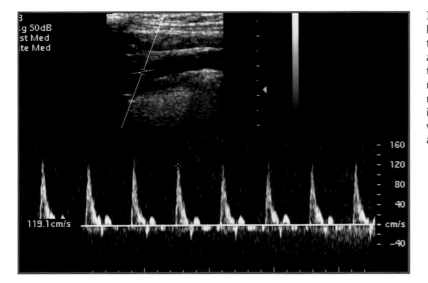

FIGURE 3-3. Doppler profile of the normal, triphasic flow of a peripheral, high-resistance artery. Doppler ultrasonography is the display of the spectrum of velocities as determined by the frequency shift of the transmitted and received ultrasound. Sound waves striking an object moving toward the sound wave have more intensity on their return, whereas objects moving away yield a smaller reflection. The frequency detected by the receiver is directly proportional to the velocity of the moving object. By interpreting the frequency shifts from the baseline transmitted frequency, waveforms or sounds can be generated [6]. The combination of B-mode and Doppler ultrasonography is called *duplex ultrasonography*.

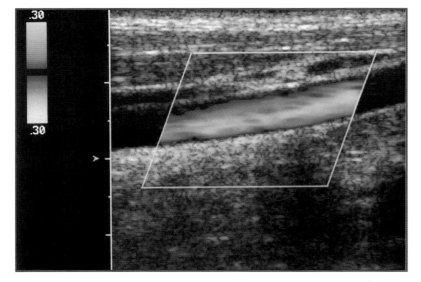

FIGURE 3-4. Color Doppler ultrasonography. Color Doppler ultrasonography is the application of color to characterize the direction and velocity of blood. The color red was arbitrarily assigned to flow toward the probe and the color blue, to flow away from the probe. Darker colors represent slower velocities, whereas brighter colors indicate higher velocity. Because blood flow is based on the cardiac cycle, variations in color are seen during each cycle. Normal blood flow is laminar or faster in the middle of the vessel (*light orange*) and slower near the endothelial wall (*red*). Laminar flow produces a smooth color image. Stenoses create turbulent flow with areas of bright, fast flow intermingled with areas of slow, dark flow [7].

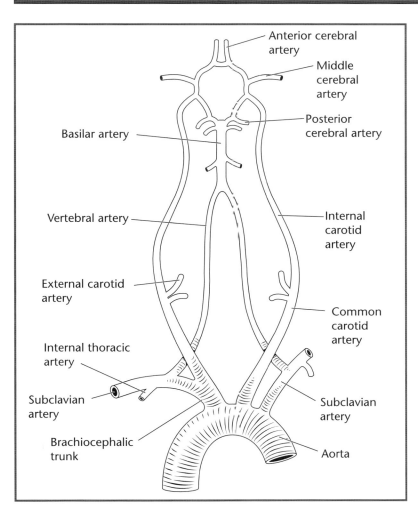

FIGURE 3-5. Normal anatomy of the carotid and major cerebral arteries. Atherosclerotic disease of the carotid arteries typically occurs at the bifurcation of the common carotid artery. At branching points, blood flow loses its laminar quality, and an alteration of the shear forces is developed. Embolization from these atherosclerotic lesions after plaque rupture is one of the prominent mechanisms of transient ischemic attacks and strokes. Disorders such as vasculitis generally produce abnormalities at locations other than branch points. Ultrasound can provide clues to the nature of the underlying disease by providing images of the localized findings.

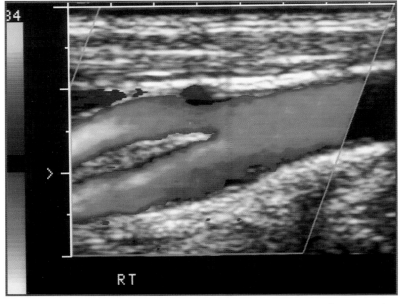

FIGURE 3-6. Bifurcation of the common carotid artery into the internal and external carotid arteries. This area is the primary focus of noninvasive vascular imaging in the neck. High-frequency ultrasound, typically 5 MHz, is used to image the shallow carotid vessels. In this image, the intima is free of irregularities by B-mode, and the color-assisted Doppler spectrum is free of flow disturbances, indicating laminar flow.

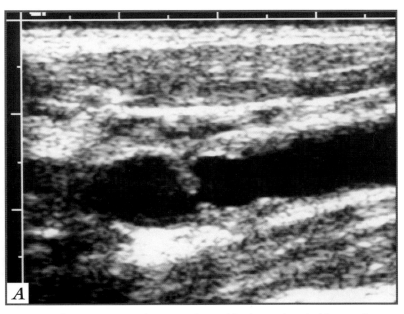

FIGURE 3-7. Important features of carotid atherosclerosis. The tendency to develop atherosclerosis at sites of bifurcation is commonly associated with disturbance of blood flow, including flow separation, low shear stress, and high tensile stress. **A,** B-mode image of the internal carotid artery (ICA) with atherosclerotic plaque projecting into the lumen.

(*Continued on next page*)

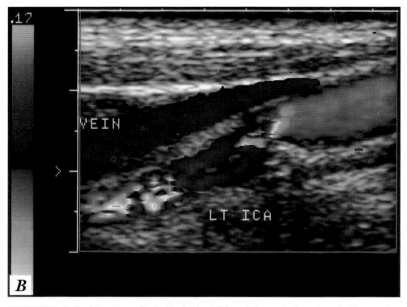

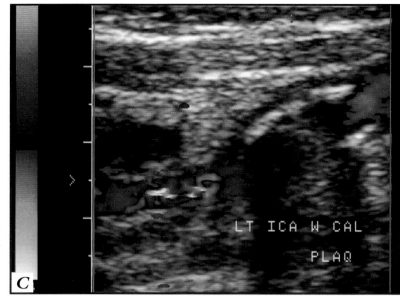

FIGURE 3-7. (*Continued*) **B**, Turbulent blood flow at the site of atherosclerotic plaque is observed with color Doppler. **C**, Calcified plaque (CAL PLAQ) results in a shadowing artefact (*arrow*), which makes it impossible to assess flow disturbances below the plaque.

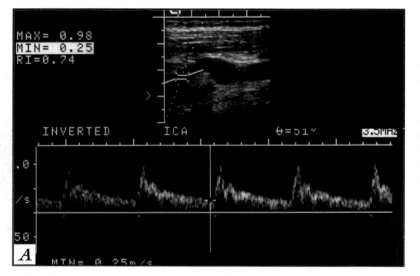

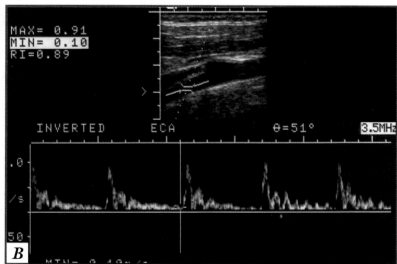

FIGURE 3-8. Pulsed-wave Doppler ultrasonography allows examination of the blood velocity within the lumen of the vessel. **A**, The flow pattern in the internal carotid artery (ICA) has unique characteristics because of the absence of branches and the low resistance of the brain's vasculature. The waveform is more smooth, and the low resistance also allows increased forward flow to occur during diastole. **B**, The external carotid artery (ECA) has waveform characteristic of high-resistance peripheral arteries, with little diastolic flow. Another means of differentiating the ECA from the ICA is to tap the temporal artery. The tapping creates a sawtooth pattern in diastole, which is transmitted to the ECA. This "temporal tap" can been seen in *B* in the last two pulse waves. The common carotid artery represents a mixture of these two patterns. Normal peak velocities in the carotid arteries are less than 1.3 m/s.

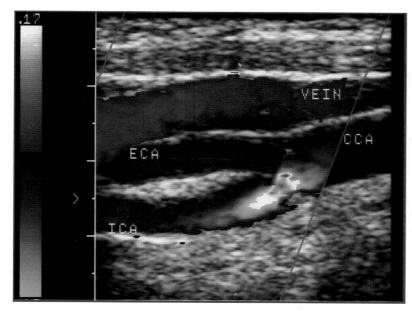

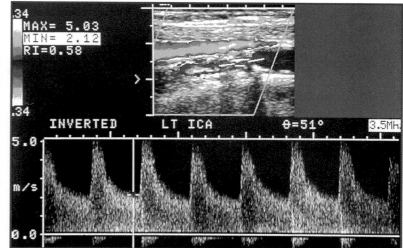

FIGURE 3-9. Thickened intima characteristic of atherosclerosis. Duplex ultrasound examination of the internal carotid artery (ICA) can demonstrate the location and composition of plaque. Significant plaque is present at the bifurcation. As seen in this image, the presence of multidirectional (*red* and *blue*) and high-velocity (*bright*) flow indicates the site of maximal narrowing. The severity of stenosis resulting from plaque cannot be accurately determined from the diameter reduction observed in the resulting B-mode image or from the color Doppler spectrum. However, blood flow velocity measurements by pulsed-wave Doppler analysis can accurately estimate the severity of the stenosis. CCA—common carotid artery; ECA—external carotid artery.

FIGURE 3-10. In the setting of a significant stenosis, the velocity of blood increases through the lesion. Velocity increases proportionally to the severity of stenosis (the continuity rule). In accordance with Poiseuille's law, the flow of a fluid through a tube remains constant. Therefore, in narrowed areas, rates of flow must increase in relation to the flow in areas of normal diameter to maintain the same forward flow. Systolic velocities above 4 m/s and diastolic velocities above 1 m/s indicate a stenosis greater than 90%. Pulsed-wave Doppler sampling demonstrates the large number of velocities in the area of the stenosis; this is referred to as *spectral broadening*. Velocities decrease significantly as stenosis progresses to subtotal occlusion, making the distinction of subtotal and total occlusion by ultrasound difficult. ICA—internal carotid artery.

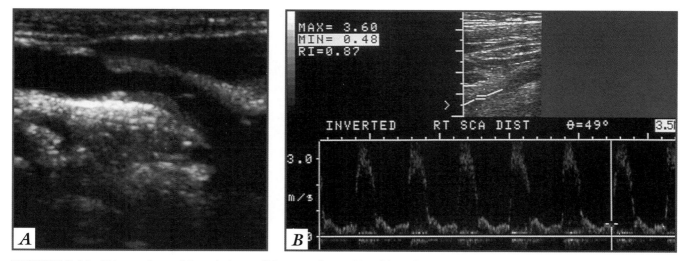

FIGURE 3-11. Takayasu's arteritis and giant cell (temporal) arteritis. Although atherosclerosis is the most common cause of cerebrovascular ischemia, vasculitides such as Takayasu's arteritis and giant cell (temporal) arteritis can also cause symptoms of cerebrovascular ischemia. Less common vasculitic causes of cerebrovascular ischemia include Wegener's granulomatosis, systemic lupus erythematosus, and polyarteritis nodosa.

A, Takayasu's arteritis is an inflammatory condition that commonly affects the aorta and its branches. The typical patient is a woman under the age of 40. Presenting complaints usually stem from ischemic syndromes, *eg,* upper extremity claudication, transient ischemic attacks, or cerebrovascular accidents. This image reveals thickening of the intimal layer of the proximal common carotid artery (CCA) in a patient with Takayasu's arteritis. Unlike atherosclerosis, the vasculitides do not commonly involve branch points.

B, Temporal arteritis, also known as giant cell arteritis, is found in older patients generally older than 50 years of age. It usually affects medium and small arteries, including the temporal, subclavian, (SCA) and ophthalmic arteries. Common findings include an elevated erythrocyte sedimentation rate, upper extremity claudication, headaches, polymyalgia, and blindness. In this image there is evidence of subclavian artery stenosis, with blood flow velocity increased to greater than 3 m/s in a patient with finger paresthesias and diminished left brachial artery pulse.

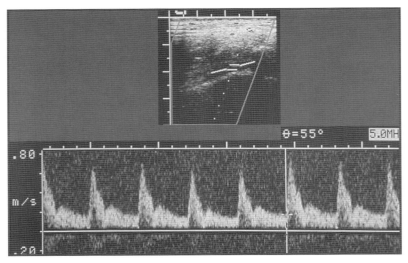

FIGURE 3-12. Ungrafted internal mammary artery showing a normal peripheral arterial waveform. In limited coronary artery bypass graft surgery, the left internal mammary artery is grafted to the left anterior descending coronary artery without proximal dissection of mammary artery graft from the chest wall. The internal mammary (thoracic) artery can be evaluated using B-mode ultrasound and pulsed-wave Doppler analysis.

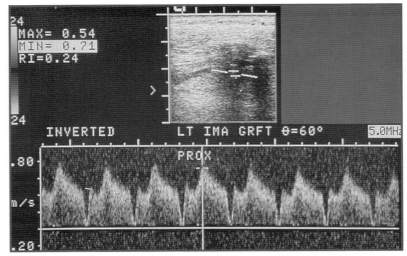

FIGURE 3-13. Pulsed-wave Doppler examination in the patent internal mammary artery graft (IMA GRFT). This image shows increased diastolic blood flow to the low-resistance coronary artery. The flow in the patent graft takes on some of the characteristics in the normal coronary artery bed, with diastolic flow greater than systolic flow, but still retains the systolic flow peak seen in the periphery.

ARTERIAL SYSTEM OF THE LOWER EXTREMITIES

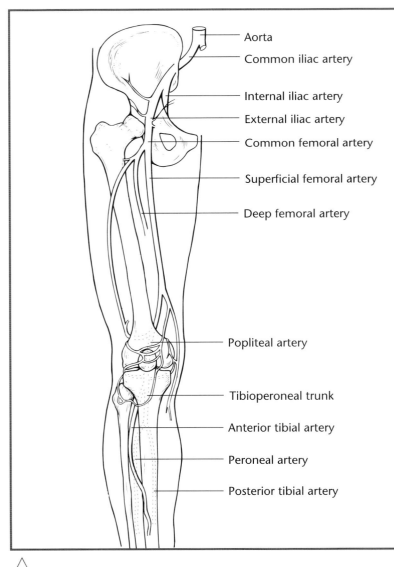

- Aorta
- Common iliac artery
- Internal iliac artery
- External iliac artery
- Common femoral artery
- Superficial femoral artery
- Deep femoral artery
- Popliteal artery
- Tibioperoneal trunk
- Anterior tibial artery
- Peroneal artery
- Posterior tibial artery

FIGURE 3-14. Lower extremity arteries. The arterial tree of the lower extremities is able to accommodate great amounts and increases in blood flow. In addition to the primary conducting system depicted, the lumbar collaterals, the lateral circumflex artery, and the internal iliac arteries provide a second avenue of blood delivery. This well-developed conduit system requires a large atherosclerotic burden to elicit symptoms of claudication. Claudication, noted in 1% to 6% of the general population, occurs at the level of the most flow-limiting stenosis [8]. The distal aorta and iliac, or inflow vessels, are involved in about 25% of patients, and these stenoses are most amenable to catheter-based therapy. Atherosclerosis affects the outflow arteries or superficial femoral, deep femoral, and popliteal arteries in more than 80% of cases. The runoff or calf vessels are affected in approximately 50% of all cases and more frequently in patients with diabetes.

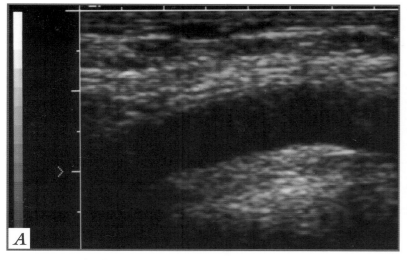

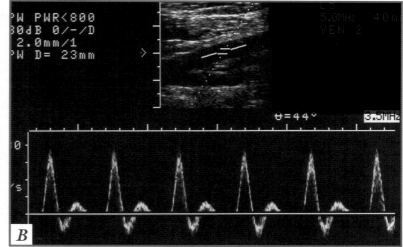

FIGURE 3-15. The normal common femoral arteries. These arteries are a site for both atherosclerotic and iatrogenic lesions. B-mode ultrasound imaging can delineate the layers of the arterial wall including the intima, media, and adventitia. The presence of a smooth, thin inner wall (**A**) indicates the absence of atherosclerotic, flow-limiting lesions. The pulsed-wave Doppler image (**B**) demonstrates the normal, narrow, triphasic flow of the high-resistance, peripheral arteries.

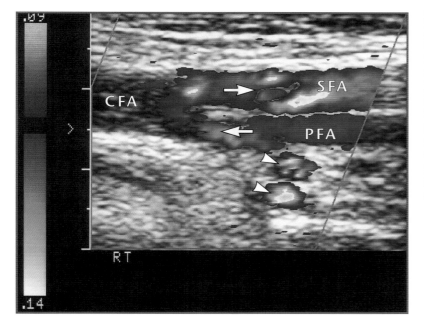

FIGURE 3-16. The diseased common femoral arteries (CFAs). Shown here is the CFA of a patient who presented to his physician with complaints of thigh and calf cramping after 200 yards of level walking. The color Doppler ultrasound image demonstrates an occluded CFA. The echogenic material within the lumen of the CFA is consistent with occlusive thrombus; no flow is detected in the distal CFA by color Doppler imaging. This occlusion impairs blood flow and creates reliance on collateral flow to meet the increased need of exercising muscles. The collateral flow into the profunda femoris artery (PFA) that then supplies the superficial femoral artery (SFA) is well represented by color-assisted Doppler ultrasonography, with high-velocity (*bright*) and multidirectional (*red* and *blue*) images. The combination of decreased supply, loss of perfusion pressure, and downstream dilatation combine to present the symptoms of ischemia. *Arrows* indicate direction of blood flow; *arrowheads* indicate collaterals.

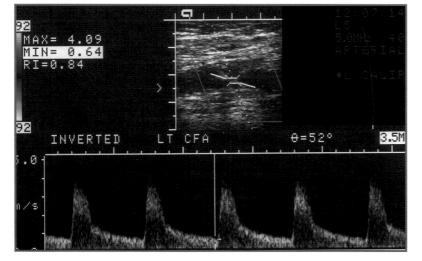

FIGURE 3-17. Pulsed-wave Doppler image revealing the abnormality of blood flow created by stenotic lesions in contrast to the triphasic, narrow band of pulsatile flow in a normal vessel. The sample volume is placed in an area of abnormal flow that has been identified by color Doppler. The maximum velocity detected, 4 m/s, is elevated. The blood cells flow haphazardly, yielding a large number of velocities on sampling (spectral broadening). CFA—common femoral artery.

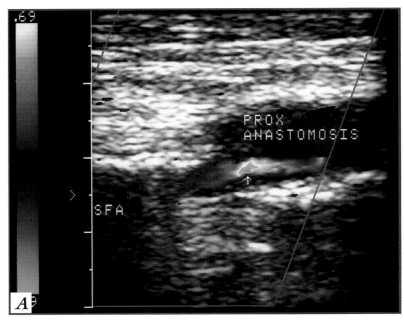

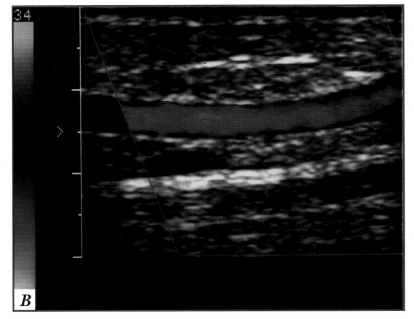

FIGURE 3-18. Surgical revascularization of the lower extremity. The presence of ischemic rest pain, nonhealing ulcers, or impending tissue loss are standard indications for lower extremity bypass grafting. Severely limiting claudication represents a gray area in which both the patient and physician must make individual decisions. Bypass grafting can be performed with saphenous vein grafts or other conduits constructed from dacron, umbilical vein, and polytetrafluoroethylene. During the past 20 years, autologous saphenous vein grafting has demonstrated superior patency and limb salvage rates in comparison with the prosthetic conduits. **A,** An occluded, plaque-laden superficial femoral artery (SFA) and patent proximal (PROX) anastomosis of a venous graft from the common femoral artery, as revealed by color-assisted Doppler ultrasonography. **B,** Normal flow in a widely patent saphenous vein graft. Bypass grafts are screened for stenosis frequently in the first year and then annually. Evidence of stenosis is acted on immediately to decrease the occurrence of graft failure.

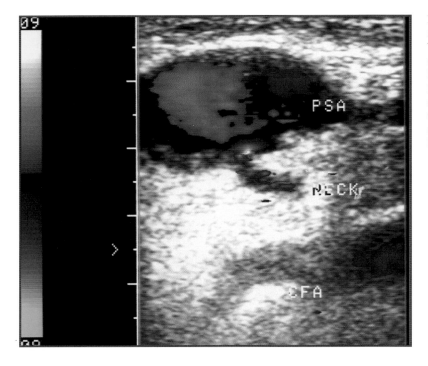

FIGURE 3-19. Pseudoaneurysm (PSA). PSA represents an uncommon but serious complication of arteriography. It occurs in less than one in 200 cases. The false aneurysm is a contained rupture of the intimal and medial layers of the vessel. The presence of flow out of the common femoral artery (CFA) into the PSA by color-assisted Doppler ultrasonography is demonstrated here. Swirling, turbulent flow is present within the PSA and in the neck, connecting the cavity to the femoral artery. The noninvasive vascular laboratory may play a therapeutic role in this case through ultrasound-assisted compression of the neck of the lesion, which may result in thrombosis of the PSA. Failing that, surgical repair is usually required.

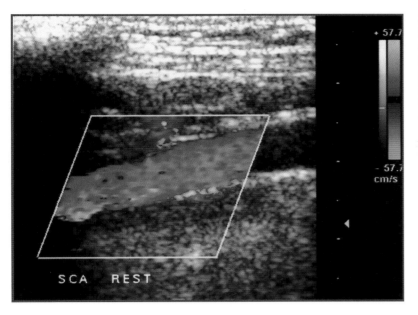

FIGURE 3-20. B-mode image demonstrating the normal, asymptomatic left subclavian artery (SCA) with the arm below the shoulder. Thoracic outlet obstruction can cause symptoms in the neck, shoulder, or upper extremity by mechanical irritation or compression of the artery, vein, or brachial plexus. The arterial variety is the least common, but potentially most serious because thromboembolic events may threaten the viability of the upper extremity. Patients usually present in their 30s to 60s and frequently have a congenital bony abnormality in the thoracic outlet.

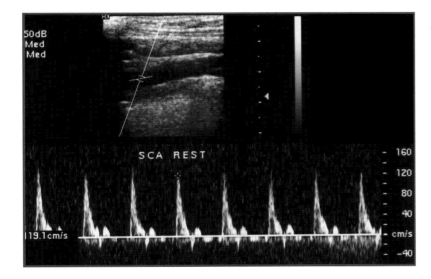

FIGURE 3-21. Normal pulsed-wave Doppler image of normal triphasic flow is present in this subclavian artery (SCA) image. The B-mode image shows normal-appearing intima and arterial diameter. Chronic compression of the SCA, usually by a cervical rib against the anterior scalene muscle and first rib, leads to injury and then to thickening of the intima. A dilated region develops beyond the site of thickening because of the turbulent flow. This may progress into a true aneurysm. Thrombus may develop at the site of intimal thickening or in an aneurysm. Thromboembolic events from the poststenotic region may lead to Raynaud's phenomenon, digital ischemia, or large vessel occlusion.

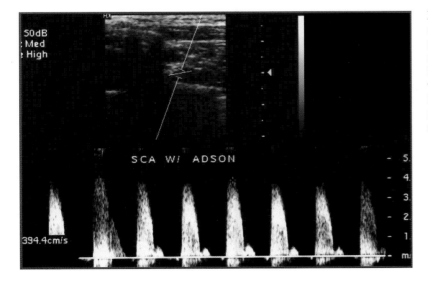

FIGURE 3-22. Duplex image acquired during performance of the Adson maneuver. Duplex ultrasonography can be used to confirm the results of physical examination. The loss of the radial pulse with thoracic outlet maneuvers demonstrates the impairment to flow. B-mode ultrasound imaging may be able to document the site of compression during maneuvers. This image demonstrates both arterial compression and a marked increase in the flow velocity. Examination demonstrating compression but no symptoms is not diagnostic of thoracic outlet syndrome. The signs of outlet obstruction can be elicited commonly by ultrasound in approximately 15% of normal patients. SCA—subclavian artery.

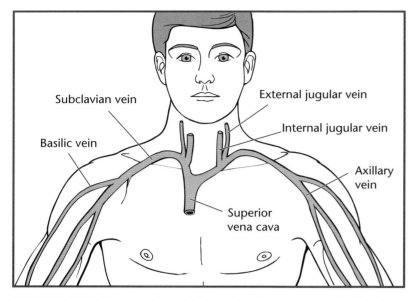

FIGURE 3-23. Venous system of the neck and upper extremity. Ninety percent of identified deep vein thromboses occur in the lower extremities. However, the noninvasive vascular laboratory is frequently called on to assess the veins of the neck and upper extremities. In the absence of venous thrombosis, a vein can be compressed with moderate external pressure that does not affect the nearby arteries. Any loss of compressibility of the neck and arm veins is consistent with venous thrombosis. The clavicle and rib cage limit the ability to compress the subclavian vein. In this case, abnormal waveforms or echogenic material within the lumen suggest thrombosis.

The inciting factors for venous thrombosis include vessel wall damage, venous stasis, and hypercoagulable states. The thrombi themselves are composed of erythrocytes, platelets, and leukocytes bound by fibrin. As they propagate centrally, venous thromboses are loosely attached to the vessel wall, creating the risk for embolic events. In the absence of embolism, the thrombosis organizes, and obstructed vessels may recanalize.

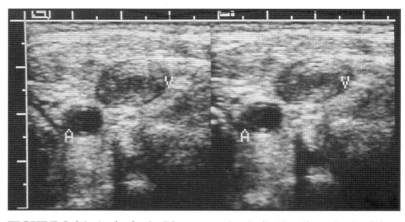

FIGURE 3-24. Lack of vein (V) compression indicating thrombosis of the internal jugular vein. The thrombus is bright, indicating that it is organized. Fresh thrombus has a composition more similar to blood, producing a dark image. Patients may complain of pain, warmth, swelling, or fullness of the neck, face, or supraclavicular fossa. Treatment is similar to that of lower extremity deep venous thromboses. The 12% to 36% incidence of pulmonary emboli underlies the importance of making this diagnosis [9]. A—artery.

Causes of Upper Extremity Vein Thrombosis

Extravascular	Intravascular
Malignancy	Central intravenous lines
Compression injury	Hypercoagulable states
Thoracic outlet obstruction	Intravenous drug use
Effort-induced (Paget-Schroetter) thrombosis	Pacing wires
	Trauma
Mediastinal fibrosis	

FIGURE 3-25. Common causes of upper extremity vein thrombosis. Axillary and subclavian vein thrombosis is an unusual cause of deep venous thrombosis, representing 1% to 2% of all deep vein thromboses.

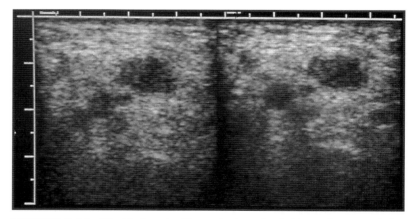

FIGURE 3-26. Effort-induced axillary vein thrombosis. Fewer than 3% of all deep venous thromboses originate in the axillary and subclavian veins. The Paget-Schroetter syndrome of effort-induced thrombosis is a venous variant of thoracic outlet obstruction. Frequently occurring in athletic young men and women, the vein is compressed between a scalene tendon and the first rib, often exacerbated by an exostosis. The unilateral swelling is usually brought on by exercise and may resolve with the formation of collaterals over several weeks. Surgical therapy is required after thrombolysis to prevent rethrombosis [10].

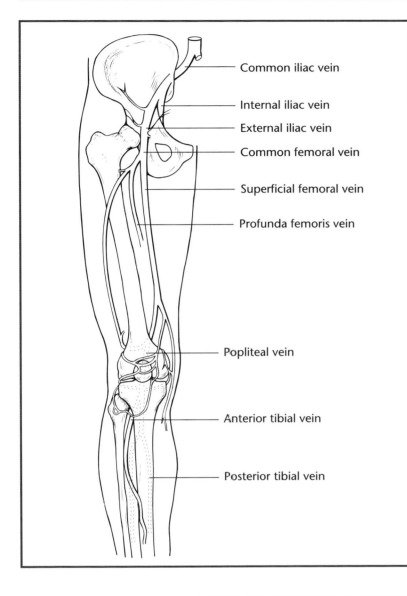

FIGURE 3-27. The normal lower extremity venous system. Venous thrombosis affects approximately one person in 1000 in the United States each year. More than 90% of all venous thrombosis occurs in the lower extremities. The location of the thrombosis is significant because of the greater risk of embolization from the proximal vessels. Making the diagnosis of deep venous thrombosis aids in preventing pulmonary embolism and mitigating the chronic-phase, postphlebitic syndrome. In addition to determining the presence of compressibility, variation in venous flow is examined with normal respiration and following Valsalva's maneuver in the common femoral vein. The absence of normal respirophasic variation in flow or venous distention following Valsalva's maneuver represents evidence for venous obstruction proximal to the common femoral vein.

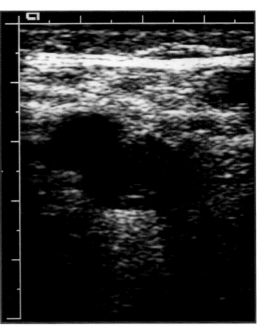

FIGURE 3-28. A common femoral vein with three markers of thrombosis. The clinical features of deep venous thrombosis include warmth, unilateral leg swelling, and erythema. A cord may be palpable and distention of superficial veins appreciated. Most importantly, the thin-walled vessel cannot be compressed. In this case, the thrombus is a combination of new (*dark*) and old and organized (*bright*) echogenic material. Finally, there is absence of flow as detected by color-assisted Doppler imaging.

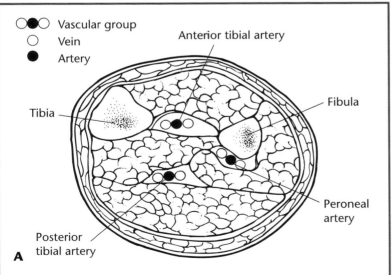

FIGURE 3-29. Calf vein anatomy shown schematically (**A**), by B-mode ultrasonography (**B**), and by color Doppler imaging (**C**). Diagnosis of thrombosis in the calf veins is more difficult than in the proximal veins. Calf vein thrombi are not easy to detect because only one of the multiple veins may be involved, and adequate venous return via the remaining patent vessels limits edema. The most common symptom of calf vein thrombosis is pain. Examination of the major calf veins requires knowledge of the calf anatomy.
(*Continued on next page*)

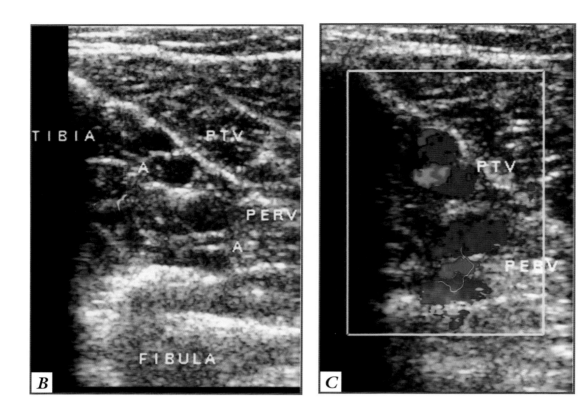

FIGURE 3-29. (*Continued*) In the B-mode and color-assisted Doppler images, the paired veins are observed with the expected relationship to the fascial plane (shown here), and can be externally compressed. Augmentation of venous flow is clearly evident in the color Doppler images. The reported sensitivity and specificity for duplex ultrasonography of the calf veins is 88% to 96% and 94% to 96%, respectively. A—artery; PERV—peroneal veins; PTV—posterior tibial veins.

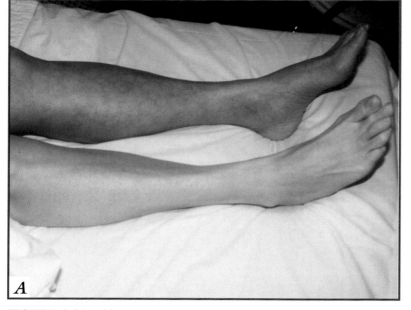

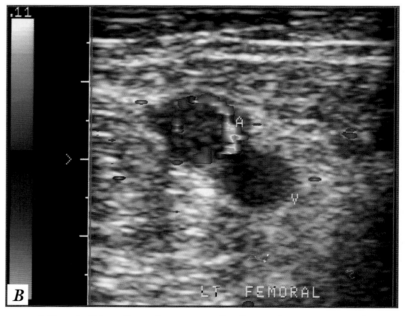

FIGURE 3-30. Phlegmasia cerulea dolens, or venous gangrene, a severe variant of deep venous thrombosis (DVT). The presentation of common DVTs may include evidence of erythema or pallor. This syndrome is caused by extensive thrombosis with marked swelling, pain, and blue discoloration. The extensive swelling can create enough pressure to limit arterial flow and yield an arterial insufficiency. Malignancy is a common co-traveler in this presentation. In this patient, the compression from edema was enough to cause thrombosis of the common femoral artery. **A,** The patient's leg with the characteristic cyanosis and edema. **B,** The accompanying duplex ultrasound image demonstrating thrombus in both the common femoral artery (A) and vein (V).

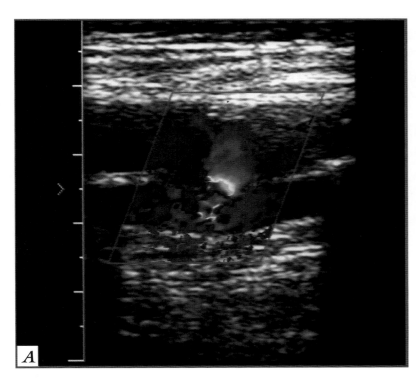

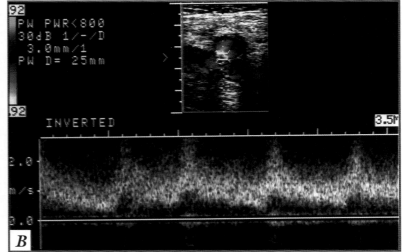

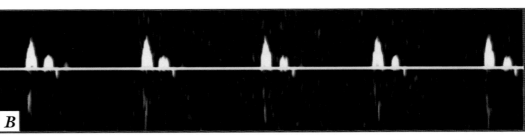

FIGURE 3-31. Arteriovenous (AV) fistula. AV fistulae may be congenital, like a cavernous hemangioma, or acquired traumatically. Injuries such as gunshot and knife wounds may disrupt the integrity of both artery and vein, yielding an abnormal connection and direction of flow. An AV fistula may have an iatrogenic cause, *eg*, intentionally for hemodialysis or unintentionally after angiography. **A** and **B** demonstrate the shunting from the arterial to the venous system. Color Doppler ultrasonography demonstrates the presence of flow connecting the artery and vein with associated turbulence. The pulsed-wave Doppler image demonstrates the velocity and volume of flow from the high- to low-pressure vascular beds.

RAYNAUD'S PHENOMENON

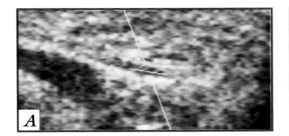

FIGURE 3-32. Raynaud's phenomenon is episodic digital vasospasm with attendant digital pallor, cyanosis, and on rewarming, rubor. The initial phase of the cold response is spasm of the digital artery and decreased perfusion of the fingers. **A** and **B**, in this image, there is a mild reduction in baseline digital artery flow with a bifid pulse waveform that is frequently observed in patients with Raynaud's phenomenon.

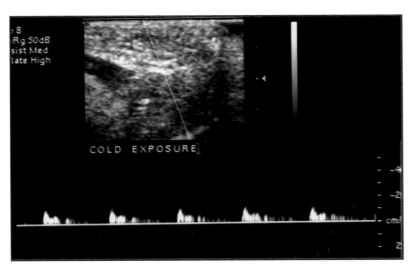

FIGURE 3-33. Duplex ultrasound of blood flow after cold exposure in Raynaud's phenomenon. Several mechanisms have been postulated to explain the digital vasospasm, including excessive sympathetic nervous efferent activity locally, abnormalities in the response of the digital arteries to normal sympathetic nervous system tone, overproduction of vasoconstrictor substances, and low digital artery flow. During the prolonged vasospasm, the capillaries and venules dilate in response to ischemia and become filled with blue, deoxygenated blood. In this image, the pulsed-wave Doppler shows the broad, monophasic, lower amplitude digital pulse wave.

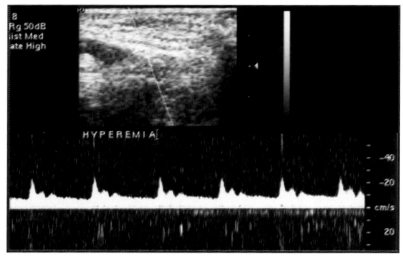

FIGURE 3-34. Duplex ultrasound of blood flow with rewarming in Raynaud's phenomenon. After rewarming, the digital vasospasm is relieved, and oxygenated blood floods the ischemic tissues, yielding red hands. In this image, the patient's Doppler waveform reveals augmented flow from baseline in both systole and diastole. Treatment of primary Raynaud's phenomenon begins with behavior modification. Patients should be instructed to maintain total body warmth, not just hand and foot warmth, in order to decrease reflex vasoconstriction. Avoidance of activities that elicit symptoms may be required. Treatment of the underlying causes of secondary Raynaud's should be initiated. Vasoactive medications specifically for the digital vasospasm should be reserved for patients with unremitting symptoms.

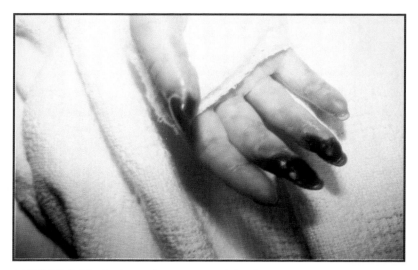

FIGURE 3-35. Prolonged vasospasm of the digital arteries with cyanosis and distal necrosis in a patient with systemic lupus erythematosus. The secondary causes of Raynaud's phenomenon include the connective tissue diseases, arterial occlusive disease, blood dyscrasias, neurologic disorders, vibration injury, chemotherapy, and vasoconstrictor medications. Secondary Raynaud's can be unilateral and is more likely to induce tissue damage.

REFERENCES

1. Criqui MH, Fronek A, Barrett-Connor E, *et al.*: The prevalence of peripheral arterial disease in a defined population. *Circulation* 1985, 71:510–515.

2. Gillum RF: Pulmonary embolism in the United States. *Am Heart J* 1987, 113:1262–1264

3. American Heart Association: *Heart and Stroke Facts*. Dallas: American Heart Association; 1991.

4. Wells P: Basic principles and Doppler physics. In *Clinical Applications of Doppler Ultrasound*. Edited by Taylor K, Burns P, Wells P. New York: Raven; 1988:1–25.

5. Creager M, O'Leary D, Doubilet P: Noninvasive vascular testing. In *Vascular Medicine*, edn 2. Edited by Loscalzo J, Creager M, Dzau V. Boston: Little, Brown and Co; 1996:415–444.

6. Polak JF: *Peripheral Vascular Sonography*. Baltimore: Williams and Wilkins; 1992.

7. Merritt CRB: Doppler color flow imaging. *J Clin Ultrasound* 1987, 15:591–597.

8. Kannel WB, Skinner JJ Jr, Schwartz MJ, Shurtleff D: Intermittent claudication: incidence in the Framingham study. *Circulation* 1970, 41:875–883.

9. Horattas MC, Wright DJ, Fenton AH, *et al.*: Changing concepts of deep venous thrombosis of the upper extremity: report of a series and review of the literature. *Surgery* 1988, 104:561–567.

10. Machleder H: Neurovascular compression syndromes of the thoracic outlet. In *Vascular Medicine*, edn 2. Edited by Loscalzo J, Creager M, Dzau V. Boston: Little, Brown and Co; 1996:1187–1208.

4

Nuclear Cardiology

Finn Mannting

During the past few years it has become clear that functional information beyond anatomic data is needed to understand and efficiently treat many patients with heart disease. The functional significance of a given anatomic abnormality varies from patient to patient depending on individual circumstances. Functional studies such as two-dimensional echocardiogram (ECHO)-Doppler and radionuclide methods supply such information. In addition to their inherent diagnostic abilities, these methods also provide highly significant prognostic information [1–3].

New developments in imaging agents and the tremendous improvement in camera technology, computers, and software have changed nuclear cardiology radically over the past 15 years, and the field is still changing. High-quality myocardial perfusion imaging with the new ^{99m}Tc-labeled agents (sestamibi and myoview) and single photon emission computed tomography (SPECT) technique is widely available. These tracers accumulate in the myocardium primarily proportionally to flow (like microspheres) and secondarily according to availability of functional myocytes. The resulting tomographic images—which are really not images of the heart in an anatomic sense but rather three-dimensional maps of myocardial blood flow at the moment of tracer administration—are provided. This tomographic technique delivers images with high anatomic resolution, as all portions of the myocardium are shown without superimposition of walls. Rest perfusion abnormalities usually represent myocardial injury, ie, loss of myocytes. Images of myocardial perfusion during stress are obtained by tracer administration during peak stress. Standardized well-established physical and pharmacologic stress protocols are available [4]. By systematic comparison of regional tracer uptake in the rest and stress studies, wall-by-wall stress-induced ischemia can be demonstrated. Computer-based quantification of SPECT myocardial perfusion data [5] has been in use for several years and has improved the method's reproducibility significantly by reducing interobserver variability in readings. In patients with left ventricular dysfunction, the possibility of improving function by revascularization has gained much interest. Identification of such viable but dysfunctional myocardium has been accomplished using ^{201}Tl and sestamibi viability protocols [6–8]. With outcome (defined as objectively demonstrated functional improvement) as the end point, these radionuclide methods have been shown to be compatible with low-dose dobutamine ECHO and slightly inferior to the more expensive metabolic imaging with positron emission tomography tracers like ^{18}F-flourodeoxyglucose [9]. First-pass radionuclide angiography for quantification of left-to-right shunts has been in use since the early days of nuclear cardiology, and is still useful in selected patients. Modern gated equilibrium radionuclide angiography (also known as equilibrium radionuclide angiocardiography, radionuclide ventriculography, and multigated angiogram), using high erythrocyte labeling efficiency methods and sophisticated computer analysis of the acquired data [10], delivers global and regional ejection fraction (EF) with unsurpassed accuracy and reproducibility. This method's role in assessment of EF and for following left ventricular function over time is well established [11].

Rapid technologic development has and will continue to provide possibilities and opportunities in nuclear cardiology that will further make it possible to measure and follow cardiac function noninvasively at reasonable cost. The key to optimal and efficient patient diagnosis and management is to combine anatomic and functional information. Radionuclide imaging, which provides the functional information, and perfusion imaging, which provides the anatomic information, assess the first step in the ischemia cascade [12].

PRINCIPLES OF CARDIAC RADIONUCLIDE IMAGING

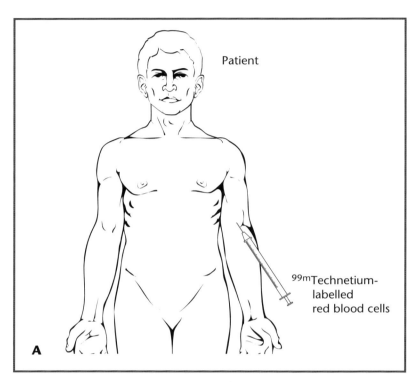

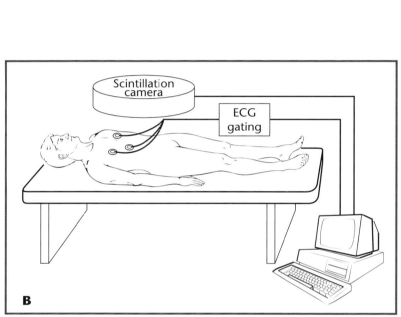

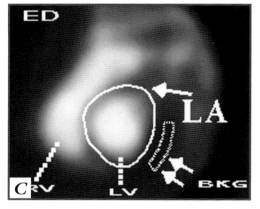

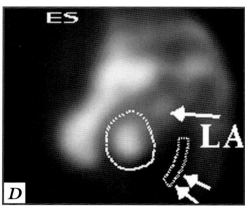

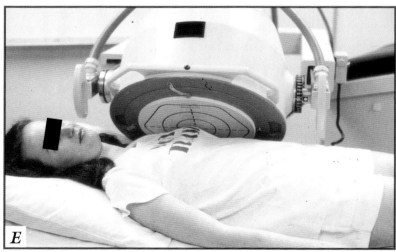

FIGURE 4-1. Basic principles of radionuclide angiography. **A,** ^{99m}Tc-labeled red blood cells are injected intravenously and circulate throughout the blood pool. **B,** Electrocardiographic (ECG) electrodes are attached to the patient and a scintillation camera is positioned over the chest. Gamma emissions over the region of interest (heart) are detected by the camera and the acquisition gated to the R wave of the ECG. Data from many cardiac cycles are obtained and averaged. An endless loop cine of an "average" cardiac cycle is then displayed for interpretation. Gated equilibrium blood pool images. **C** and **D,** Frames representing end-diastole (ED) and end-systole (ES). An automatic edge detection algorithm was applied for definition of the edges. Left atrium (LA) is correctly excluded from the left ventricular (LV) region of interest. Background region (*arrows*) is in standardized position and covers representative background area (BKG) (**C**). **E,** Typical single-head camera used for first-pass and radionuclide ventriculography studies. Here the camera is positioned in left anterior oblique 45° position. RV—right ventricle. (Parts A, B, C, and D *courtesy of* Gerald G. Blackwell and Gerald M. Pohost; part E *courtesy of* Frans J. Th. Wackers.)

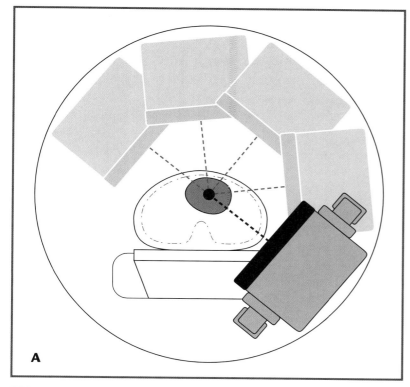

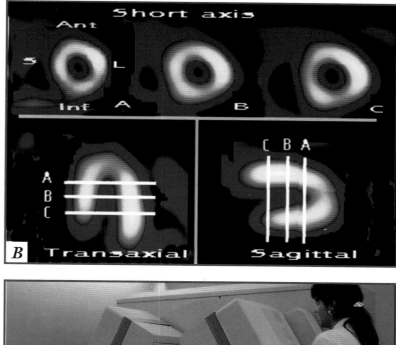

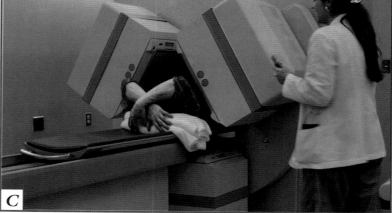

FIGURE 4-2. Basic concept of single photon computed tomography (SPECT). Gamma camera images are obtained from many angles around the patient. **A,** Computed tomography. **B,** Images of myocardial perfusion reconstructed into short axis, transaxial, and sagittal cuts. **C,** Modern three-headed gamma camera suitable for myocardial perfusion studies. Multihead cameras with medium-sized fields of view are advantageous for cardiac SPECT studies. Cameras with medium-sized heads (in cranial-caudal direction) can get closer to the patient's chest, and multiple heads reduce the acquisition time significantly. (Part A *courtesy of* Frans J. Th. Wackers.)

Radionuclides and Methods in Nuclear Cardiology

Study Type	Tracer Agent	Study Name	Assessment of
Flow	^{99m}Tc pertechnetate	First-pass	LV and RV EF
		Shunt	QP/QS
Function	^{99m}Tc-labeled RBC	RVG (or MUGA, ERNA)	LV- and RVEF
Perfusion viability	201-T1	Rest-stress perfusion	Scar/ischemic
		Viability protocol	Scar/viability
Perfusion	^{99m}Tc sestamibi	Rest-stress perfusion	Scar/ischemic (LVEF wall motions)
Viability	^{99m}Tc sestamibi	Rest perfusion	Scar/viability (LVEF, wall motions)
Perfusion	^{99m}Tc myoview	Rest-stress perfusion	Scar/ischemic (LVEF, wall motions)
Viability	^{99m}Tc myoview	Rest perfusion	Scar/viability (LVEF, wall motions)
Metabolic	FDG	Myocardial viability	Glucose metabolism

FIGURE 4-3. Radionuclides and methods in nuclear cardiology. EF— ejection fraction; ERNA—equilibrium radionuclide angiocardiography; FDG— ^{18}F-fluorodeoxyglucose; LV—left ventricle; MUGA—multigated angiogram; QP—pulmonary flow; QS—systemic flow; RBC—red blood cells; RV—right ventricle; RVG—radionuclide ventriculography.

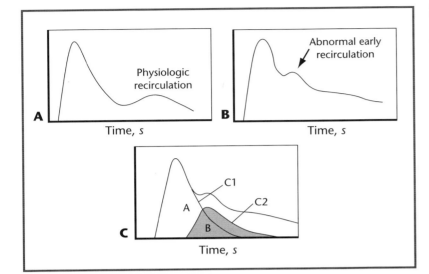

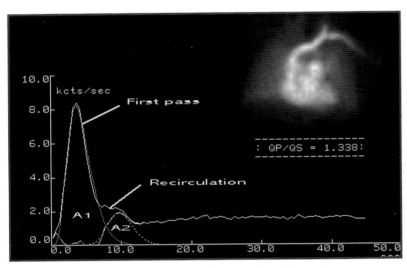

FIGURE 4-4. First-pass curves showing changes in tracer content in the lungs over time after intravenous injection of tracer bolus. **A,** Normal time activity curve. The tracer reaches the lungs as a slightly diluted bolus; a physiologic recirculation occurs later, mainly caused by the quick return of coronary and pulmonary venous blood. **B,** If a left-to-right shunt is present, an abnormal early recirculation will take place (*arrow*). The size of this abnormal recirculation curve is a function of the shunt size. **C,** By fitting the initial portion of the original first-pass curve to a gamma variate function (thus producing an idealized first-pass curve [C1]) and subtracting this curve from the original curve, the recirculation curve caused by a shunt will become apparent. This curve is also fitted to a gamma variate function, giving an idealized recirculation curve (C2). The areas under the curves are then integrated (A and B) and entered into the equation (A/A-B) = QP/QS, which is the ratio of pulmonary flow to systemic flow. This ratio is of course normally 1.0; if greater than 1.3, a shunt is considered present, and if greater than 2.0, the shunt is considered clinically significant (the pulmonary flow is double the systemic flow).

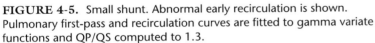

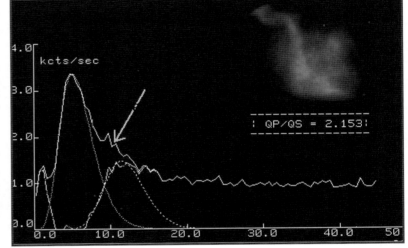

FIGURE 4-5. Small shunt. Abnormal early recirculation is shown. Pulmonary first-pass and recirculation curves are fitted to gamma variate functions and QP/QS computed to 1.3.

FIGURE 4-6. Medium-sized shunt. Large abnormal early recirculation is noted (*arrow*). QP/QS computed to 2.2. Right-heart catheterization showed large atrial septal defect, oxymetric QP/QS: 2.4.

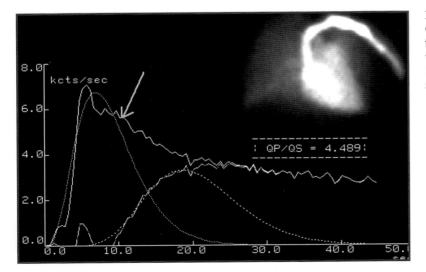

FIGURE 4-7. Large shunt. Very large abnormal early recirculation. Gamma variate fit was performed giving a QP/QS of 4.5; however, the fitting and the computation model are not valid in a very large shunt like this in which the curves are distorted. Computed QP/QS values larger than 3.0 are therefore only reported as greater than 3.0. Catheterization demonstrated large ventricular septal defect.

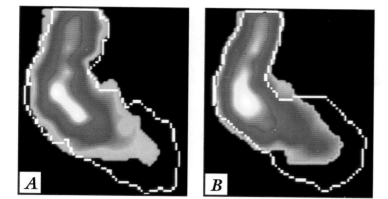

FIGURE 4-8. Abnormal first-pass radionuclide angiograms at rest and during exercise. In this patient, resting left ventricular ejection fraction (LVEF) is 60% (**A**), and peak exercise LVEF is 45% (**B**), with uniformly decreased regional wall motion. An abnormal response is defined as either a decrease greater than 5%, or no change in LVEF compared with baseline. In patients with a high baseline LVEF (*ie,* 70% or greater), only a decrease in LVEF is considered an abnormal response. (Legend *from* Wackers [13]; figure *courtesy of* Frans J. Th. Wackers.)

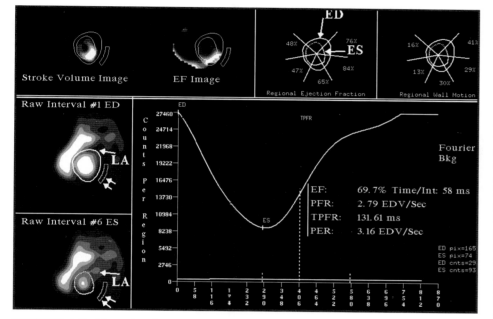

FIGURE 4-9. Normal radionuclide ventriculography (RVG). A gated dynamic study consisting of 24 frames per cardiac cycle is shown. An analytic software package was applied. First the left ventricular (LV) edge on the end-diastole (ED) image is defined, then the LV edge on the end-systole (ES) image, both by means of a fast automatic second deridivate method (*left column, middle* and *bottom images*). A background region (*arrows*)

is automatically placed below and to the left of LV. A volume-equivalent, Fourier-fitted time activity curve is then generated (*lower right field*), and ejection fraction (EF) calculated from this curve using the following equation:

$$EF = (ED\ volume - Bkg\ volume)\ (ES\ volume - Bkg\ volume) / (ED\ volume - Bkg\ volume).$$

The volume units in this equation can be replaced with amount of labeled blood expressed as counts. The EF calculation is thus based directly on changes in amount of tracer and therefore is not dependent on any volume model. Peak filling rate (PFR), time to peak filling rate (TPFR), and peak ejection rate (PER) are also calculated. Functional images illustrating the stroke volume distribution and regional EF are displayed in the *upper left field*. The *upper right fields* show the ED and ES edges overlaid for objective assessment of regional wall motion. Regional EF and regional radial shortening are also computed and shown. The dynamic display of these images is usually shown as an endless-loop "movie" simultaneously with the data shown on the screen, allowing for visual estimation of wall motions. The reproducibility of EF assessments with modern RVG is very high owing to the automatic edge detection, and the method is accurate even in dilated hearts and in hearts with unusual form. The accuracy, independence of volume equations, and high reproducibility make RVG the method of choice for measuring effect of intervention, effect of treatment, and natural changes over time. Bkg—background; LA—left atrium.

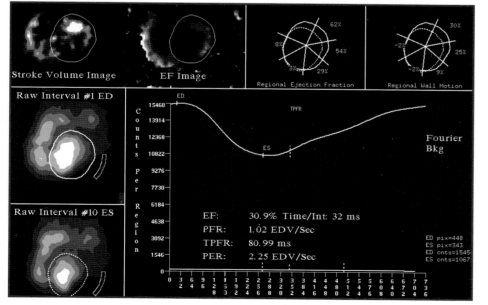

FIGURE 4-10. Radionuclide ventriculogram in a 45-year-old man with a history of two myocardial infarctions (MIs), now presenting with progressing dyspnea. Left ventricular (LV) ejection fraction (EF) is 31%. The LV is moderately dilated. Objective wall motion analysis (*left column, middle* and *bottom images*) shows good contractions in the lateral wall and akinesis in the apex and septum. The anterior wall was akinetic in the study obtained in the anterior projection. Volume-equivalent, Fourier-fitted activity curve is shown in the *lower right*. Thus, neither the computed regional function nor the dynamic images (*upper left*) revealed any evidence of LV aneurysm, but they did show severe regional wall motion abnormalities consistent with several prior MI's. Bkg—background; ED—end-diastole; ES—end-systole; PER—peak ejection rate; PFR—peak filling rate; TPFR—time to peak filling rate.

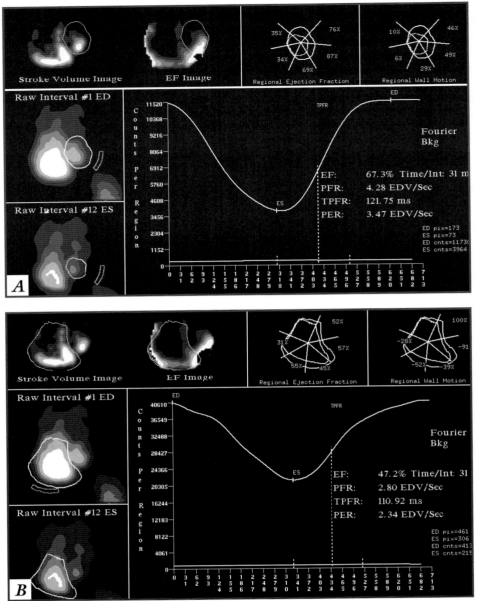

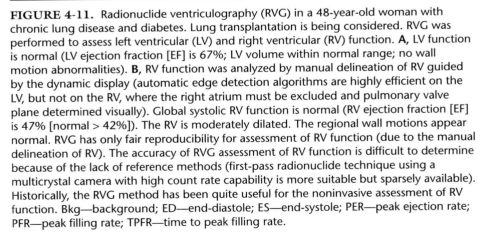

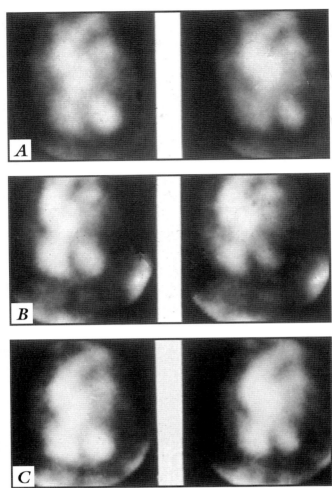

FIGURE 4-11. Radionuclide ventriculography (RVG) in a 48-year-old woman with chronic lung disease and diabetes. Lung transplantation is being considered. RVG was performed to assess left ventricular (LV) and right ventricular (RV) function. **A,** LV function is normal (LV ejection fraction [EF] is 67%; LV volume within normal range; no wall motion abnormalities). **B,** RV function was analyzed by manual delineation of RV guided by the dynamic display (automatic edge detection algorithms are highly efficient on the LV, but not on the RV, where the right atrium must be excluded and pulmonary valve plane determined visually). Global systolic RV function is normal (RV ejection fraction [EF] is 47% [normal > 42%]). The RV is moderately dilated. The regional wall motions appear normal. RVG has only fair reproducibility for assessment of RV function (due to the manual delineation of RV). The accuracy of RVG assessment of RV function is difficult to determine because of the lack of reference methods (first-pass radionuclide technique using a multicrystal camera with high count rate capability is more suitable but sparsely available). Historically, the RVG method has been quite useful for the noninvasive assessment of RV function. Bkg—background; ED—end-diastole; ES—end-systole; PER—peak ejection rate; PFR—peak filling rate; TPFR—time to peak filling rate.

FIGURE 4-12. Abnormal equilibrium radionuclide angiography (ERNA) at rest (**A**), at peak exercise (**B**), and immediately after exercise (**C**). This illustration shows an abnormal rest and exercise ERNA (also referred to as *radionuclide ventriculography* [RVG], *multi-gated acquisition* [MUGA], or *gated blood pool imaging*). Radioactivity is shown in *white*. The end-diastolic (ED) and end-systolic (ES) left anterior oblique still frames are shown. Left ventricular ejection fraction (LVEF) at rest is 75% with normal left ventricular wall motion. The right ventricle, pulmonary artery, and aorta, which are normal, can be noted. At peak exercise, LVEF decreased to 54% with apical akinesis. LVEF improved to 74% immediately after exercise. Regional wall motion is best interpreted by displaying the images as an endless loop cine on a computer screen. (Legend *from* Wackers [13]; figure *courtesy of* Frans J. Th. Wackers.)

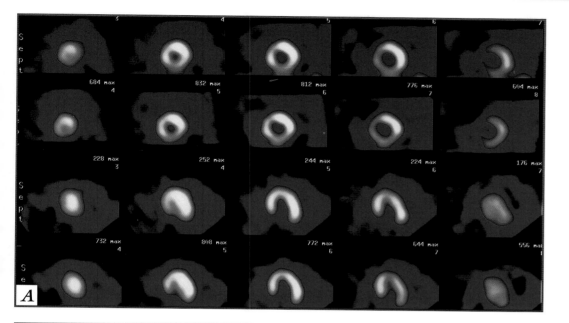

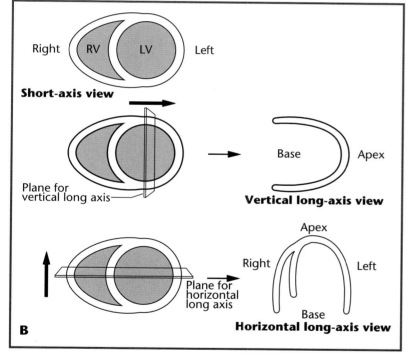

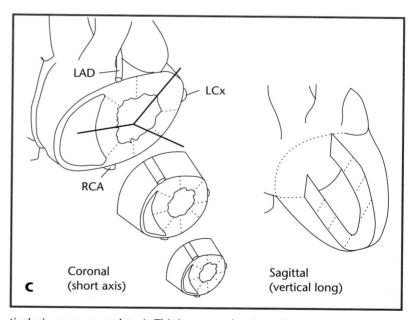

FIGURE 4-13. A, Normal myocardial perfusion scan using a standard rest-stress protocol. Eight mCi ^{99m}Tc-labeled sestamibi was administered at rest (*upper row*), and a second higher dose (24 mCi) was administered at peak stress 3 hours after the rest injection. Images were acquired 30 to 60 minutes after the tracer administration to allow for liver clearance. The single photon emission computed tomography (SPECT) technique was used. The data were reconstructed to coronal (*upper two rows*) and transaxial (*lower two rows*) cuts. The original slice thickness is 6 mm; three slices are added to reduce random noise and to produce clinically relevant myocardial volumes. Fairly homogeneous tracer uptake is noted in all walls, except for the inferior wall where the tracer uptake is slightly reduced in typical attenuation artefact pattern. Notice in the transaxial images that the septum is shorter than the free lateral wall; the septum at the base is there-fore not visualized or has reduced uptake (*fifth* and *fourth image,* respec-

tively, in *rows one* and *two*). This is a normal variant; there is considerable variability in the length of the muscular septum. **B,** SPECT reconstructed slices. The display of reconstructed SPECT myocardial perfusion slices has a standard format. Three sets of slices are displayed: short-axis slices (from apex to base), horizontal long-axis slices (from inferior wall to anterior wall), and vertical long-axis slices (from septum to lateral wall). **C,** Model of left ventricular (LV) myocardium. The LV is divided into basal, middle, and apical thirds. Each third is further divided into eight segments, and the apex (the most distal portion without cavity) is considered a segment, for a total of 25 segments. The three major coronary arteries are marked, and the general vascular territories illustrated. LAD—left anterior descending coronary artery; LCx—left circumflex coronary artery; RCA—right coronary artery; RV—right ventricle. (Legend for part B *from* Wackers [13]; figure for part B *courtesy of* Frans J. Th. Wackers.)

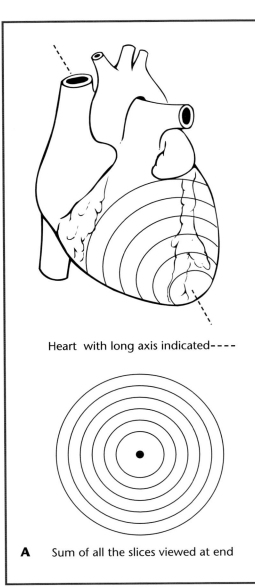

Heart with long axis indicated----

A   Sum of all the slices viewed at end

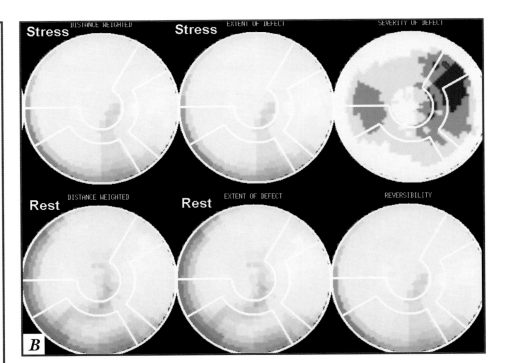

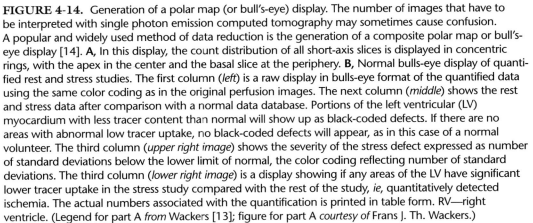

FIGURE 4-14. Generation of a polar map (or bull's-eye) display. The number of images that have to be interpreted with single photon emission computed tomography may sometimes cause confusion. A popular and widely used method of data reduction is the generation of a composite polar map or bull's-eye display [14]. **A,** In this display, the count distribution of all short-axis slices is displayed in concentric rings, with the apex in the center and the basal slice at the periphery. **B,** Normal bulls-eye display of quantified rest and stress studies. The first column (*left*) is a raw display in bulls-eye format of the quantified data using the same color coding as in the original perfusion images. The next column (*middle*) shows the rest and stress data after comparison with a normal data database. Portions of the left ventricular (LV) myocardium with less tracer content than normal will show up as black-coded defects. If there are no areas with abnormal low tracer uptake, no black-coded defects will appear, as in this case of a normal volunteer. The third column (*upper right image*) shows the severity of the stress defect expressed as number of standard deviations below the lower limit of normal, the color coding reflecting number of standard deviations. The third column (*lower right image*) is a display showing if any areas of the LV have significant lower tracer uptake in the stress study compared with the rest of the study, ie, quantitatively detected ischemia. The actual numbers associated with the quantification is printed in table form. RV—right ventricle. (Legend for part A *from* Wackers [13]; figure for part A *courtesy of* Frans J. Th. Wackers.)

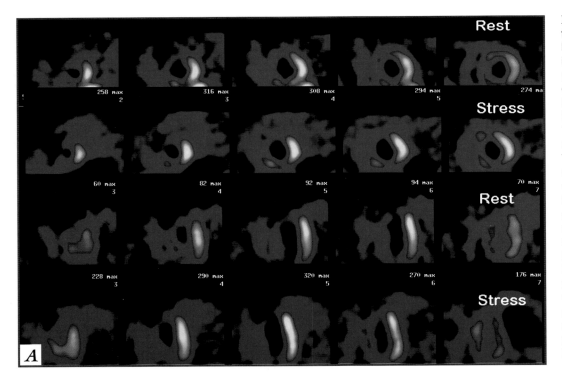

FIGURE 4-15. A, Myocardial perfusion scan from a 42-year-old man (67 in, 180 lbs) with a history of recent large anterior wall myocardial infarction (MI), and possibly previous MI, now presenting with severe shortness of breath, cold extremities, and occasional exertional chest pain. Stress test: 6:00 minutes standard Bruce protocol; heart rate, 78 → 169; blood pressure, 110 → 140; rate-pressure product, 15.500. Test stopped due to dyspnea and fatigue but no chest pain. ST-T abnormalities at baseline, accentuation with stress. Findings: no tracer uptake in apex, anterior wall, and septum at baseline, consistent with transmural MI (12 of 25 segments, left anterior descending coronary artery territory). Marked reduced uptake in the inferior and inferior-lateral walls, consistent with severe but not transmural injury (six of 25 segments, right coronary artery). During stress minimal ischemia in a few segments in the inferior-lateral wall (*dots*). The lateral wall is well perfused at baseline and during stress, and serves as reference in both studies. Both studies are composed of relative images; it is therefore impossible to assess if there is ischemia in the lateral wall.

(*Continued on next page*)

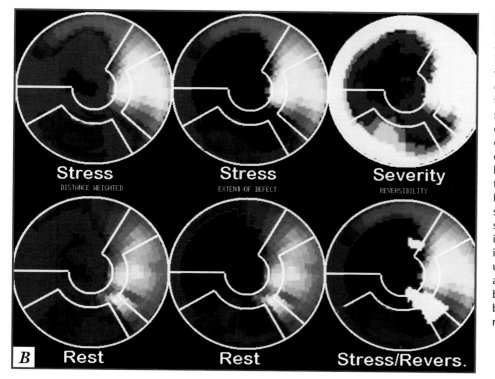

FIGURE 4-15. (*Continued*) **B,** Quantification and bulls-eye display of the quantified data. The extent of the perfusion abnormalities at baseline is displayed in the *lower row*. The first bulls eye is raw data; in the second, the data are compared with normal database (abnormal areas flagged in *black*). The extent of perfusion abnormalities during stress is displayed in the *upper row*. The severity of the perfusion abnormalities are shown in the third bulls eye, *upper row*, expressed in standard deviations below the lower limit of normal and shown color coded. Areas of the left ventricular myocardium with significantly lower tracer uptake (flow) during stress compared with baseline are computed and flagged in *white* and displayed on top of the stress extent bulls eye display (*lower right bulls eye*). Both the visual and the quantified data point to very large and severe injury (about 60% of the myocardium) with minimal stress-induced ischemia in a very small volume myocardium inferior laterally (< 5% of the myocardium). The tracer uptake in the apex, septum, and anterior wall is so low that it is very unlikely that revascularization will improve function in these areas. Even in the inferior wall, the tracer uptake clearly is below the 50% level, which has been shown to be the level below which myocardium rarely gain function after successful revascularization.

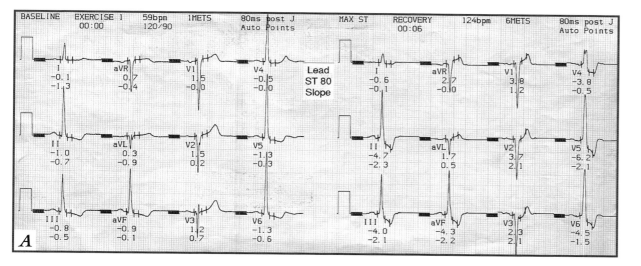

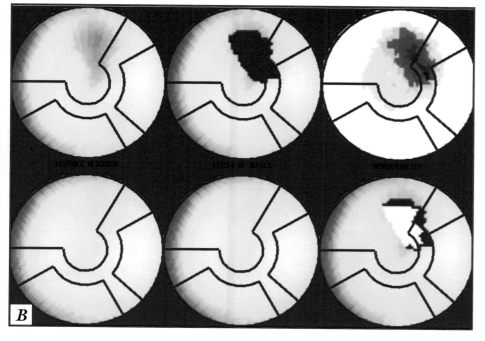

FIGURE 4-16. A 65-year-old hypertensive man who had undergone coronary angioplasty was referred for exercise testing. **A,** The standard 12-lead rest electrocardiogram (ECG) revealed an inferior-wall myocardial infarct with voltage criteria for left ventricular (LV) hypertrophy and a strain pattern (not shown). The rest torso 12-lead ECG (baseline) as compared with the standard rest 12-lead ECG (not shown) resulted in a right-axis shift that minimized Q-wave amplitude in the inferior lead group. The patient exercised to a peak heart rate of 124 bpm and reached a peak blood pressure of 168/98 mm Hg. At that point, the test was stopped because of dyspnea and chest discomfort; a work-load of 6 metabolic equivalents had been reached. Profound downsloping ST-segment depression is noted in the inferior and anterolateral lead groups (*arrows*) with QRS widening. LV hypertrophy is a relatively common cause of false exercise ECG responses for coronary disease presence and extent, and exercise myocardial perfusion imaging should be considered initially if the ECG is being performed for diagnostic or prognostic purposes. **B,** Selected tomographic views (using thallium) during and after a 4-hour delay. There are no areas of hypoperfusion, and LV mass is increased. (Legend for part A *from* Chaitman [15]; figure for part A *courtesy of* Bernard R. Chaitman.)

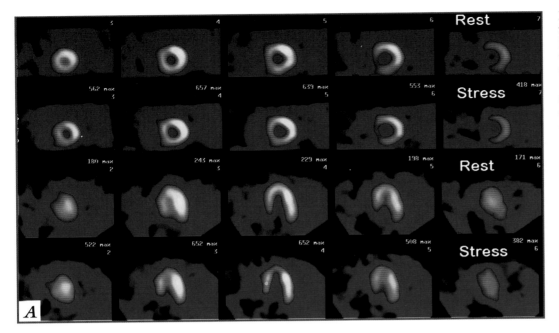

FIGURE 4-17. A, Myocardial perfusion scan from a 64-year-old man (68 in, 200 lbs) with a history of increasing exertional chest pain. Stress test: 5:00 minutes standard Bruce protocol; heart rate, 60 → 115 (85% = 132); blood pressure, 130 → 140; rate-pressure product, 16.200. Test stopped due to typical chest pain. Normal baseline electrocardiogram (ECG), 1 to 2 mm upsloping ST during stress, 1 to 2 horizontal ST depression in II, III, aVF, and V4 to V6 3 minutes into recovery. Findings: normal rest perfusion study. Stress-induced mild ischemia in the apex and apical septum (three of 25 segments, left anterior descending coronary artery). This is best seen in the transaxial images (row 4 compared with row 3). Apex is difficult to evaluate in coronal slices but is well seen in long-axis, sagittal, or, as here, transaxial cuts. ECG is notoriously bad at localizing ischemia. B, Quantification and bulls-eye display of the above data. Minor nondiagnostic findings in the rest study (lower row, middle image). Significantly larger and more severe findings in the stress images (upper row, middle image). The changes from rest to stress are significant, as shown in the third image, lower row, where portions of the myocardium with rest to stress changes larger than predefined threshold are indicated in white overlay on the stress image.

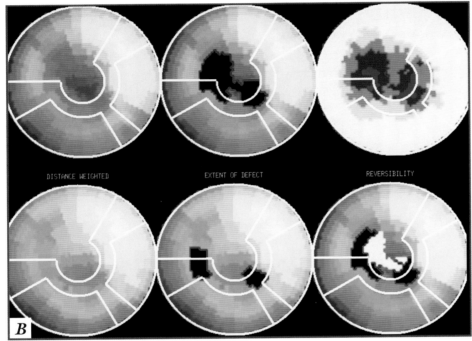

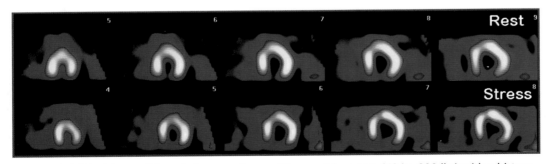

FIGURE 4-18. Myocardial perfusion scan from a 60-year-old woman (69 in, 200 lbs) with a history of large myocardial infarction (MI) several years ago, now presenting with atypical chest pain. Stress test: 7:30 minutes standard Bruce protocol; heart rate, 60 → 130 (85% = 127); blood pressure, 160 → 220; rate-pressure product, 27.900. Test stopped due to leg fatigue, no chest pain. Abnormal baseline electrocardiogram with Q wave in inferior leads; no ST changes with stress. Findings: fixed marked reduced (at the level of the background) perfusion defect in the inferior wall from base to apex and stretching into posterior septum (seven of 25 segments, right coronary artery territory). No ischemia detected at the high cardiac workload achieved. No significant tracer uptake in the inferior wall, which is consistent with transmural MI. An echocardiogram 1 year prior showed akinesis in the inferior wall. The present study shows no remaining viable myocardium in the inferior wall; it is therefore very unlikely that any functional improvement would occur if revascularized [6–8], and there is no stress-induced ischemia at high workload in any territory. Thus there is no indication for further evaluation.

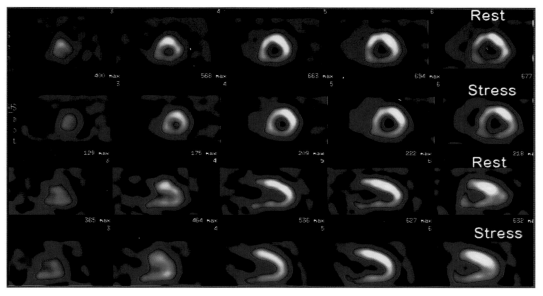

discomfort. Electrocardiogram showed ST-T abnormalities at rest, and no additional changes with stress were found. Findings: fixed mild reduced uptake in the inferior wall from apex to base and stretching into posterior septum (seven of 25 segments, right coronary artery territory). No ischemia detected at the high cardiac workload achieved. Reduced tracer uptake in the inferior wall due to attenuation is common, especially in men and in patients with enlarged hearts. In this patient, the sagittal long-axis images reveal inhomogeneous tracer uptake in the inferior wall, and involvement of the posterior septum is clear in the coronal slices. These findings make myocardial injury much more likely than just attenuation artefact. The degree of reduction in tracer uptake is mild; therefore, there is considerable amount of remaining myocardium, findings consistent with a nontransmural injury. The patient had single-vessel coronary artery bypass graft 6 years prior; a recent coronary angiogram showed 90% stenosis of native right coronary artery with patent graft. Left ventricular angiography revealed an ejection fraction of 50% and mild inferior wall hypokinesis.

FIGURE 4-19. Myocardial perfusion scan from a 65-year-old man (67 in, 190 lbs) with a history of recent-onset chest pain. Stress test: 4:00 minutes standard Bruce protocol; heart rate, 90 → 143 (85% = 132); blood pressure, 150 → 160; rate-pressure product, 22.900. Test stopped due to atypical chest

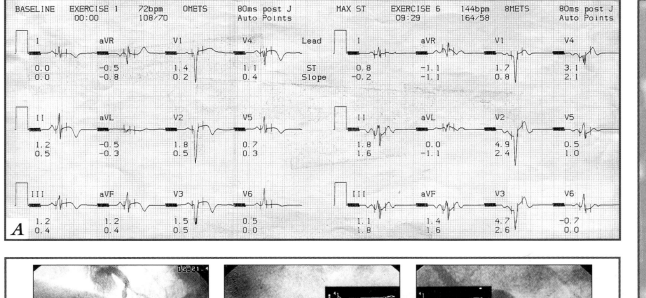

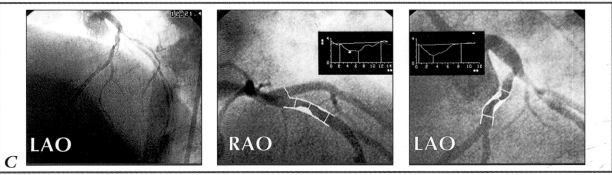

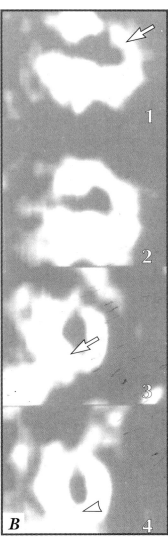

FIGURE 4-20. A 42-year-old man had an anteroseptal myocardial infarction 1 week before risk stratification with peak creatine kinase (CK) of 3767 and CK-MB of 243. The postinfarct course was uneventful. **A,** The rest electrocardiogram (baseline) demonstrated a recent anterior wall myocardial infarct with ischemic T-wave inversion in the inferior and anterolateral leads. The patient was able to exercise to 8 metabolic equivalents (reaching 81% of the age-predicted maximum) when the test was stopped because of leg fatigue. The patient had no chest discomfort, and no arrhythmia was noted. At peak exercise (maximum ST), an additional 3.1 (4.9–1.8) mm of ST-segment elevation at ST-80 is noted in lead V_2 with 0.7 mm of ST-segment depression in lead V_6 and pseudonormalization of T waves. One minute before exercise was stopped, 22 mCi of sestamibi was injected intravenously, and the heart was imaged using a tomographic camera. The exercise images were compared with those obtained at rest after 8 mCi of ^{99m}Tc sestamibi. **B,** The stress tomographic images (*1* and *3*) reveal a reduction in counts in the anteroapical region of the heart, and the rest images (*2* and *4*) show partial fill-in in the apical and inferoapical region of the heart. *Arrows* indicate reduction in counts; *arrowhead* indicates partial fill-in. **C,** Quantitative coronary angiography (QCA) revealing a diameter narrowing of 60% in the proximal left anterior descending coronary artery with impaired distal flow reserve of 1.42 after 12 μg of intracoronary adenosine. (*Continued on next page*)

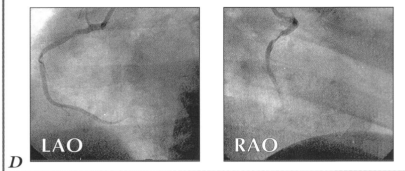 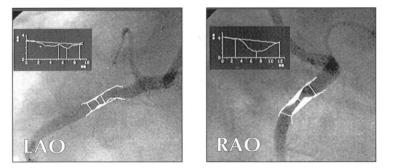

FIGURE 4-20. (*Continued*) **D,** The proximal right coronary artery has an eccentric 63% diameter narrowing with normal distal flow velocity and normal distal flow reserve of 2.9 after 6 µg of intracoronary adenosine. QCA and measurement of coronary flow reserve distal to intraluminal narrowings are helpful in explaining why some intermediate lesions with luminal narrowings of 50% to 70% cause exercise-induced ischemic responses. LAO—left anterior oblique; RAO—right anterior oblique. (Legend *from* Chaitman [15]; figure for part A *courtesy of* Bernard R. Chaitman; figures for parts B, C, and D *adapted from* Kern and coworkers [16]; with permission.)

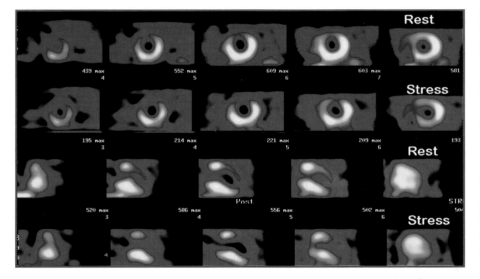

FIGURE 4-21. Myocardial perfusion scan from a 69-year-old man (62 in, 140 lbs) with a history of anterior wall myocardial infarction (MI) now presenting with postinfarction unstable angina. Stress test: 9:00 minutes standard Bruce protocol; heart rate, 90 → 136 (85% = 122); blood pressure, 115 → 160; rate-pressure product, 24.000. Test stopped due to fatigue, no chest pain. Electrocardiogram showed ST-T abnormalities at rest and accentuation with stress. Findings: in the rest study, very little or no tracer uptake is found in the apex, whereas the apical two thirds of the anterior wall and anterior septum shows moderate reduced uptake. These findings are consistent with transmural MI in the apex and nontransmural injury in the anterior wall and anterior septum (11 of 25 segments, left anterior descending coronary artery [LAD] territory). During stress, moderate severe ischemia develops in residual myocardium in the anterior wall and septum, and some peri-infarct ischemia is also evident at the edges of the injury (six of 25 segments show ischemia). Coronary angiogram showed 70% proximal LAD stenosis followed by 50% midstenosis, and 70% left circumflex coronary artery stenosis. The functional significance of the LAD disease in this patient would have been difficult to predict from pathoanatomy alone.

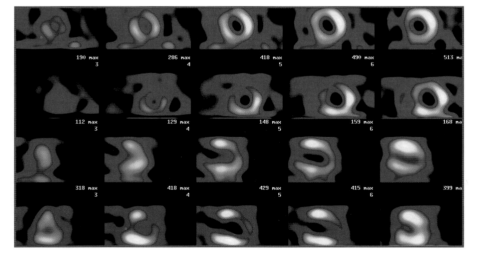

FIGURE 4-22. Myocardial perfusion scan from a 53-year-old man (71 in, 217 lbs) with a family history of coronary artery disease, now presenting with congestive heart failure and electrocardiographic evidence of anterior myocardial infarction (MI); no history of chest pain. Stress test: 5:25 minutes standard Bruce protocol; heart rate, 84 → 131 (85% = 142); blood pressure, 115 → 155; peak rate-pressure product, 20.300. Test stopped due to fatigue and dyspnea but no chest pain. ST-T abnormalities at rest, pseudonormalization during stress. Findings: fixed moderate reduced uptake in apex, the apical half of the anterior wall, and the apical third of septal-inferior-lateral walls—consistent with mainly nontransmural MI (nine of 25 segments, left anterior descending coronary artery [LAD]). Severe stress-induced ischemia in the residual myocardium in the apex, anterior wall, septum, and apical third of the lateral and inferior walls (14 of 25 segments). By quantification the extent of the ischemia is about 40% to 45% of the total myocardium, and the ischemia severity score is very high. Coronary angiogram: LAD 90% stenosis, right coronary artery 40% to 50%, left circumflex coronary artery normal, anterior wall hypokinesis, left ventricular ejection fraction 54%. Echocardiography: hypokinesis/akinesis of the anterior septum and apical anterior wall. This is a high-risk patient [2]. The baseline ECG revealed a prior MI. The stress test results (ECG and symptoms) did not disclose the severity of the disease.

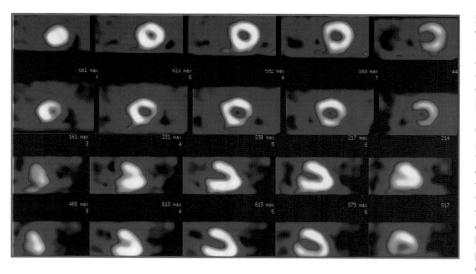

FIGURE 4-23. Myocardial perfusion scan from a 61-year-old woman (66 in, 165 lbs) with a history of coronary artery disease, multiple percutaneous transluminal coronary angioplasties, and laser angioplasty of proximal left anterior descending coronary artery (LAD) with initial good result; now presenting with recurrent typical exertional chest pain (CP). Stress test: 4:57 minutes standard Bruce protocol; heart rate, 53 → 88 (85% = 134); blood pressure, 130 → 135; peak rate-pressure product, 11.800. Test stopped due to typical CP; echocardiography shows 1-mm ST depression. Findings: no rest perfusion abnormalities. During stress, moderate severe ischemia in the lateral wall from apex to base (six of 25 segments, typical left circumflex coronary artery [LCx] territory). Quantification confirms the visual impression; the extent of ischemia is computed to 20% of total myocardium. Coronary angiogram: LAD 40% stenosis, LCx totally occluded distally, obtuse marginal branch 95% stenosis, right coronary artery small and totally occluded. Thus, LCx and RCA are both occluded. Both the lateral and the inferior still show normal perfusion at rest. This appearance can be explained by sufficient collateral flow at rest, but insufficiency of the collateral flow during stress first manifested in the lateral wall.

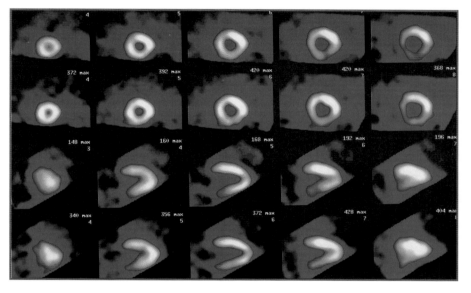

FIGURE 4-24. Myocardial perfusion scan from a 32-year-old woman (65 in, 170 lbs) with a history of chest pain (CP) and syncope episodes. Recently diagnosed small myocardial infarction (MI) by enzymes. Stress test: 9:00 minutes standard Bruce protocol; heart rate, 62 → 105 (85% = 159; blood pressure, 115 → 130. Test stopped due to typical CP, no ST-T changes. Findings: at baseline, mild reduced uptake in the basal third of the inferior and inferior-lateral segments (*upper row, last two images* and *third row, third and fourth images*) consistent with nontransmural MI (three of 25 segments, right coronary artery [RCA]). Although no stress-induced ischemia was detected, the achieved workload was low (on β-blocker therapy). Coronary angiogram showed 85% stenosis in nondominant RCA; a stent was placed. It is difficult to detect mild perfusion abnormalities in the inferior wall due to the commonly observed attenuation artefact in this region. The sagittal images (*third and fourth rows, fourth image*) are quite convincing. Note the abrupt change in tracer content, very unlike the smooth attenuation artefacts; also note how the adjacent posterior septum and the inferolateral wall seem to be slightly involved.

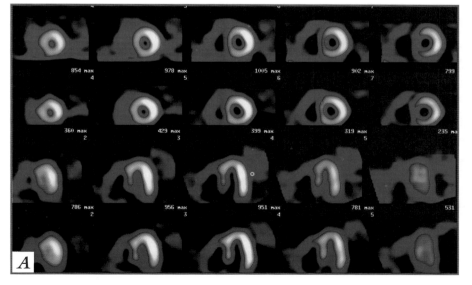

FIGURE 4-25 Myocardial perfusion scan from a 56-year-old man (66 in, 220 lbs) with no history of chest pain (CP). Left bundle branch block (LBBB) incidentally detected at screening for life insurance. Stress test: standard adenosine protocol (140 µg/kg/min for 6 minutes, tracer administration at 3 minutes); heart rate, 60 → 72; blood pressure, 135 → 130. No CP or arrhythmia. LBBB at baseline and during the test. **A,** Findings: at baseline, mild reduced uptake in septum from apex to base (*upper row, 7 o'clock to 11 o'clock positions*). No hypoperfusion detected during vasodilatation stress test. Therefore, there is no evidence of functional significant coronary artery disease (CAD). LBBB may lead to hypoperfusion in the septum secondary to increased intramural pressure generated by the abnormal septal contraction. This increased intramural pressure reduces the effective coronary perfusion pressure. Such hypoperfusion is usually limited to the septum and involves the middle portions of the septum, as in this patient. The "perfusion" abnormality is often enhanced with increase in heart rate. If stress test protocols in which the heart rate increases during the test are used, the perfusion abnormality may become more prominent and it may be impossible to discriminate between CAD with ischemic LBBB and nonischemic LBBB and functional septal hypoperfusion. Pharmacologic vasodilatation is thus the preferred stress protocol in patients with LBBB.

(Continued on next page)

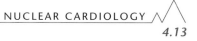

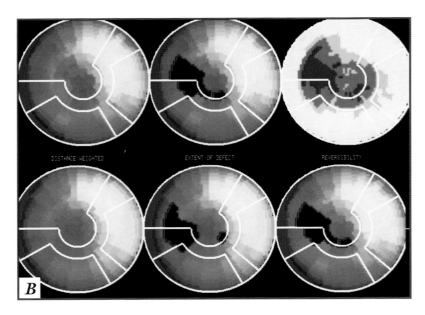

FIGURE 4-25 (*Continued*) **B,** Quantification and bulls-eye display. Notice that the perfusion abnormality is limited to the septum; the free anterior wall and apex are not involved. The latter would have favored ischemic LBBB. In addition, stress-induced hypoperfusion is detected quantitatively.

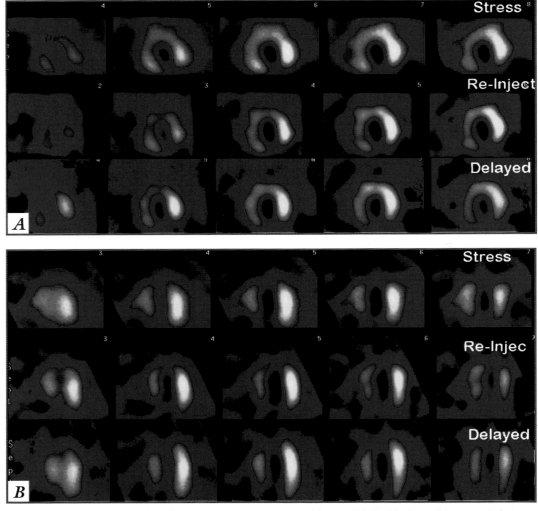

FIGURE 4-26. Myocardial perfusion scan from a 51-year-old man (70 in, 250 lbs) with recent inferior wall myocardial infarction (MI), acute thrombolysis instituted in emergency room on arrival, enzymes moderately elevated. Coronary angiogram 2 days prior to the study showed "clean right coronary artery (RCA), good flow" (< 30% stenosis) and 70% to 80% left anterior descending coronary artery (LAD) stenosis. The acute thrombolysis was believed to be successful. Stress test: 6:46 minutes modified Bruce protocol; heart rate, 69 → 99; blood pressure, 110 → 130; rate-pressure product, 13.000. Test stopped due to dyspnea; no chest pain. ST-T abnormal at baseline; no additional changes. Two clinical questions were raised: is there stress-induced ischemia, and how much viable myocardium is in the inferior wall? To answer both questions, a ^{201}Tl protocol was used: First, 3 mCi was injected at peak stress and images obtained 15 minutes poststress. Next, 1.5 mCi was reinjected 3 hours later and images obtained 15 minutes postinjection. Finally, delayed images were obtained 4 hours after reinjection. **A,** Coronal slices. **B,** Transaxial slices. Findings: no tracer uptake in the inferior wall from the base to the apex or in the apex are seen in any of the studies, consistent with transmural MI (seven of 25 segments, RCA). Moderate reduced tracer uptake in the septum and anterior wall in all three studies was found consistent with nontransmural MI (11 of 25 segments, LAD). No stress-induced ischemia was detected; if anything, only mild reverse changes were present in the septum and anterior wall (very high tracer uptake in the lungs may contribute to these findings). The inferior wall and apex do not appear to contain viable myocardium, and there is no late fill-in. The apical third of the septum and adjacent anterior wall contains an insignificant amount of viable myocardium, and there is no late fill-in. However, the basal two thirds of the septum and adjacent anterior wall contain a significant amount (at the level of 60% of maximum myocardial uptake) of viable myocardium, which potentially could regain function (if dysfunctional) by revascularization. The thrombolytic treatment was obviously not successful; it was probably started later in the event than anticipated. There was very good flow in RCA at the follow-up angiogram, yet no tracer uptake in the inferior wall! This again demonstrates that although ^{201}Tl and the Tc-based agents are flow tracers, they only accumulate locally if there are myocytes with preserved cellular function in the area. Follow-up echocardiogram 2 weeks later showed akinesis in the inferior wall and apex and extensive hypokinesis in the septum and anterior wall.

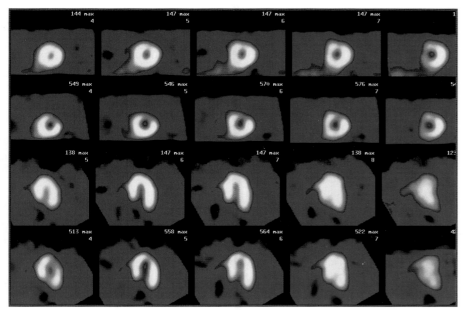

FIGURE 4-27. Myocardial perfusion scan from a 67-year-old woman (60 in, 125 lbs) with a history of atypical chest pain. Results of a planar myocardial perfusion study done in another institution were inconclusive. Stress test: 9:00 minutes standard Bruce protocol; heart rate, 62 → 170; blood pressure, 150 → 180; rate-pressure product, 30.600. Test stopped due to dyspnea and neck tightness (this patient's angina equivalent), 2-mm upsloping ST depression during stress, 1-mm downsloping ST depression in recovery. Findings: at baseline, very small area in the anterior wall (*upper row, images three and four, between the 12 o'clock and 1 o'clock positions*) showing mild reduced uptake consistent with but not diagnostic for injury. During stress, moderate severe ischemia in the anterior wall (*12 o'clock to 1 o'clock positions*) from the apex to the base, about four of 25 segments. The location is between the left anterior descending coronary artery and the left circumflex coronary artery territory; first obtuse marginal branch (OM$_1$) or ramus are most likely arteries. Coronary angiogram: 90% stenosis in OM$_1$; otherwise, only minimal arteriosclerosis. The history, pain type, and echocardiogram response were all atypical. The volume of myocardium involved is small (between 10% and 15%) but still detectable if the degree of ischemia is high, and this patient was very motivated on the treadmill.

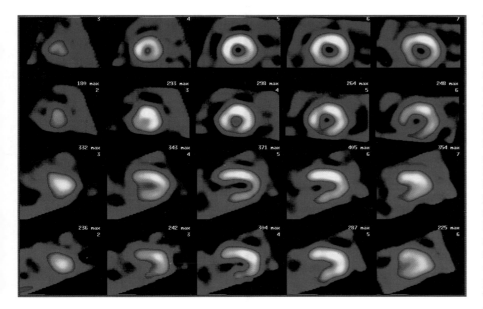

FIGURE 4-28. Myocardial perfusion scan from an 83-year-old man (68 in, 178 lbs) with a history of chest pain (CP) but no known myocardial infarction (MI). He was previously very active. Recently diagnosed small MI by enzymes, stuttering course with unstable angina, now pain-free and ready for discharge. An echocardiogram (ECHO) shows ejection fraction (EF) of about 30%, severe hypokinesis and akinesis in the inferior wall, and mild to moderate hypokinesis in the lateral wall. Stress test: standard dobutamine protocol (5 µg/kg/min for 3 minutes, gradually increasing to 40 µg/kg/min); heart rate, 50 → 109; blood pressure, 130 → 150; rate-pressure product, 16.000. No CP, left bundle branch block at baseline. Findings: moderate increased left ventricular (LV) volume. Mild reduced tracer uptake in the inferior wall and posterior septum, consistent with mild nontransmural MI (four of 25 segments, right coronary artery [RCA]). Mild-to-moderate severe stress-induced ischemia in the residual myocardium in the inferior wall and posterior septum (five of 25 segments, RCA). There is a striking discrepancy between the echocardiogram findings less than 12 hours earlier and the rest perfusion images, which show only mild abnormalities. There were no changes in the clinical picture and no CP for days. The most reasonable explanation for these seemingly paradoxical findings would be that the patient has "stunned myocardium," defined as prolonged postischemic dysfunction, *ie*, there is flow and tracer uptake but temporarily no function. LV angiography 3 weeks later revealed an EF of 70% and minor wall motion abnormalities, confirming the stunned myocardium hypothesis.

 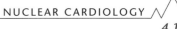

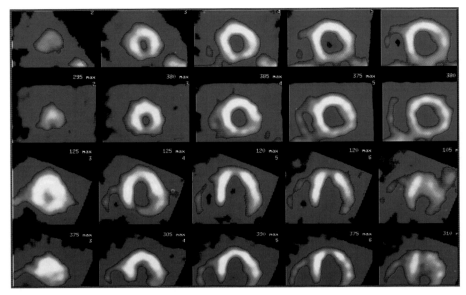

FIGURE 4-29. Myocardial perfusion scan from a 67-year-old man (69 in, 251 lbs) with no history of cardiac disease. Supposedly successful surgery for carcinoid 4 years prior. Patient presented with recent onset of severe dyspnea and palpitations. New

left bundle branch block (LBBB) and left anterior hemiblock on baseline echocardiogram (ECG) believed to be consistent with coronary artery disease. Clinical impression: fragile and high risk. Stress test: 3:20 minutes standard Bruce protocol; heart rate, 92 → 164 (85% = 130); blood pressure, 165 → 165; rate-pressure product, 27.100. Test stopped due to dyspnea, no chest pain. Baseline ECG: LBBB and LAH. Findings: marked increased left ventricular (LV) volume (+ 5 standard deviation above the upper limit of normal, weight taken into consideration). At baseline, mild-to-moderate decreased uptake in the inferior wall and in the basal third of the lateral wall, consistent with mild nontransmural myocardial infarction. No stress-induced ischemia. There is striking discrepancy between LV volume and the minor fixed perfusion abnormalities, which should not lead to LV dilatation of this degree. Overall picture diagnostic for LV volume overload condition such as cardiomyopathy (CMP) or left-sided valve disease. There is only slightly increased right ventricular uptake; thus carcinoid valve disease is unlikely. Follow-up echocardiography disclosed marked general hypokinesis of dilated CMP type. When all processing steps are standardized, the image dimensions will be constant; thus information about LV cavity size with diagnostic and prognostic implications [17] can be obtained from myocardial perfusion studies.

MYOCARDIAL VIABILITY IMAGING

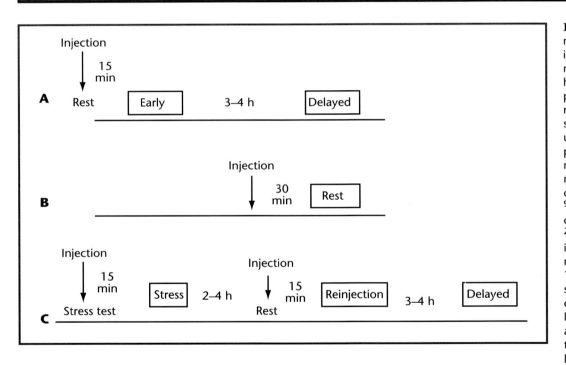

FIGURE 4-30. Viability protocols. **A,** The classic rest-delayed protocol [6]. At rest, 3 mCi ^{201}Tl is injected, and rest imaging is started about 15 minutes later. Delayed images are acquired 3 to 4 hours later. Whereas the rest images describe rest perfusion, fill-in in delayed images indicates hibernating myocardium. Segments in the delayed study with less than 50% of the maximum tracer uptake are unlikely to regain function. **B,** Viability protocol for the ^{99m}Tc-based agents. At rest, 20 mCi is injected, and imaging starts about 30 minutes later [7]. Recent studies from several centers confirm that the delayed ^{201}Tl and the rest ^{99m}Tc give similar information concerning viability on a segment-by-segment basis [8]. **C,** Complete ^{201}Tl protocol for assessment of stress-induced ischemia and myocardial viability. At peak stress, 3 mCi ^{201}Tl is injected, and stress imaging is started 15 minutes later. A reinjection dose (one half the stress dose) is given 2 to 4 hours after the stress dose and reinjection imaging started 15 minutes later. Delayed images are obtained 3 to 4 hours after the reinjection. The first part (stress vs reinjection) will disclose stress-induced ischemia, and the latter part (reinjection and delayed images) demonstrates viability.

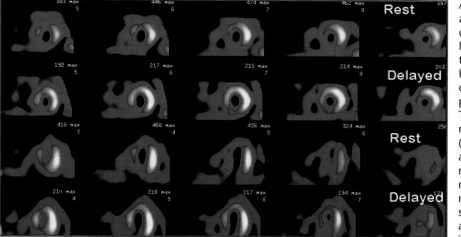

FIGURE 4-31. Myocardial perfusion scan from an 82-year-old man (65 in, 155 lbs) with a long history of coronary artery disease (CAD), several myocardial infarctions, and exertional chest pain. Whereas congestive heart failure (New York Heart

Association class 3) is progressing, the angina is stable and acceptably controlled. Left ventricular (LV) ejection fraction by echocardiography about 30%, severe general hypokinesis except for the lateral wall; there is no evidence of valve disease. The clinical question is, could revascularization improve LV function? If the patient has a significant amount of hibernating myocardium (defined as chronic ischemic dysfunctional myocardium), then LV function potentially could improve if such myocardium were revascularized. The rest-delayed ^{201}Tl viability protocol was used. Findings: at rest, no tracer uptake in the inferior wall and posterior septum (right coronary artery [RCA]), and marked reduced uptake in the anterior septum and anterior wall (left anterior descending coronary artery [LAD]). In the delayed images, the tracer clearly accumulated in the anterior septum and anterior wall, indicating viable myocardium in the LAD territory. The inferior wall and posterior septum (RCA) show only mild changes, and the tracer content is at a low level. Even the apex shows significant tracer accumulation in the delayed images. Thus, although there is strong evidence of a significant volume of viable hibernating myocardium in the LAD territory, the RCA territory is unlikely to benefit functionally from revascularization.

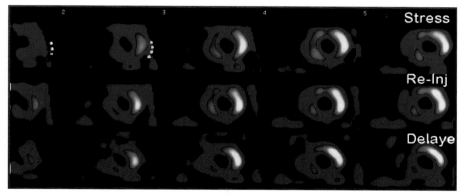

FIGURE 4-32. Myocardial perfusion scan from a 60-year-old man (68 in, 200 lbs) with a long history of ischemic heart disease, multiple myocardial infarctions (MIs), exertional chest pain (CP), and congestive heart failure. The failure component has lately become dominant and is now New York Heart Association class 4. Coronary angiogram: left anterior descending coronary artery (LAD) 90%, left circumflex coronary artery 65%, right coronary artery occluded. Left ventricular ejection fraction is about 25% by echocardiography, which also demonstrated extensive and severe wall motion abnormalities. Clinical question: is there stress-induced ischemia or hibernating

myocardium that would justify revascularization, and if so, where? The combined stress–rest–delayed imaging protocol was chosen to address both questions. Stress test: 4:00 minutes standard Bruce protocol; heart rate, 88 → 148 (85% = 140); blood pressure, 120 → 120; rate-pressure product, 17.800. Test stopped due to dyspnea, no CP. Abnormal baseline electrocardiogram, no additional ST-T abnormalities. Findings: the reinjection study serves as the baseline (rest) study and revealed marked reduced uptake in the anterior septum plus anterior wall (LAD) and in the posterior septum and inferior wall, consistent with severe and extensive injury in these walls (17 of 25 segments are involved). The delayed images show no evidence of late fill-in to indicate hibernating myocardium in these walls, which appear to be a mixture of transmural and nontransmural myocardial infarctions; there is very little viable myocardium, which is unlikely to improve in function if revascularized. When comparing the reinjection (rest) and the stress images, mild stress-induced ischemia is found in the apical third of the lateral wall (marks) albeit in a small-volume myocardium (two of 25 segments). The overall impression is, therefore, that there is neither chronic ischemic myocardium nor stress-induced ischemia in a large enough volume to justify high-risk revascularization surgery.

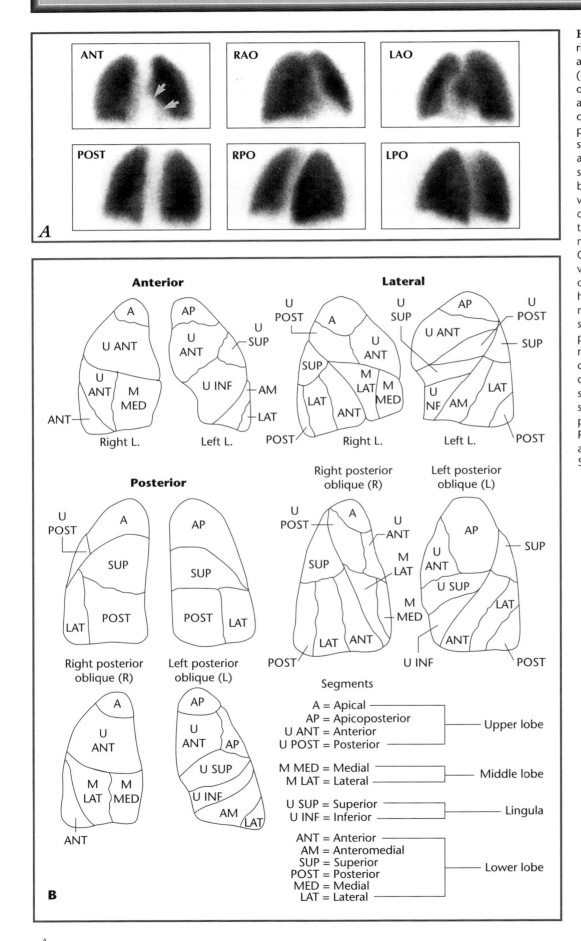

FIGURE 4-33. A, Six-view scan using the anterior (ANT) and posterior (POST) oblique views in addition to the anterior (ANT) and posterior (POST) ones. Many centers use both lateral and oblique projections to complement the anterior and posterior views. The anterior view should correlate roughly with the chest radiograph. No perfusion is expected in the region of the cardiac silhouette (*arrows*). The aortic knob is often visualized as well. On the posterior view, the activity should taper toward the bases as the lungs become thinner in the posterior sulci. On lateral views (not shown), about one third of the activity comes from the contralateral lung (shine-through), so that areas of actual absent perfusion may be displayed as only decreased perfusion. On the left lateral and left anterior oblique (LAO) views, the heart is evident as a large defect anteriorly. Most patients with pulmonary embolism have full-segmental defects, although the wide normal variation in the size and shape of segments must be taken into account. Most patients with pulmonary embolism also have multiple and bilateral emboli. More perfusion defects from emboli are seen in the lower lobes in comparison with the upper lobes, and more are seen in the right lung than in the left lung. **B,** The segmental lung anatomy [19,20]. LPO—left posterior oblique; RAO—right anterior oblique; RPO—right posterior oblique. (Legend *from* Skibo and Goldhaber [21]; figure *courtesy of* Lorraine Skibo and Samuel Z. Goldhaber.)

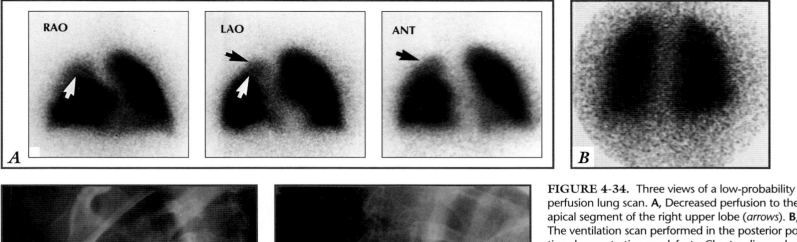

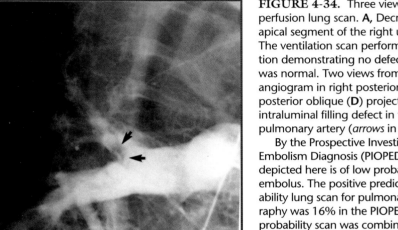

FIGURE 4-34. Three views of a low-probability perfusion lung scan. **A,** Decreased perfusion to the apical segment of the right upper lobe (*arrows*). **B,** The ventilation scan performed in the posterior position demonstrating no defects. Chest radiography was normal. Two views from the right pulmonary angiogram in right posterior oblique (**C**) and left posterior oblique (**D**) projections show a persistent intraluminal filling defect in the upper lobe pulmonary artery (*arrows in D*).

By the Prospective Investigation of Pulmonary Embolism Diagnosis (PIOPED) criteria [22], the scan depicted here is of low probability for pulmonary embolus. The positive predictive value of a low-probability lung scan for pulmonary embolus at angiography was 16% in the PIOPED study. When a low-probability scan was combined with a low clinical suspicion for embolus, the likelihood of pulmonary embolus at angiography was only 4%. However, nearly half the patients with the combination of low-probability lung scans and a high clinical suspicion of pulmonary embolism were found to have pulmonary embolism at angiography. (*See* Fig. 4-32 for abbreviations.) (Legend *from* Skibo and Goldhaber [21]; figure *courtesy of* Lorraine Skibo and Samuel Z. Goldhaber.)

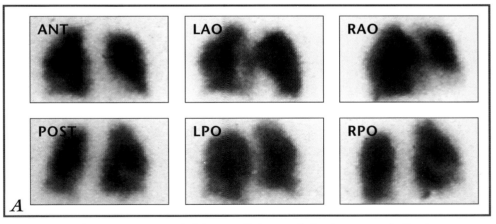

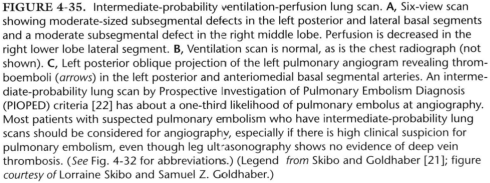

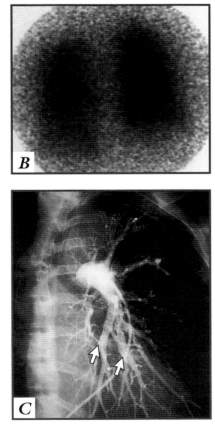

FIGURE 4-35. Intermediate-probability ventilation-perfusion lung scan. **A,** Six-view scan showing moderate-sized subsegmental defects in the left posterior and lateral basal segments and a moderate subsegmental defect in the right middle lobe. Perfusion is decreased in the right lower lobe lateral segment. **B,** Ventilation scan is normal, as is the chest radiograph (not shown). **C,** Left posterior oblique projection of the left pulmonary angiogram revealing thromboemboli (*arrows*) in the left posterior and anteriomedial basal segmental arteries. An intermediate-probability lung scan by Prospective Investigation of Pulmonary Embolism Diagnosis (PIOPED) criteria [22] has about a one-third likelihood of pulmonary embolus at angiography. Most patients with suspected pulmonary embolism who have intermediate-probability lung scans should be considered for angiography, especially if there is high clinical suspicion for pulmonary embolism, even though leg ultrasonography shows no evidence of deep vein thrombosis. (*See* Fig. 4-32 for abbreviations.) (Legend *from* Skibo and Goldhaber [21]; figure *courtesy of* Lorraine Skibo and Samuel Z. Goldhaber.)

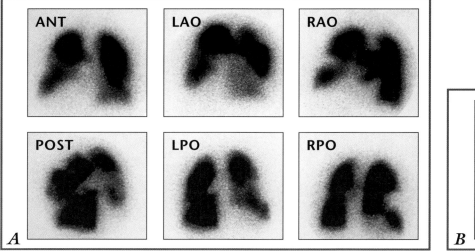

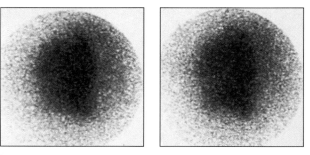

FIGURE 4-36. High-probability ventilation-perfusion lung scan. A clinical and diagnostic pearl is that high-probability lung scans are almost always abnormal bilaterally. Only extremely rarely is perfusion to one lung entirely normal in a patient with scintigraphic evidence of pulmonary embolism. **A,** Six-view scan showing absent perfusion in the right middle lobe and the superior segment of the left lower lobe. A moderate subsegmental defect is present in the apical-posterior segment of the left upper lobe. A nonsegmental defect is present in the right base. **B,** Ventilation scan obtained in the left posterior oblique projection was normal, as was the chest radiograph (not shown). **C,** Pulmonary angiogram with main pulmonary artery injection showing thromboemboli (*arrows*) in the right upper lobe, right interlobar, and left interlobar pulmonary arteries. In the Prospective Investigation of Pulmonary Embolism Diagnosis (PIOPED) study [22], most patients (102 of 116 patients) with high-probability lung scans had angiographic evidence of pulmonary embolism, yielding a positive predictive value of 88%. High-probability scans were shown to be 97% specific but, surprisingly, only 41% sensitive. Relying only on high-probability lung scans for diagnosis of pulmonary embolism would allow more than half (59%) of the pulmonary emboli to go unrecognized. (*See* Fig. 4-32 for abbreviations.) (Legend *from* Skibo and Goldhaber [21]; figure *courtesy of* Lorraine Skibo and Samuel Z. Goldhaber.)

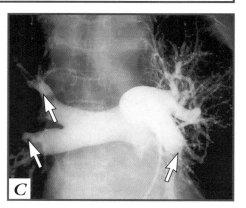

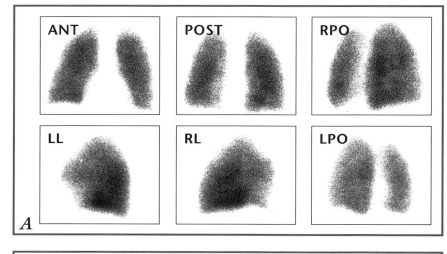

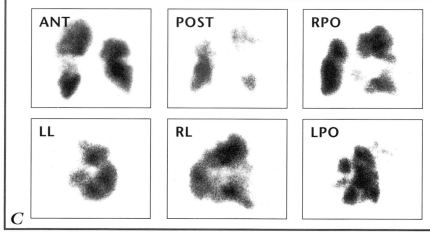

FIGURE 4-37. **A,** Normal six-view perfusion lung scan. **B,** Perfusion lung scan in primary pulmonary hypertension (PPH). **C,** Perfusion lung scan in a patient with chronic thromboembolic pulmonary hypertension (CTEPH). Ventilation scan was normal. Ventilation-perfusion lung scanning provides an excellent, low-risk, noninvasive means of distinguishing between pulmonary hypertension due to potentially operable CTEPH and obliterative, small-vessel pulmonary hypertension [23–26]. In chronic thromboembolic disease, at least one (and, more commonly, several) segmental or larger mismatched defect is present. In PPH, the perfusion scan is either normal or has a mottled appearance consisting of patchy, subsegmental abnormalities. Although the ventilation-perfusion lung scan can suggest the diagnosis of CTEPH, it is incapable of confirming the diagnosis or establishing surgical feasibility. Any process that occludes major pulmonary arteries, either through external compression (fibrosing mediastinitis, mediastinal tumors) or intraluminal obstruction (thrombus, tumor) will result in similar defects. (*See* Fig. 4-32 for abbreviations.) (Legend *from* Fedullo and coworkers [27]; figure *courtesy of* Richard N. Channick.)

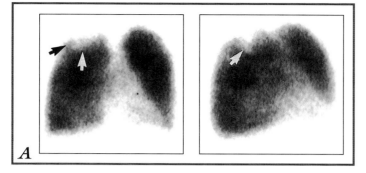

A

FIGURE 4-38. Pulmonary disease and perfusion defects in emphysema. **A,** Anterior and right anterior oblique views from a six-view perfusion scan showing a segmental defect in the apical portion of the right upper lobe (*arrows*). **B,** Corresponding angiogram revealing a bulla (*arrowhead*) in the right upper lobe corresponding to the perfusion defect. Pulmonary vessels (*arrow*) appear draped around the bullae. No evidence of pulmonary embolism was seen. **C,** In another patient, a frontal chest radiograph reveals diminished vascularity in both lungs. **D,** Pulmonary perfusion scan with diffuse heterogeneous perfusion with several small subsegmental defects. On the ventilation scan, the steady state (**E**) and last washout image at 2 min (**F**) show diffuse air-trapping. **G,** A left pulmonary angiogram in the left posterior oblique projection was performed because of high clinical suspicion of pulmonary embolism, but demonstrates no evidence of pulmonary embolism.

In chronic bronchitis and emphysema, perfusion scans often demonstrate patchy, uneven tracer activity. Multiple nonsegmental perfusion defects may be present due to bullae or an unventilated lung distal to a mucous plug [19]. Ventilation scans are the key to interpretation of abnormalities seen at perfusion scanning in primary pulmonary disease. The initial breath images reflect regional ventilation rates if a maximum inspiratory effort is obtained. Equilibrium images display the aerated volume of lung. Washout images can only be obtained with the inert gases, and, normally, activity should be cleared within 2 to 3 min. The washout phase is most sensitive for air-trapping [19]. (*See* Fig. 4-32 for abbreviations.) (Legend *from* Skibo and Goldhaber [21]; figure *courtesy of* Lorraine Skibo and Samuel Z. Goldhaber.)

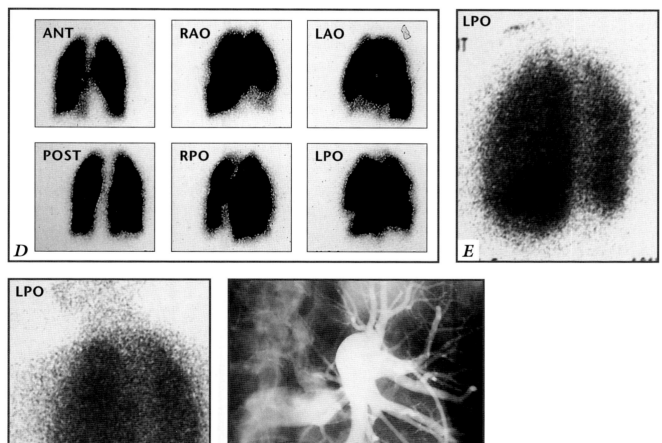

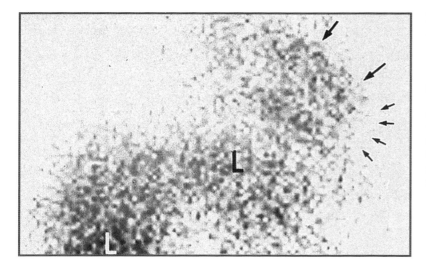

FIGURE 4-39. Nuclear imaging in the diagnosis of myocarditis. Antimyosin ^{111}In scintigraphy is a useful modality for the initial evaluation of patients with suspected myocarditis. This image depicts diffuse global uptake of radiolabeled antimyosin antibody by the left ventricle (*large arrows*) in an anterior planar image. The apical region has been relatively spared (*small arrows*). This patient presented with a syndrome masquerading as myocardial infarction with chest pain and elevations in creatine kinase MB isoenzymes. The left ventricle was dilated and hypocontractile. *L* denotes the normal hepatic activity of the labeled antibody. Compared with endomyocardial biopsy, antiomyosin antibody imaging was 83% sensitive and 53% specific for the diagnosis of myocarditis [28]. (Legend *from* Hare [29]; figure *adapted from* Narula and coworkers [30]; with permission.)

NEW IMAGING METHOD: GATED SINGLE PHOTON EMISSION COMPUTED TOMOGRAPHY

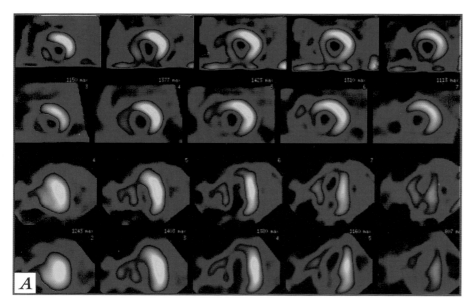

FIGURE 4-40. Myocardial perfusion scan from a 55-year-old man (70 in, 200 lbs) with a history of at least one myocardial infarction (MI), now presenting with unstable angina. Stress test: 4:00 standard Bruce protocol; heart rate, $50 \rightarrow 110$; blood pressure, $120 \rightarrow 130$; rate-pressure product, 13.500. Test stopped due to typical chest pain. Abnormal baseline electrocardiogram, accentuation of ST-T abnormalities with stress. **A,** Findings: moderate-to-severe reduced uptake in the anterior and posterior septum, apex, and inferior wall from base to apex consistent with mixed transmural and nontransmural MI in probably two vascular territories (left anterior descending coronary artery and right coronary artery); about 10 of 25 segments involved. Stress-induced ischemia in residual myocardium mainly in the posterior septum and the inferior wall, five of 25 segments.

   B, Gated single photon emission tomography (SPECT) [31]. Transversal view, end-diastolic frame (*left*) and end-systolic frame (*right*). The *green mask* indicates the end-diastolic edge; *yellow-red*, the endocardial demarcation. These images were originally displayed in dynamic mode for wall motion assessment; here only the end-diastolic and end-systolic images are shown. The end-systolic image demonstrates akinesis in the septum and apex, with good wall motions in the lateral wall.

(*Continued on next page*)

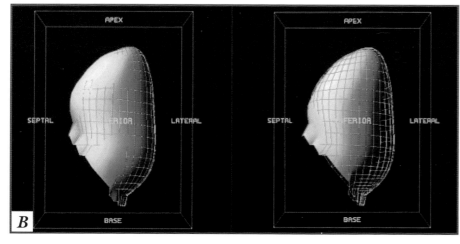

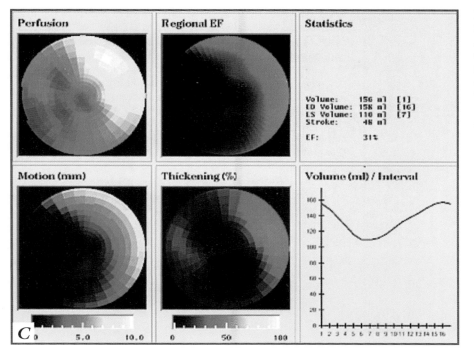

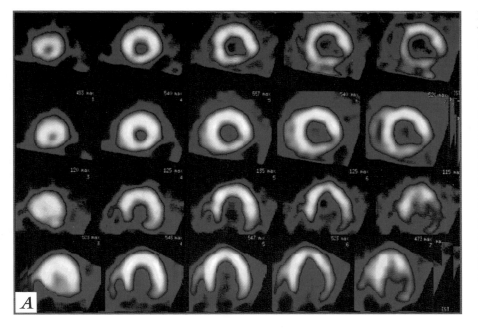

FIGURE 4-40. (*Continued*) **C,** Bulls-eye display of perfusion, regional wall motions in millimeters, regional ejection fraction (EF), and regional systolic thickening. Volumes, global EF, and left ventricular volume curve are shown in the *right column*. EF is moderate, reduced at about 31%. Myocardial perfusion studies using gated SPECT technique deliver perfusion data *plus* functional information in the form of regional function and global EF [32,33]. In this patient, matching perfusion and functional abnormalities (findings consistent with coronary artery disease) were revealed.

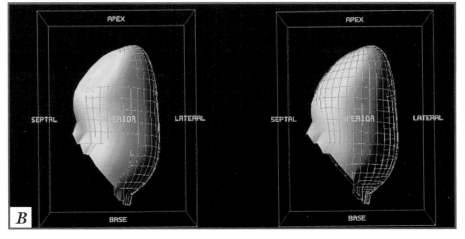

FIGURE 4-41. Myocardial perfusion scan in a 45-year-old woman (64 in, 124 lbs) with long-standing insulin-dependent diabetes mellitus. She had a 6-month history of exertional chest discomfort and dyspnea, which is increasing lately. Clinical signs of congestive heart failure were observed. Stress test: 5:20 standard Bruce protocol; heart rate, 81 → 142; blood pressure, 110 → 130; rate-pressure product, 18.500. Test stopped due to dyspnea and chest discomfort. Left bundle branch block at baseline. **A,** Findings: marked increased left ventricular (LV) volume. Moderate reduced uptake in the basal two thirds of the inferior lateral wall consistent with nontransmural myocardial infarction (three of 25 segments) (left circumflex coronary artery). No stress-induced ischemia detected in the stress images. **B,** Gated single photon emission computed tomography: end-diastolic frame (*left*) and end-systolic (*right*). The *green mask* is the end-diastolic edge; *red-yellow* is the endocardial demarcation in the end-systole. Note that the septum and anterior and inferior walls basically are akinetic; the apex and the lateral walls are markedly hypokinetic. These findings are striking in the cine display of the all the frames from the cardiac cycle.

(*Continued on next page*)

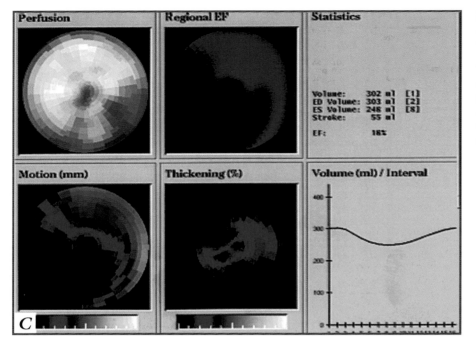

FIGURE 4-41. (*Continued*) **C,** The bulls-eye display of perfusion, motion, regional ejection fraction (EF), and wall thickening confirms strictly objectively a minor perfusion abnormality and marked general wall motion abnormalities. LV-EF is about 18%. Thus, whereas the clinical presentation was highly suspicious for coronary artery disease and ischemic cardiomyopathy, the perfusion-function imaging reveals a picture of mismatching perfusion and function, a pattern consistent with a LV volume overload condition (cardiomyopathy and valvular disease, such as aortic and mitral regurgitation, are first on the list of possible causes). Dilated cardiomyopathy was the final clinical diagnosis.

REFERENCES

1. Krawczynska EG, Weintraub WS, Garcia EV, *et al.*: Left ventricular dilatation and multivessel coronary artery disease on thallium-201 SPECT are important prognostic indicators in patients with large defects in the left anterior descending distribution. *Am J Cardiol* 1994, 74:1233–1239.

2. Iskandrian A, Chae S, Heo J, *et al.*: Independent and incremental prognostic value of exercise single photon emission computed tomographic (SPECT) thallium imaging in coronary artery disease. *J Am Coll Cardiol* 1993, 22:665–670.

3. Moss A, Goldstein R, Hall W, *et al.*: Detection and significance of myocardial ischemia in stable patients after recovery from an acute coronary event [editorial]. *JAMA* 1993, 269:2379.

4. Abdulmassih S, Iskandrian A, Mario SV, Jaekyeong H: Pharmacologic stress testing: mechanism of action, hemodynamic responses, and results in detection of coronary artery disease. *J Nuclear Cardiol* 1994, 1:94–111.

5. Maddahi J, Van Train K, Prigent F, *et al.*: Quantitative single photon emission computed thallium-201 tomography for detection and localization of coronary artery disease: optimization and prospective validation of a new technique. *J Am Coll Cardiol* 1989, 14:1689–1699.

6. Dilsizian V, Rocco TP, Freedman NM, *et al.*: Enhanced detection of ischemic but viable myocardium by the reinjection of thallium after stress-redistribution imaging. *N Engl J Med* 1990, 323:141–146.

7. Udelson JE, Coleman PS, Metherall J, *et al.*: Predicting recovery of severe regional ventricular dysfunction: comparison of resting scintigraphy with 201T1 and 99mTc-sestamibi. *Circulation* 1994, 89:2552–2561.

8. Kauffman GJ, *et al.*: Comparison of rest thallium-201 imaging and rest technetium-99m sestamibi imaging for assessment of myocardial viability in patients with coronary artery disease and severe left ventricular dysfunction. *J Am Coll Cardiol* 1996, 27:1592–1597.

9. Bax JJ, Cornel JH, Visser FC, *et al.*: Prediction of recovery of myocardial dysfunction after revascularization: comparison of F-14 fluoro-deoxyglucose/thallium-201 SPECT, thallium-201 stress-reinjection SPECT and dobutamine echocardiography. *J Am Coll Cardiol* 1996, 28:558–564.

10. Wackers FJ, Terrin ML, Kayden DS, *et al.*: Quantitative radionuclide assessment of regional ventricular function after thrombolytic therapy for acute myocardial infarction: results of phase I thrombolysis in myocardial infarction (TIMI) trial. *J Am Coll Cardiol* 1989; 13:998–1005.

11. Palmeri ST, Bonow RO, Myers CE, *et al.*: Prospective evaluation of doxorubicin cardiotoxicity by rest and exercise radionuclide angiography. *Am J Cardiol* 1986, 58:607.

12. Braunwald E, Rutherford JD: Reversible ischemic left ventricular dysfunction: evidence for the "hibernating myocardium." *J Am Coll Cardiol* 1986, 8:1467–1470.

13. Wackers FJTh: Stress radionuclide imaging for detecting and assessing prognosis of coronary artery disease. In *Atlas of Heart Diseases: Chronic Ischemic Heart Diseases*, vol 5. Edited by Braunwald EB, Beller GA. Philadelphia: Current Medicine; 1995.

14. Tamaki N, Yonekura Y, Mukai T, *et al.*: Stress thallium-201 transaxial emission computed tomography: quantitative versus qualitative analysis for evaluation of chronic heart disease. *J Am Coll Cardiol* 1984, 4:1213–1221.

15. Chaitman BR: Exercise electrocardiographic stress testing. In *Atlas of Heart Diseases: Chronic Ischemic Heart Diseases*, vol 5. Edited by Braunwald EB, Beller GA. Philadelphia: Current Medicine; 1995.

16. Kern MJ, Flynn MS, Caracciolo EA, *et al.*: Use of translesional coronary flow velocity for interventional decisions in a patient with multiple intermediately severe coronary stenoses. *Cathet Cardiovasc Diagn* 1993, 29:148–153.

17. Krawczynska EG, Weintraub WS, Garcia EV, *et al.*: Left ventricular dilatation and multivessel coronary artery disease on thallium-201 SPECT are important prognostic indicators in patients with large defects in the left anterior descending distribution. *Am J Cardiol* 1994, 74:1233–1239.

18. Klein JL, Garcia EV, DePuey EG, *et al.*: Reversibility bull's eye: a new polar bull's eye map to quantify reversibility of stress-induced SPECT thallium-201 myocardial perfusion defects. *J Nucl Med* 1990, 31:1240–1246.

19. Mettler FA, Guiberteau MJ: *Essentials of Nuclear Medicine*, edn 3. Philadelphia: WB Saunders; 1991.

20. Fogelman I, Maisey M: *An Atlas of Clinical Nuclear Medicine*. St. Louis: Mosby; 1988.

21. Skibo L, Goldhaber SZ: Diagnosis of acute pulmonary embolism. In *Atlas of Heart Diseases: Cardiopulmonary Diseases and Cardiac Tumors*, vol 3. Edited by Braunwald EB, Goldhaber SZ. Philadelphia: Current Medicine; 1995.

22. The PIOPED Investigators: Value of the ventilation/perfusion scan in acute pulmonary embolism. *JAMA* 1990, 263:2753–2759.

23. Fishmann AJ, Moser KM, Fedullo PF: Perfusion lung scans vs pulmonary angiography in evaluation of primary pulmonary hypertension. *Chest* 1983, 84:679–683.

24. Moser KM, Page GT, Ashburn WL, *et al.*: Perfusion lung scans provide a guide to which patients with apparent primary pulmonary hypertension merit angiography. *West J Med* 1988, 148:167–170.

25. D'Alonzo GE, Bower JS, Dantzker DR: Differentiation of patients with primary and thromboembolic pulmonary hypertension. *Chest* 1984, 85:457–461.

26. Lisbona R, Kreisman H, Novales-Diaz J, *et al.*: Perfusion lung scanning: differentiation of primary from thromboembolic pulmonary hypertension. *AJR Am J Roentgenol* 1985, 144:30.

27. Fedullo PF, Auger WR, Channick RN, *et al.*: A multidisciplinary approach to chronic thromboembolic pulmonary hypertension. In *Atlas of Heart Diseases: Cardiopulmonary Diseases and Cardiac Tumors*, vol 3. Edited by Braunwald EB, Goldhaber SZ. Philadelphia: Current Medicine; 1995.

28. Goldhaber SZ, Vaughan De, Markis JE, *et al.*: Acute pulmonary embolism treated with tissue plasminogen activator. *Lancet* 1986, 2:886–889.

29. Hare JM: The etiologic basis of chronic heart failure. In *Atlas of Heart Diseases: Cardiac Function and Dysfunction*, vol 4. Edited by Braunwald EB, Colucci WS. Philadelphia: Current Medicine; 1995.

30. Narula J, Khaw BA, Dec GW, *et al.*: Recognition of acute myocarditis masquerading as acute myocardial infarction. *N Engl J Med* 1993, 328:100–104.

31. Mannting F, Morgan-Mannting MG: Gated SPECT with technetium-99m-sestamibi for assessment of myocardial perfusion abnormalities. *J Nucl Med* 1993, 34:601–608.

32. DePuey EG, Nichols K, Dobrinsky C: Left ventricular ejection fraction assessed from gated technetium-99m-sestamibi SPECT. *J Nucl Med* 1993, 34:1871–1876.

33. Germano G, Kiat H, Kavanagh PB, *et al.*: Automatic quantification of ejection fraction from gated myocardial perfusion SPECT. *J Nucl Med* 1995, 36:2138–2147.

CHAPTER 5

Digital Echocardiography

James D. Thomas

Echocardiography has been very useful in the diagnosis of cardiovascular disease. However, two of its major limitations are that it typically relies on analog storage technology (*eg*, videotape recording) and usually is interpreted in only a qualitative or semiquantitative sense. Digital storage and analysis of echocardiograms would improve the utility of echocardiography in the following ways: 1) studies could be examined more quickly, rather than searching through videotape for the appropriate views; 2) serial examinations are easy, because prior studies can be placed in adjacent computer windows for comparison; 3) echocardiographic data are available throughout the hospital (and beyond), allowing nonechocardiographic clinicians to have access to the primary imaging data on their patients; 4) calibration data may be built into the image file, allowing true quantitation of ventricular function and valvular disease; 5) digital images may be replicated repeatedly without the degradations seen when videotape is copied; 6) there is no image degradation over time, as occurs with videotape storage; and 7) digital storage facilitates telemedicine, with significant impact on remote provision of cardiac imaging as well as fostering clinical trials and continuing medical information.

Although digital storage of echocardiograms has been possible for some time, recent developments are accelerating this trend. The first of these developments is the acceptance by the medical and industrial community of the Digital Imaging and Communications in Medicine (DICOM) standard for echocardiographic data exchange. This standard, which dictates the way images are exchanged (either by disk or over a network), allows for the imbedding of patient identification and calibration data, so that quantitative algorithms can be applied directly to the echocardiographic image. Although mature products supporting the DICOM standard are just emerging, it is anticipated that this will become widely available from echocardiographic and workstation vendors over the next few years. The second major development has been the validation of clinical and digital compression technology for use with echocardiography images. Echocardiography generates approximately 30 MB of data per second, or 20 GB for a typical 10-minute study, which is completely impractical for digital storage or transmission. Through careful choice of which data to store (several cardiac cycles from multiple imaging windows), it is possible to significantly reduce the data requirements. Furthermore, compression using the Joint Photographic Expert Group (JPEG) algorithm at a compression ratio of 20:1 has been shown to be clinically acceptable, and other compression algorithms are currently under evaluation. Finally, the remarkable progress in computer technology over the past 30 years is continuing to fuel the move toward digital echocardiography. Digital echocardiography requires high-speed network transmission, inexpensive high-capacity storage, powerful processors, and graphics facilities for rapid review. In all of these areas, advances in computer technology are making digital echocardiography equipment cheaper and more powerful each year.

Although digital echocardiography will benefit all examinations, allowing data to be transferred instantaneously around the hospital or to a colleague in another city, some areas of quantitation will be particularly improved with this technique. Digital echocardiograms should allow the application of edge-detection algorithms that will better be able to quantify regional wall motion and overall ventricular function. Calibration can also be applied to color Doppler maps of intracardiac velocity. Using these velocities in a quantitative way will allow better characterization of regurgitant flow rate (using the proximal convergence analysis) and of ventricular filling using color M-mode echocardiography.

Benefits of Routine Digital Echocardiography

Random access to all views on a patient examination
Easy side-by-side comparison with prior studies
Echocardiographic review throughout the hospital
Study reproduction without image degradation
Easier quantitation using stored calibration
Remote transmission of echocardiograms for telediagnosis
Integration with other medical data on a disk for a
  "unit patient record"
Off-line computer analysis and image processing
Long-term archival without data deterioration

FIGURE 5-1. Benefits of routine digital storage and transfer of echocardiograms. First, the echocardiogram could be reviewed more quickly because specific views on the echocardiogram can be accessed randomly without having to search through videotape. Digital storage also allows prior studies to be retrieved easily for side-by-side comparison with the current study, which is critical for judging interval change in cardiovascular function. Because digital echocardiograms are stored centrally on a server, they would be available for review throughout the hospital both by cardiologists and general clinicians and can be copied multiple times without any image degradation, which is a particular problem with the copying of videotape. It is also possible to store calibration factors in the file to specify the spatial, temporal, and velocity calibration on the image, allowing automated quantitation. A major impetus for digital storage is the remote transmission of echocardiograms for telemedicine purposes or to integrate them with other medical data on a disk for a unit patient record, which the patient would be able to take with him or her on transfer to another hospital. Digital images are also suitable for off-line computer analysis and image processing and may be archived indefinitely without data deterioration. Videotape suffers an inevitable degradation in image quality as the magnetized iron coating realigns itself spontaneously on the tape [1].

Expectations of Functionality

Nonechocardiographer or clinician
  Diagnostic quality images
  Rapid access and display with other data
Clinical echocardiographer
  Onscreen calibration of two-dimensional, Doppler,
    and color flow
  Comprehensive analysis package
  Rapid access to prior reports and studies
Echocardiographic researcher
  As much quantitative data as possible
  Not confined to video format (ρ-ϑ display, RF data,
    raw Doppler data)

FIGURE 5-2. Expectations of functionality. It is important to recognize that digital echocardiography means different things to different users. For the nonechocardiographer or clinician, the need is for good-quality images that can be reviewed alongside expert interpretations. For the clinical echocardiographer, there is a need for onscreen calibration of two-dimensional, spectral Doppler, and color-flow Doppler data integrated with a comprehensive analysis package and rapid access to prior reports and images. For the echocardiography researcher, there is a need for even more quantitative data and storage formats beyond the standard video output, such as scan-line storage, radiofrequency (RF) storage, and the raw Doppler data [2].

THE DICOM STANDARD

Definition of DICOM

A set of rules to specify how medical images are exchanged
  over a network or stored digitally on a disk
A result of a 10-year collaboration among the NEMA, ACR,
  ASE, ACC, and others
A way to store echocardiographic images along with patient
  and other relevant information

FIGURE 5-3. Definition of Digital Imaging and Communications in Medicine (DICOM). One of the critical ingredients for making routine digital echocardiography a reality is the development of image storage formats that are standardized for use by vendors and professional societies. For medical imaging, the DICOM standard has emerged as the worldwide standard for storage. DICOM is simply a set of rules to specify how medical images are exchanged over a network or stored digitally on a disk. These rules should not affect the end-user at all, but are simply there to allow vendors to store their files in a standardized way. DICOM was developed through a more than 10-year collaboration between the National Electrical Manufacturers Association (NEMA) and various professional societies such as the American College of Radiology (ACR), American College of Cardiology (ACC), American Society of Echocardiography (ASE), and many others. It is simply a way to store echocardiography images along with patient and other relevant information [3].

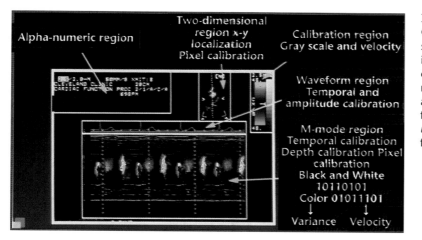

FIGURE 5-4. Regional calibration in ultrasound. The Digital Imaging and Communications in Medicine (DICOM) standard for ultrasound allows the storage of sophisticated calibration data within the image file. For example, in an echocardiogram, one might have a temporal sweep area, such as the color M-mode area, in the center of the image on this frame. For this region, the temporal calibration along the horizontal axis, spatial calibration along the vertical axis, and velocity calibration from the colors may be specified. Additional regions, such as the two-dimensional finder image in the *upper right corner* of the image, may be specified with separate calibration factors [3].

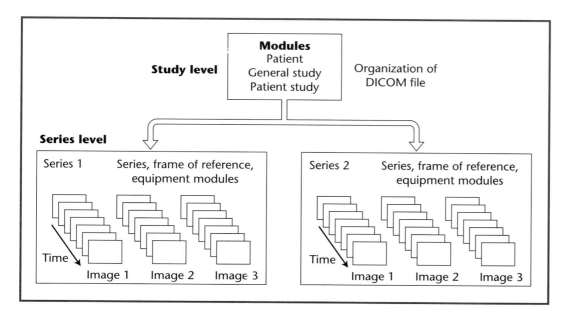

FIGURE 5-5. Organization of a Digital Imaging and Communications in Medicine (DICOM) file. One of the useful aspects of DICOM is the way it allows patient studies to be organized in a database. For example, an image may be assigned to a specific patient and a specific study. Within that study there may be several series of images that represent different stages of the examination, such as pre- and post-exercise, pre- and post-pump for intraoperative echocardiograms, or various stages of an interventional procedure. Note that an image may be either a single frame or a loop of frames, most commonly representing a cardiac cycle [3].

Media Considerations for Digital Formatting in Echocardiography

1.44-MB floppy disk
  Ubiquitous; useful for highly condensed studies and
    selected views
3.5- and 5.25-in magneto-optical drives
  Cost-effective storage, incremental write capability,
    rapidly improving storage capacity and transfer speed
Writable CD-ROM
  Very low media costs, ubiquitous reading drives
  Limited multisession capability and transfer rate
Videotape
  More useful for archival than exchange

FIGURE 5-6. Media considerations. The Digital Imaging and Communications in Medicine (DICOM) standard was initially designed for the network exchange of radiographic images, such as computed tomography, magnetic resonance imaging, and plain films. In cardiology, however, there has been much greater interest in storage of examinations on a disk that could accompany the patient on transfer. For angiography, the only acceptable medium is the writable CD-ROM, which has very low media costs and has drives available for reading on virtually all contemporary computers. However, it does not have rewritable capability and has a fairly slow transfer rate. In echocardiography, in addition to the CD-ROM, it is permissible to store studies on 1.4-MB floppy disks, which are useful for small studies such as stress echocardiograms. For larger studies, 3.5- and 5.25-in magneto-optical disks are suitable for moving echocardiographic data from the echocardiograph to a workstation. Because they are rewritable, they may be used over and over again. Finally, for actual archival of echocardiographic data, digital tape may be most suitable because it is the cheapest storage medium available. Note that the DICOM standard is designed specifically for information *exchange*, not for archival, and individual users and vendors must decide on the best way to actually store the data for long-term purposes in a given facility. Thus, digital tape may be the most appropriate archival medium for echocardiography, although it is not on the list of accepted media for information exchange [3].

Proposed Application Profiles for the DICOM Standard in Cardiology

Angiography
  Standard: 512 × 512 × 8 bit monochrome × 4800 frames
  High resolution: 1024 × 1024 × 10 bit × 1000 frames
Echocardiography
  Image display (ID): required data elements only (types 1,
    1C, 2, and 2C), supports viewing images qualitatively
  Spatial calibration (SC): includes elements to calibrate
    lengths, areas, intervals (scrolling displays), and velocity
    (spectral displays)
  Combined calibration (CC): includes elements to extract
    velocity from color pixels

FIGURE 5-7. Digital Imaging and Communications in Medicine (DICOM) application profiles in angiography and echocardiography. For network transmission of medical images, a negotiation can take place, leading to an image format that both the sending and receiving computers can support. For disk-based transfer, however, such features must be agreed on ahead of time through the use of *application profiles*. For angiography, there is currently a single application profile, specifying the storage of angiographic images based on a 512 × 512 pixel matrix and 8-bit gray-scale depth. This allows approximately 4800 frames to be stored on a standard CD-ROM. A high-resolution application profile is being developed with better spatial and gray-scale fidelity but fewer frames stored on the disk. In echocardiography, application profiles are based on the degree of calibration data contained. For simple image display, only enough data are included to show the image on the screen. For the spatial calibration profile, spatial and temporal calibration data are included. For the combined calibration profile, sufficient calibration data are included to allow quantitative reconstruction of velocity maps from color Doppler images [3].

Current Activities of the DICOM Ultrasound Committee

Results reporting
  Quantitative data
  Standardized reports
Unification with SNOMED nomenclature
Alternate storage formats
  Three- and four-dimensional data, polar storage,
    audio Doppler
Alternate compression approaches
  Currently RLE (lossless) and JPEG (lossy)
  Multiframe: MPEG-1, MPEG-2
  Wavelets, fractals

FIGURE 5-8. Current activities of the Digital Imaging and Communications in Medicine (DICOM) Ultrasound Committee. The DICOM Ultrasound Committee has already standardized the formatting in which echocardiographic images will be stored, but there are a number of enhancements to the standard that are underway. The most active of these is the development of a results-reporting module, which would allow the transfer of measured data from echocardiography machine to workstation and may eventually allow the issuance of standardized reports from various echocardiographic laboratories. As part of this, all medical imaging modalities are unifying their nomenclature with the Standardized Nomenclature of Medicine (SNOMED) lists from the College of American Pathology. In addition, there is interest in developing standardized storage formats for data types other than the video-based images currently used. Among these alternate formats are three- and four-dimensional datasets, polar storage (in which each scan-line is stored in its original acquisition order), and more robust Doppler formats. Finally, there is interest in studying alternate compression approaches that may be applicable to echocardiography. Currently, only the lossless run-length–encoding algorithm Packbits and the lossy Joint Photographic Expert Group (JPEG) algorithm are supported in DICOM, but there is interest in testing the applicability of Motion Picture Expert Group (MPEG)-1, MPEG-2, and wavelet encoding. RLE—run-length encoding.

The Importance of DICOM

Avoiding battles over standards
Avoiding mistakes of the past
  Beta vs VHS
  NTSC vs PAL vs SECAM

FIGURE 5-9. The Importance of Digital Imaging and Communications in Medicine (DICOM). The key importance of DICOM is not that it is a perfect standard, but that it is one that has been agreed on by manufacturers and users around the world. With this standard in place, the echocardiographic community may hope to avoid the mistakes of the past, such as the battle between Beta and VHS video formats in the early 1980s and the continuing incompatibility of video formats around the world (NTSC vs PAL vs SECAM).

One of the ways of ensuring vendor compliance to a new standard is to stage public demonstrations at major professional meetings, where any areas of ambiguity in the standard may be identified and eliminated. A combined DICOM demonstration of echocardiography, angiography, and nuclear medicine was staged for the American College of Cardiology. The demonstration included the issuance of a disk with over 100 loops of cardiac images and software to view them.

The DICOM standard is intended to be a living document, with enhancements added from time to time, while still preserving backwards compatibility with the original standard. This standard has already been endorsed by The American College of Cardiology, The American Society of Echocardiography, and The European Society of Cardiology, and has strong support in Japan. Some of these societies have special needs (*eg*, Kanji characters in Japanese), but these needs can be met with minor additional options to the standard, allowing one worldwide approach to the storage of echocardiography images.

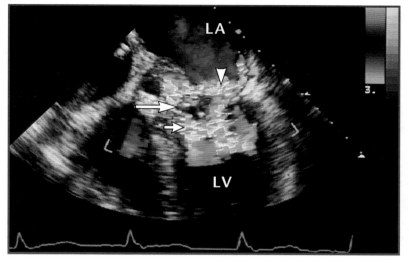

FIGURE 5-10. Digital echocardiogram. This sample digital echocardiogram from the 1996 American College of Cardiology DISC'96 demonstration shows aortic valve endocarditis (*long arrow*) with severe aortic insufficiency (*short arrow*) and an aorto-to-left atrium fistula (*arrowhead*).

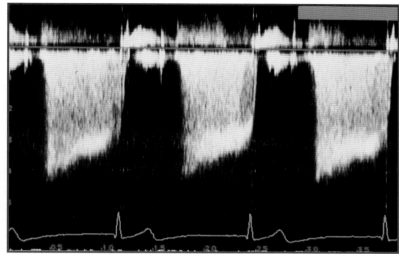

FIGURE 5-11. Digital Doppler echocardiogram. In this sample image from the DISC'96 Digital Imaging and Communications in Medicine (DICOM) demonstration at the American College of Cardiology, a continuous-wave Doppler jet of aortic insufficiency is interrogated, yielding a dense spectral envelope with relatively slow pressure half-time, indicating only mild to moderate regurgitation. Digital storage of spectral Doppler data would allow automated edge detection techniques to quantify peak gradient and pressure half-time.

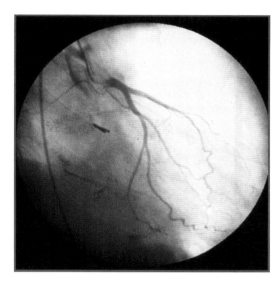

FIGURE 5-12. Digital angiography. This sample image from the American College of Cardiology DISC'96 demonstration shows a left coronary angiogram, demonstrating the potential for multimedia storage of digital cardiologic data.

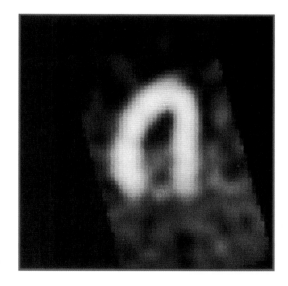

FIGURE 5-13. Digital nuclear cardiology. This sample image from the American College of Cardiology DISC'96 demonstration shows a single photon emission computed tomography image demonstrating normal perfusion. The Digital Imaging and Communications in Medicine (DICOM) standard allows angiograms, echocardiograms, and nuclear studies to reside on a single piece of media (writable CD-ROM).

COMPRESSION ECHOCARDIOGRAMS

FIGURE 5-14. Storage requirements for digital echocardiograms. As this matrix demonstrates, digital echocardiographs require a huge amount of storage. For a full-resolution (512 × 512) matrix with full color (24 bit) 230.4 MB is required for 10 s of video.

Storage Requirements for Digital Echocardiograms (10s [30 fps] of video)

	128 matrix, *MB*	256 matrix, *MB*	512 matrix, *MB*
8-bit gray	4.8	19.2	76.8
16-bit color	9.6	38.4	153.6
24-bit color	14.4	57.6	230.4

Choices for Clinical Compression of Echocardiographic Data

None (640 × 480 × 30 fps × 24-bit color)
  30 MB/s; 20 GB per 10-min study
Clinical
  Single cycle loops only (50×)
  Systole only (2×–3×)
  Quad screen (4×)
  8–16 bit color (1.5-3×)
  Half resolution (4×)
  Potential savings: 7200:1 (3 MB per study)

FIGURE 5-15. The need for clinical compression. The greatest limitation of digital echocardiography is the enormous storage requirements. Full-motion video contains approximately 640 pixels across the screen, 480 lines down the screen, 30 frames/s, and 24 bits to fully represent the color. At this rate, 30 MB/s is required for storage or 20 GB for a 10-minute study, over 14,000 1.4-MB floppy disks! It is clear that very aggressive clinical editing is necessary to make digital echocardiography feasible. For example, by storing only single cardiac cycle loops rather than recording long sequences from a single vantage, up to 50-fold reduction in data can be achieved. For stress-echocardiography studies, systole alone may be sufficient for diagnosis, saving one half to two thirds of the data. For some applications, storage in a quadscreen will obtain an additional fourfold compression. It is often possible to use fewer bits for color representation and may be possible to store some images at reduced resolution. Combining all of these clinical compression options would produce a very dramatic reduction in the size of an echocardiography examination [4].

Choices of Digital Echocardiographic Compression

None
  Easy programming and indexing of disk
Lossless (Packbits RLE in DICOM)
  No pixel alteration
  2–3:1 for gray scale; up to 7:1 for color Doppler
JPEG (single-frame lossy compression)
  Standardized in DICOM
  20:1 appears safe for clinical images
Multiframe compression (MPEG, H.261, wavelets)
  Much higher compression (100:1–1000:1)
  Not in DICOM
  Clinical validation lacking

FIGURE 5-16. Digital echocardiographic compression. Even with the significant savings that can be achieved through clinical compression of echocardiographic data, there is still a need for further reduction in data, both for storage and speed of transmission. To achieve this, digital compression must be used, whereby each image is stored with fewer bytes of data. Digital compression is divided into two basic types: 1) "lossless," in which there is no change whatsoever in the image (but only relatively modest compression levels are achieved [2:1 or 3:1]); and 2) "lossy," in which some alteration in the appearance of the image occurs (hopefully, without clinical impact) and much higher compression ratios are possible. In the ultrasound standard for Digital Imaging and Communications in Medicine (DICOM), images may be stored either uncompressed, with lossless compression using the Packbits run-length encoding algorithm or with the Joint Photographic Expert Group (JPEG) lossy algorithm. Clinical studies have demonstrated that 20:1 JPEG compression does not appear to affect the diagnostic interpretation of echocardiograms. More sophisticated compression algorithms operate on multiple frames at a time and exploit the redundancy between echocardiographic images. Such algorithms as Motion Picture Expert Group (MPEG) and H.261 provide much higher compression ratios, but they are not standardized in DICOM, and clinical validation of these compression modalities has not been completed [4]. RLE—run-length encoding.

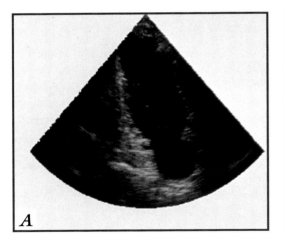 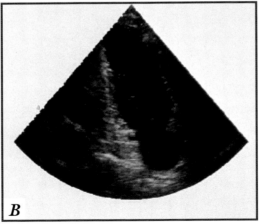

A *B*

FIGURE 5-17. Impact of Joint Photographic Expert Group (JPEG) compression on image quality. In this apical two-chamber view of the left ventricle and left atrium, the uncompressed image (**A**) requires 216 kilobytes for storage. The same image after JPEG compression (**B**) at 34:1 ratio now requires only 6 kilobytes. Very close inspection may reveal subtle block artefacts reflecting the 8 × 8 pixel blocks used for JPEG encoding. Overall, however, there is little degradation of the image [5].

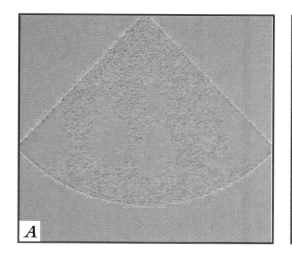

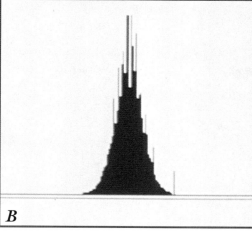

FIGURE 5-18. Difference image (**A**) and histogram (**B**) for uncompressed and compressed echocardiograms. One way to assess the impact of digital compression on an image is to subtract the compressed from the original image and display the difference both as an image and as a histogram of the pixel values. Whereas lossless compression will result in a featureless gray image, clinically acceptable lossy compression algorithms should have essentially random variations in gray, narrowly clustered around a value of 0. In this image, a 35:1 Joint Photographic Expert Group (JPEG) image is subtracted from the uncompressed image, resulting in a difference image in which the features of this apical echocardiogram are just barely discernible. The histogram shows no significant shift in values, with an acceptable SD of 8 [5]. The mean shift is 0.18, and the median shift is 0.

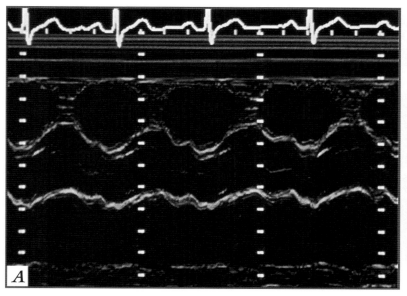

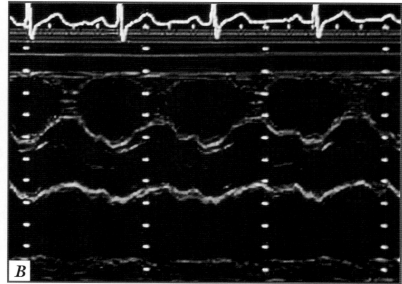

FIGURE 5-19. Impact of Joint Photographic Expert Group (JPEG) compression M-mode echocardiograms. Image showing an M-mode through the aortic root and left atrium. Uncompressed image (**A**) and a 23:1 JPEG image (**B**). Very slight blurring can be seen of especially sharp interfaces, such as the calibration markers, but in general there is no significant loss of information [5].

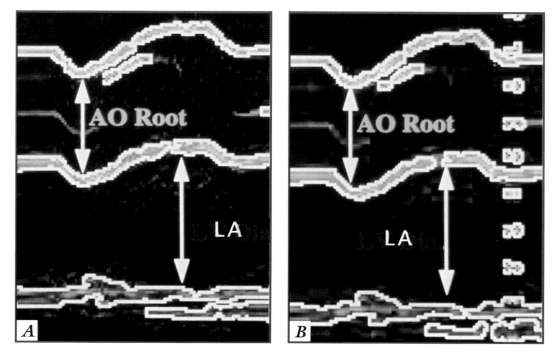

FIGURE 5-20. Impact of Joint Photographic Expert Group (JPEG) compression on automated edge detection. One of the concerns with JPEG compression is that the 8×8 pixel blocks used in the compression may lead to inappropriate edge detection when automated algorithms are applied to the image. This image shows an M-mode echocardiogram to which an automated edge detection algorithm has been applied both to the uncompressed image (**A**) and a 23:1 JPEG compressed image (**B**). It is evident that no significant shift in the edge localization had occurred due to the compression [5]. AO—aorta; LA—left atrium.

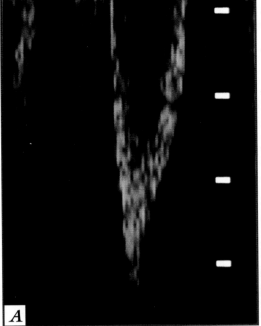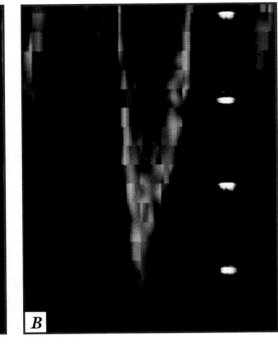

FIGURE 5-21. Impact of Joint Photographic Expert Group (JPEG) compression on spectral Doppler. Image demonstrating a pulsed Doppler spectrum for flow in the left ventricular outflow tract. Uncompressed image (**A**) and a 27:1 JPEG image (**B**) demonstrating excellent fidelity to the original [5].

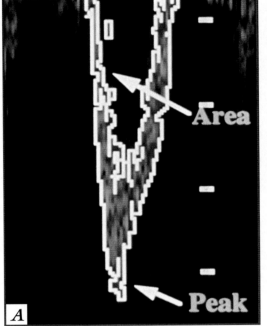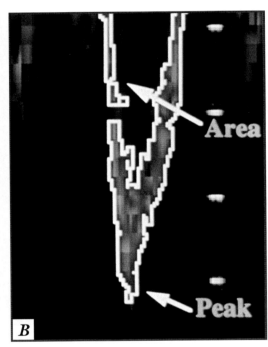

FIGURE 5-22. Impact of Joint Photographic Expert Group (JPEG) compression on automated edge detection. Shown here is a pulsed Doppler spectrum of left ventricular outflow tract flow with an automated edge detection algorithm applied. **A,** The uncompressed image. There is no significant difference in the peak and enclosed area of the pulsed Doppler, despite 27:1 compression (**B**) [5].

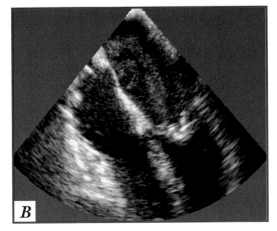

FIGURE 5-23. Digital Echo Record Access (ERA) study. The largest trial of compression in echocardiography was the Digital ERA trial, conducted at the 1994 American Society of Echocardiography Scientific Sessions in San Francisco, CA. Each participant was asked to view two moving echocardiography loops side by side on a computer screen. One of these images was derived from a videotaped echocardiogram that had been digitized; the other was a direct digital storage. The digital echocardiograms were stored either uncompressed or with 10:1 or 20:1 Joint Photographic Expert Group (JPEG) compression. Viewers were asked to compare the loops on the basis of image quality and diagnostic content [6].

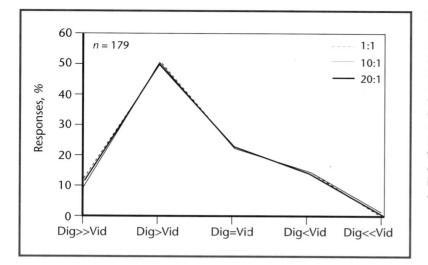

FIGURE 5-24. Impact on image quality in the Digital Echo Record Access (ERA) study. As shown in this image from the Digital ERA study, there was a highly significant preference ($P < 0.001$) for the digital (Dig) videos rather than the digitized videotape (Vid) images. Further, careful observation reveals that there are actually three lines on this graph representing the uncompressed, 10:1, and 20:1 compressed images, indicating no effect of compression on the preference for digital images. Similar findings were observed for diagnostic content. Thus it is evident that digital echocardiography images are higher in quality than videotape images, and Joint Photographic Expert Group (JPEG) compression at 20:1 appears acceptable for routine clinical use. Limitations of this study included the absence of color Doppler images and the fact that only a few pathologies were included [6]. >—better than; >>—much better than; <—worse than; <<—much worse than.

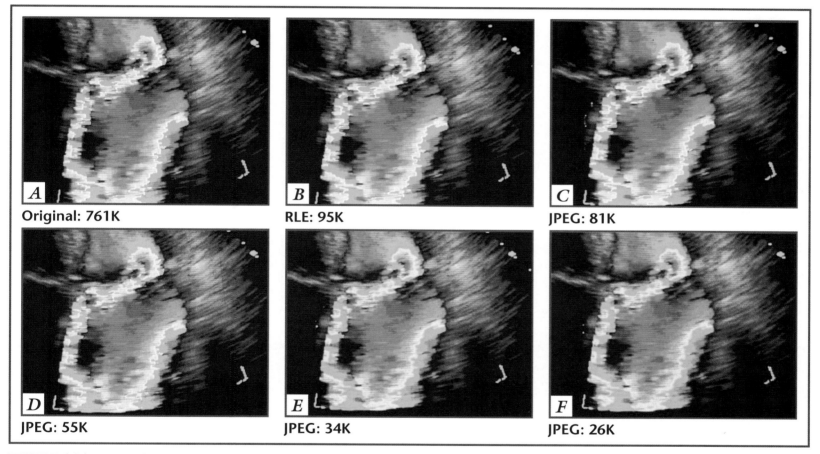

FIGURE 5-25. Impact of Joint Photographic Expert Group (JPEG) compression on color Doppler echocardiograms. In this montage of six echocardiography frames, varying compression levels are used, with the uncompressed image in **A** and a lossless run-length encoded (RLE) image in **B**. **C** to **F**, Increasing degrees of JPEG compression, with barely noticeable degradation at the highest compression levels. Note that because of the special nature of color Doppler echocardiograms (with the color sector occupying only a small part of the whole image), lossless compression is unusually effective.

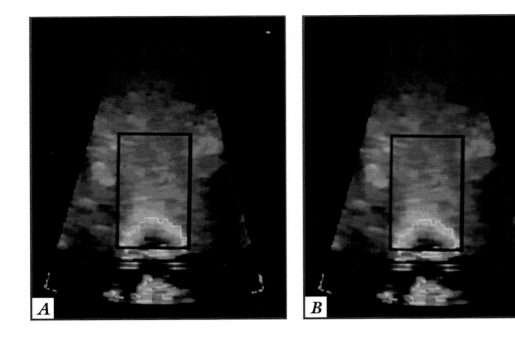

FIGURE 5-26. Impact of Joint Photographic Expert Group (JPEG) compression on quantitative color Doppler echocardiography. Increasingly, the actual velocities encoded within color Doppler maps are being used for quantification of forward and regurgitant flow. An *in vitro* representation of a proximal flow convergence region is shown, uncompressed (**A**) and following 24:1 JPEG compression (**B**). Although very slight shifts in colorization may have occurred, the original appearance has not been altered [7].

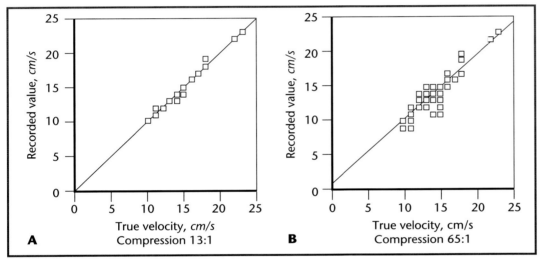

FIGURE 5-27. Impact of Joint Photographic Expert Group (JPEG) compression on quantitative color velocity. Using the color bar as a reference, it is possible to translate color Doppler maps into velocity maps. This image demonstrates the impact that JPEG compression has on the ability to recover quantitative velocities. The results following 13:1 compression, with near perfect representation of velocity (**A**). Even after 65:1 compression, there is good fidelity to the original velocities (**B**) [7].

PRACTICAL ASPECTS OF DIGITAL ECHOCARDIOGRAPHY

Development of the Desktop System

	1992	1996	1998
Processor	80486	P6	P7
Speed, *MHz*	33	180	400
Memory, *MB*	8	32	64
Hard drive	340 MB, 15 ms	3000 MB, 11 ms	8000 MB, 5 ms
Video	16 bit, 1 MB	64 bit, 2 MB	64 bit, 8 MB
Software	Win 3.0	Win95, OfficePro	Win 98 (?)
Extras	None	8X CD-ROM	10 GB CD
Cost, *dollars*	3895	2609	2499
Value (PC=1)	100	1500	4000

FIGURE 5-28. Computer improvements. In addition to the adoption of the Digital Imaging and Communications in Medicine (DICOM) standard, the move toward digital echocardiography has been significantly encouraged by the ongoing improvement in cost performance ratio of computer systems. This image shows typical high-end computer systems as quoted from magazine advertisements in 1992 and 1996, with projections to 1998. From 1992 to 1996, the processor advanced two generations, with a five-fold increase in speed, a fourfold increase in memory, and near 10-fold improvement in hard disk storage, with corresponding improvements in video and software, and the addition of an 8× (1.2 MB/s) CD-ROM reader, all accompanied by a fall in price of over $1000 or a 15-fold improvement in price and performance. With no slowing of this trend in sight, there should be even further improvements before the end of the century [8]. PC—personal computer.

Choices in Echocardiographic Export

Video capture
  Applicable to existing equipment, but separate calibration
    and patient management information needed
Optical disk
  Full digital fidelity but separate database needed;
    applicable to portable studies
Direct network connection
  Integrated image and patient database possible,
    but difficult to retrofit existing equipment
Hard disk to network
  Possible to combine stationary and portable studies

FIGURE 5-29. Choices in echocardiographic export. In the transition from an analog to a digital echocardiographic laboratory, a variety of strategies must be used to get the digital data out of existing and new equipment. For older equipment that has no digital output capabilities on its own, the only real choice is "frame-grabbing" images from the video port. Although some loss of fidelity may be anticipated during this process, the results are actually quite acceptable, provided the image is digitized directly from the video port of the echocardiograph, rather than from videotape (the source of most of the distortion). Currently, several vendors offer true digital output onto a magneto-optical disk. This offers all the fidelity and quantitation opportunities of digital echocardiographic data, but must be transferred to a workstation for long-term storage and retrieval. The rewritable nature of magneto-optical disks makes them applicable to a "sneaker net" for gathering portable echocardiographic studies onto a server. Very soon, we anticipate direct network output from echocardiographic instruments using the Digital Imaging and Communications in Medicine (DICOM) protocol to negotiate the sending of images into a central server. With this development, there should be significant improvements in the efficiency of performing and reviewing echocardiographic studies. Finally, for portable studies in the future, it will be possible to store all data internally on a hard disk for later downloading onto a network [8].

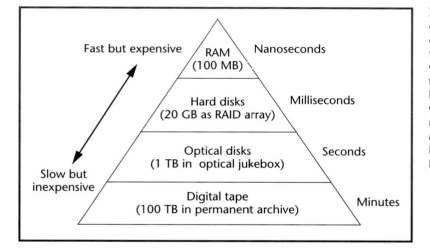

FIGURE 5-30. Hierarchical storage in medical imaging. For maximal efficiency in the storage of digital echocardiography images, it is necessary to develop a hierarchical, pyramid-shaped storage architecture. At the top of the pyramid are very fast but relatively expensive storage modalities that will allow all recent echocardiograms to be retrieved in a matter of seconds for review and approval. Older studies then would be transferred to slower but vastly cheaper storage modalities such as digital tape. A useful strategy would be to arrange for studies stored on digital tape to be moved to rapid-access media as soon as a patient is admitted to the hospital or if another echocardiographic examination is scheduled for the next day [4]. RAID—redundant array of inexpensive disks; RAM—random access memory; MB—megabite; TB—terabyte.

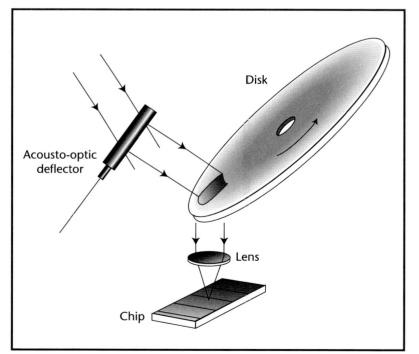

FIGURE 5-31. Advances in digital storage. Over the next decade, we can anticipate the development of several new storage technologies that will dramatically increase the capabilities of current systems. Among the possibilities is the holographic three-dimensional optical disk, whereby an entire image will be encoded holographically on a small piece of an optical disk the size of a CD-ROM. Such a disk potentially could hold as much as 1 terabyte of data, but it is only in the laboratory development stage at this time.

Advantages of Digital Transmission

Remote consultation in difficult cases
Expedite appropriate management
  Transfer, thrombolysis, pericardiocentesis
Reduce repetition of tests
  Primary data can accompany patient
Foster clinical trials
  Rapid dissemination of data
Continuing medical education
  Teaching cases on central server

FIGURE 5-32. Advantages of digital transmission. There are a number of important reasons for developing the capability for long-distance transmission of digital echocardiograms. Primarily, global telemedicine would be possible: it would allow remote consultation with experts in difficult cases and expedite appropriate management, such as patient transfer, thrombolysis, pericardiocentesis, or other intervention. This would have important implications in medical economics because it would reduce the needless repetition of tests, because the primary data could accompany the patient on transfer. Two advantages outside the direct patient care realm include the improved efficiency of clinical trials, whereby studies could be reviewed in a Core Lab shortly after being acquired, and continuing medical education, in which physicians in remote locations could review cases posted centrally on a digital server [9].

Echocardiographic Telemedicine Choices

Fax machine
  Applicable to M-mode, and so on, but low fidelity
Express mail
  Used for 99% of current echo telemedicine
Direct file transfer
  Convenient for non–real-time review; should be increasingly
    feasible with DICOM standardization
Real-time review (teleconferencing)
  Useful for interactive review and acquisition, but not (yet)
    part of DICOM standard; convenience a concern

Choices in Telecommunications

POTS
  Ubiquitous, cheap, modems up to 28.8 kbps
ISDN
  2 × 64 kbps line; can mix video, voice and data; $65/month
  or more
T1
  1.54 Mbps; full video; $800/month + $100/hour
Internet
  Great for data, e-mail, image files; CU-SeeMe; "free"
Future network trends
  Asynchronous transmission mode: 622 Mbps
  "Son of Internet:" 3 Gbps

FIGURE 5-33. Options for integrating echocardiography into telemedicine systems. Currently, most echocardiographic telemedicine is done by fax machine or express mail. The fax machine is useful for transferring reports and possibly some M-mode and spectral Doppler data, but is far too low-fidelity for actual images. Express mail is actually quite effective, allowing the transfer of complete echocardiography studies within a day in a very cost-efficient manner; in fact, it is the standard against which new digital methodologies should be judged. For digital transfer, there are two philosophical approaches: direct file transfer and real-time review. In direct file transfer, a study is performed remotely, and the images are stored for the complete study. This file is then forwarded via the Internet or other network to the remote station, where it may be reviewed by the consulting cardiologist at a convenient time. This closely matches the model for videotape review in most current echocardiographic practices. In real-time review, however, the images are played directly over a network to the reviewing physician as they are being acquired. This allows interaction between the consulting and sending sites; it is important for pediatric cardiology, transesophageal echocardiography, and intraoperative echocardiography. It has the disadvantage, however, of requiring immediate availability of the consulting physician whenever a remote study is being acquired [9]. DICOM—Digital Imaging and Communications in Medicine.

FIGURE 5-34. Choices in telecommunications. A revolution is occurring in telecommunication, with more widespread availability of high-speed digital transfer technologies. Many residential services and small hospitals are still limited to analog telephone service (ie, POTS [plain old telephone service]) and the use of analog modems. Unfortunately, these are too slow for practical use in tele-echocardiography. For example, a typical complete echocardiographic study, even with some degree of Joint Photographic Expert Group (JPEG) compression, may occupy 35 MB of storage. At a transfer speed of 28.8 kilobits/s (kbps; rarely achieved in actuality, even for a modem of this speed), the transfer would require 10,000 s or almost 3 hours. Increasingly, ISDN (integrated sound and data network) end-lines are available, allowing integrated voice and data transfer at rates up to 128 kbps. This would reduce the transfer time for the typical echocardiographic study fivefold, to approximately 36 minutes. More acceptable would be transfer over high speed T1 lines, capable of data rates of 1.54 megabits/s (Mbps). At this speed, the file could be transferred within about 3 min. Unfortunately, T1 lines generally are not available on demand and must be leased on a monthly basis at fairly high charge. The Internet is a potential mechanism for transferring echocardiographic files, although many servers refuse to handle a file as large as 35 MB. For isolated images and small loops, however, it provides an essentially free service. There are issues to be resolved, such as preserving patient confidentiality as images pass through multiple servers on the way to the recipient. There are also low-cost teleconferencing options such as CU-SeeMe, although these are quite low fidelity for echocardiography studies. With future developments in the Internet, however, much higher data rates can be anticipated, as the Internet backbone will be increased to data-rates of 3 to 10 gigabits/s (Gbps). Cable modems may allow high-speed review over cable television lines.

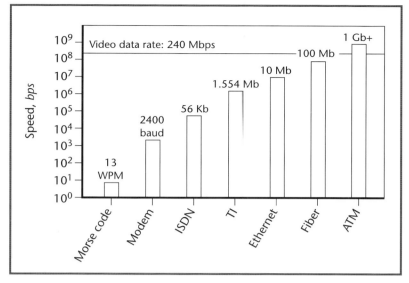

FIGURE 5-35. Choices in telemedicine speed. This figure illustrates (on a logarithmic scale) the increase in digital transfer speed over the past century. Also shown is the data rate for full uncompressed video. It should be recognized that with relatively modest compression, broadcast-quality video can be sent at data rates between 5 and 10 Mbps, which should make feasible direct digital echocardiographic transfers over existing technology in the near future. ATM—asynchronous transmission mode; ISDN—integrated sound and data network; WPM—words per minute.

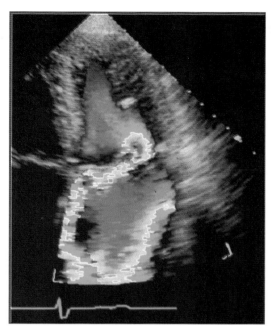

FIGURE 5-36. Echocardiography in manned space flight. In the ultimate test of echocardiographic telemedicine, the United States will transport a commercial echocardiograph to the International Space Station via space shuttle for permanent installation in the year 2000 to study changes in the cardiovascular system in microgravity. Transmission of digital echocardiography data over the relatively narrow communication bandwidth from the space station will require careful application of compression technology and selection of the key data to send. It is anticipated that data will be stored and transmitted in the Digital Imaging and Communications in Medicine (DICOM) format.

APPLICATIONS OF DIGITAL ECHOCARDIOGRAPHY

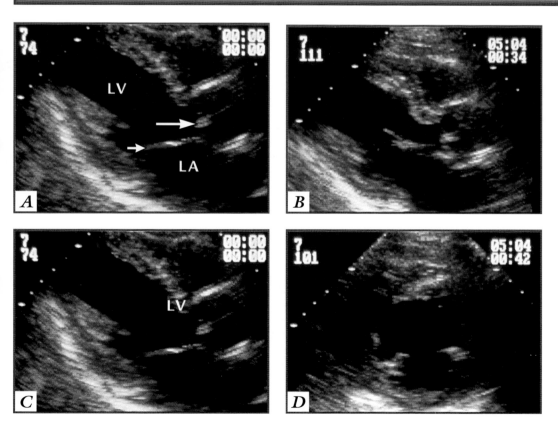

FIGURE 5-37. Stress echocardiography. The initial application of digital echocardiography has been in the analysis of stress echocardiography images. As shown here, parasternal long-axis (**A** and **B**) and short-axis (**C** and **D**) images are shown pre- (**A** and **C**) and post-exercise (**B** and **D**), allowing the identification of stress-induced wall motion abnormalities. *Long arrow* in *A* indicates aortic valve; *short arrow* in *A* indicates mitral valve. LA—left atrium; LV—left ventricle.

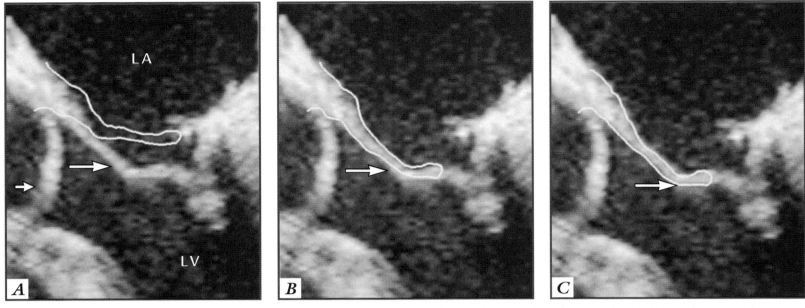

FIGURE 5-38. Automated edge detection. With the availability of digital echocardiography images, it is possible to perform automated edge detection algorithms. In this example, the location of the mitral leaflet on the preceding frame is shown (**A**), and the algorithm uses the velocity data of mitral valve (*long arrow*) motion to project itself onto the new position of the mitral leaflet (**B**). Finally, using a template for mitral leaflet shape, refinement is made to the localization of the leaflet (**C**) [10]. *Short arrow* in *A* indicates aortic valve. LA—left atrium; LV—left ventricle.

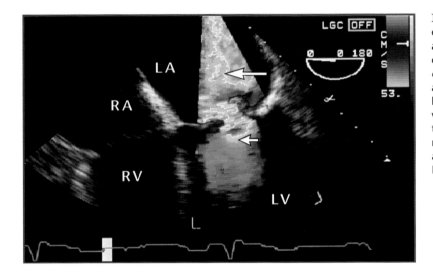

FIGURE 5-39. Proximal acceleration in mitral regurgitation. In this transesophageal image, a large jet of mitral regurgitation is seen entering the left atrium (*long arrow*). This jet is turbulent and difficult to use in quantitation of regurgitation, but the proximal convergence zone (*short arrow and rings of color* just on the ventricular side of the valve) is much better behaved, allowing flow rate to be quantified. Assuming this flow to form concentric hemispheric shells of decreasing radius and increasing velocity, a contour with velocity V at radius r will yield a flow rate of $Q = 2\pi r^2 V$. Dividing Q by the peak velocity of the jet (from continuous-wave Doppler) yields the regurgitant flow orifice area. Digital storage of these velocities is critical for automated assessment of proximal convergence zones [11]. LA—left atrium; LV—left ventricle; RA—right atrium; RV—right ventricle.

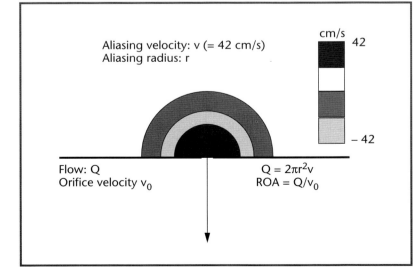

FIGURE 5-40. Quantification of valvular regurgitation. Digital echocardiography allows the color Doppler images to be used as velocity maps rather than simply spatial representations of jets. The proximal convergence theory analyzes the acceleration of blood proximal to an orifice, identifying a contour at radius r where the blood is moving at velocity V (typically identified by aliasing of the color). At this point, assuming the contour to be hemispherical, one obtains a flow rate $Q = 2\pi r^2 V$ and a regurgitant orifice area given by Q/V_0, where V_0 is the peak velocity through the valve by continuous-wave Doppler [11].

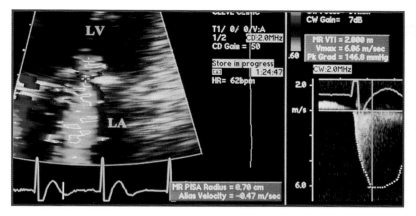

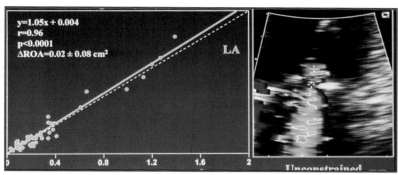

FIGURE 5-41. Proximal convergence analysis. In this example of moderate mitral regurgitation, analysis of the proximal convergence zone demonstrates a regurgitant orifice area of 0.24 cm². The necessary data for this calculation (two-dimensional imaging and continuous-wave Doppler spectrum) can be obtained from a single imaging window.

FIGURE 5-42. Quantification of regurgitant flow. The proximal convergence method has been shown to be quite accurate in quantifying regurgitant orifice area, particularly for convergence zones that are unconstrained by surrounding walls [12].

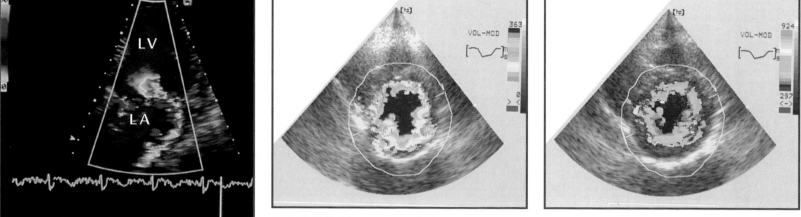

FIGURE 5-43. Constrained proximal convergence flow. In this patient with a flail mitral leaflet, the proximal convergence zone is constrained by an adjacent wall and displaced outward, resulting in an overestimation of flow rate if the simple proximal convergence formula was used [12]. LA—left atrium; LV—left ventricle.

FIGURE 5-44. Automated edge tracking (systole). By thresholding on the back-scattered ultrasound intensity on each image, it is possible to track endocardial movement throughout systole [13].

FIGURE 5-45. Automated edge tracking (diastole). By thresholding on the back-scattered ultrasound intensity on each image, it is possible to track outward endocardial movement throughout diastole [13].

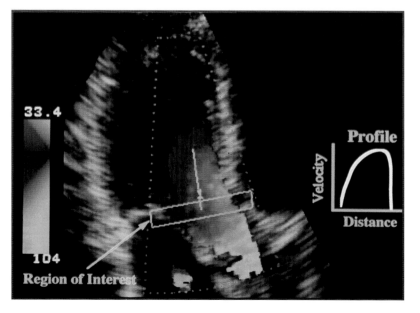

FIGURE 5-46. Automated cardiac output measurement. By integrating the color Doppler velocities across the left ventricular outflow tract and throughout systole, it is possible to calculate cardiac stroke volume [14].

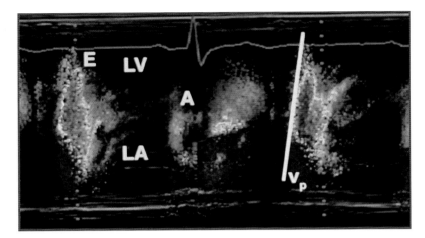

FIGURE 5-47. Color Doppler M-mode of left ventricular (LV) in-flow. Image demonstrating the propagation of flow from the left atrium (LA) to the LV through the mitral valve during diastole, showing the early-filling wave (E) and late-filling wave with atrial contraction (A). The slope of this propagation wave, termed the *propagation velocity* (V_p) is different from the velocities contained within the E-wave (E) and relates closely to LV relaxation. Automated processing of digital Doppler velocities contained within such color M-mode maps may allow noninvasive quantification of intraventricular pressure gradients [15,16].

REFERENCES

1. Thomas JD, Nissen SE: Digital storage and transmission of cardiovascular images: is now the time to invest [editorial]? *Heart* 1996, 76:13–17.

2. Thomas JD, Khandheria B: Digital formatting standards in medical imaging: a primer for echocardiographers. *J Am Soc Echocardiogr* 1994, 7:100–104.

3. Thomas JD: The DICOM image formatting standard: what it means for echocardiographers. *J Am Soc Echocardiogr* 1995, 8:319–327.

4. Thomas JD: Digital archiving of echocardiograms. *Coronary Artery Disease* 1995, 6:4–9.

5. Karson TH, Chandra S, Morehead A, *et al.*: JPEG compression of digital echocardiographic images: impact on image quality. *J Am Soc Echocardiogr* 1995, 8:306–318.

6. Karson TH, Zepp RC, Chandra S, *et al.*: Digital storage of echocardiograms offers superior image quality to analog storage even with 20:1 digital compression: results of the Digital ERA (Echo Record Access) study. *J Am Soc Echocardiogr* 1996, 9:769–778.

7. Thomas JD, Chandra S, Karson TH, *et al.*: Digital compression of echocardiograms: impact on quantitative interpretation of color Doppler velocity. *J Am Soc Echocardiogr* 1996, 9:606–615.

8. Thomas JD: Digital storage and retrieval: the future in echocardiography. *Heart* 1997, 78(suppl I)19–22.

9. Dewey CF, Thomas JD, Kunt M, Hunter IW: The prospects for telediagnosing using ultrasound. *Telemedicine* 1996, 2:87–100.

10. Mikic I, Krucinski S, Thomas JD: Segmentation and tracking of mitral valve leaflets in echocardiographic sequences: active contours guided by optical flow estimates. *SPIE Medical Imaging.* Newport Beach, CA; February 10–15, 1996; proceedings no. 2710:311–320.

11. Vandervoort PM, Rivera JM, Mele D, *et al.*: Application of color Doppler flow mapping to calculate effective regurgitant orifice area: an in vitro study with initial clinical observations. *Circulation* 1993, 88:1150–1156.

12. Pu M, Vandervoort PM, Griffin BP, *et al.*: Quantification of mitral regurgitation by the proximal convergence method using transesophageal echocardiography: clinical validation of a geometric correction for proximal flow constraint. *Circulation* 1995, 92:2169–2177.

13. Mor-Avi V, Vignon KP, Koch R, *et al.*: Segmental analysis of color kinesis images: new method quantification of the magnitude and timing of endocardial motion during left ventricular systole and diastole. *Circulation* 1997, 95:2082–2097.

14. Sun JP, Stewart WJ, Pu M, *et al.*: Automated cardiac output measurement by spatiotemporal integration of color Doppler data: in vitro and clinical validation. *Circulation* 1997, 95:932–939.

15. Garcia MJ, Ares MA, Asher C, *et al.*: Color M-mode velocity propagation: an index of early ventricular filling that, combined with pulsed Doppler peak E velocity may estimate capillary wedge pressure. *J Am Coll Cardiol* 1997, 29:448–454.

16. Greenberg NL, Vandervoort PM, Thomas JD: Estimation of instantaneous diastolic transmitral pressure difference from color Doppler M-mode echocardiography. *Am J Physiol* 1996, 271:H1267–H1276.

CHAPTER 6

Advanced Coronary Imaging

Robert N. Piana ~ Scott Kinlay

Selective coronary angiography remains the principal method used to image coronary arteries today, nearly four decades after the development of this technique by Sones in 1959. Coronary angiography originally served as a diagnostic tool to identify significant stenoses in the epicardial arteries. However, diagnostic angiography soon spawned the development of percutaneous catheter-based techniques to treat critical coronary stenoses once identified. The rapid proliferation of percutaneous coronary interventional techniques in recent years has occurred in parallel with continued progress in the basic understanding of native and transplant coronary atherosclerosis, acute coronary syndromes, and restenosis. Together these forces have stimulated the development of new modalities for coronary imaging that can provide more detailed information on coronary anatomy and function than is possible with traditional coronary angiography.

Perhaps the greatest impact of the more advanced coronary imaging modalities has been their contribution to clinical research. Coronary angioscopy has confirmed the central role of thrombus and plaque rupture in unstable angina and myocardial infarction [1,2]. These observations have supported the use of antiplatelet, antithrombotic, and thrombolytic therapies in specific acute coronary syndromes. Quantitative coronary angiography (QCA) has helped elucidate the mechanisms underlying the benefits of cholesterol lowering in atherosclerosis. This sensitive technique has documented that

the improvements in coronary lumen size with cholesterol reduction therapy, although statistically significant, are relatively small in absolute terms [3]. Nevertheless, these modest changes are associated with much greater reductions in adverse clinical events [4]. This disparity between modest angiographic regression and significant clinical benefit has promoted interest in changes in the content and structure of coronary atherosclerotic plaque caused by lipid lowering. Therefore, techniques such as intravascular ultrasound (IVUS), optical coherence tomography, and magnetic resonance imaging are now actively under investigation for this purpose. Other studies using QCA have found that cholesterol lowering can improve coronary vasomotor function [5,6]. The focus of research in atherosclerosis regression has therefore evolved from a purely structural paradigm to one that considers the cellular dysfunctions of atherosclerotic plaques.

Intravascular ultrasound imaging has been applied extensively in cardiology to characterize coronary pathology and to guide coronary interventions. Clinical studies using IVUS imaging have confirmed the presence of compensatory enlargement, a concept originally advanced by Glagov *et al.* [7] based on pathologic specimens. This process reveals the dynamic nature of atherosclerosis, in which the whole vessel at the site of early atheroma enlarges to accommodate the growing plaque and thereby reduces encroachment on the lumen. IVUS imaging has also identified cases of maladaptive shrinkage of the coronary artery, which may accelerate luminal narrowing and contribute to either restenosis after coronary interventions [8] or progressive arteriopathy in cardiac transplant recipients [9]. IVUS imaging has also helped to document the diffuse nature of coronary artery disease (CAD), which often is not apparent by conventional angiography, particularly in transplant atherosclerosis [10,11]. This finding has bolstered support for pharmacologic approaches to arresting and stabilizing plaque growth, including the aggressive control of blood lipids in those with CAD and in heart transplant recipients.

In interventional cardiology, IVUS imaging has provided insight into the mechanisms by which different devices increase the diameter of the arterial lumen. Balloon angioplasty predominantly results in stretching and expansion of the total artery and plaque compression and fracture [12,13]. Whereas directional coronary atherectomy is more selective at removing noncalcified plaque, rotational coronary atherectomy selectively removes calcified and more rigid plaque [14]. These differences have led to the concept of "lesion-specific therapy" and may justify the more widespread use of IVUS imaging if clinical outcomes can be improved with this approach. IVUS imaging has also played a major role in refining the technique of intracoronary stent placement. A high rate of inadequate stent expansion can be

documented with IVUS imaging when inflation pressures standard for balloon angioplasty are used to achieve angiographic criteria for success [15,16]. IVUS imaging has shown that high-pressure balloon inflations are required to accomplish optimal apposition of the stent struts against the wall of the artery and to maximally increase the lumen area [15,16]. In conjunction with the use of antiplatelet agents, high-pressure balloon inflations have revolutionized intracoronary stenting by obviating the need for anticoagulation and reducing bleeding and thrombotic complications [17,18]. Although angiography cannot determine adequate stent deployment, the routine use of high-pressure balloon inflations achieves this result with such consistency that today IVUS imaging is not required in most cases of intracoronary stenting.

Presently, advanced coronary imaging techniques and quantitative analysis remain research tools in most institutions, despite their many contributions to our current understanding of CAD. They entail increased time on the part of the operator, and device costs are significant. The use of certain advanced techniques may increase in the future if their application results in improved clinical outcomes such as averting plaque rupture or reducing restenosis, particularly if these technologies are deemed cost-effective.

PITFALLS OF CORONARY ANGIOGRAPHY

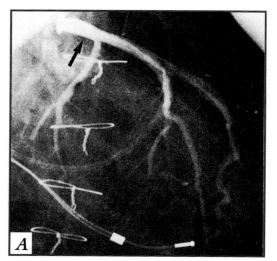

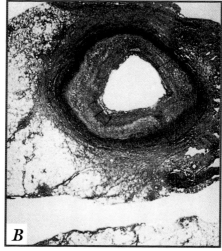

FIGURE 6-1. Angiographically silent disease: correlation of angiography with histopathology. **A,** Coronary angiogram demonstrating a normal-appearing left main coronary segment (*arrow*) in a cardiac transplant recipient. The patient died 4 days later. **B,** Histologic section of the left main coronary artery, demonstrating significant concentric atheromatous plaque. These images illustrate the important concept that angiography gives information about the arterial lumen but little, if any, information about disease of the arterial wall. Angiography may thus provide a poor estimate of the extent of atherosclerosis in coronary arteries. (Legend *adapted from* Powers [19]; figure *from* Johnson and coworkers [20]; with permission.)

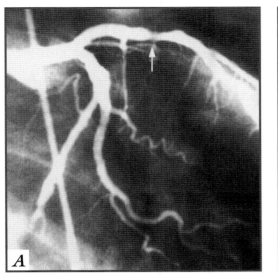
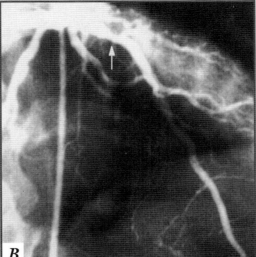

FIGURE 6-2. Intracoronary thrombus. The coronary angiogram is relatively insensitive to the presence of intracoronary thrombus. This angiogram is from an elderly woman who had sustained an anterior myocardial infarction with S-T elevation 2 days earlier and who underwent cardiac catheterization for postinfarction angina. **A,** Coronary angiography demonstrates some haziness in the proximal left anterior descending coronary artery in the right anterior oblique-caudal view (*arrow*), raising the question of intracoronary thrombus. Intraluminal thrombus would be consistent with the patient's clinical presentation, particularly given the absence of other critical coronary stenoses. However, the right anterior oblique-cranial view (**B**) does not suggest thrombus at this site (*arrow*), and neither view fulfills the rigorous angiographic definition of thrombus as an intraluminal filling defect outlined on three sides by contrast medium. Comparative studies have demonstrated the superiority of angioscopy and intravascular ultrasound imaging to coronary angiography for the detection of intracoronary thrombus [2].

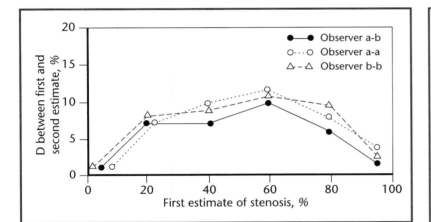

FIGURE 6-3. Visual interpretation of coronary angiography: issues of accuracy and precision. Visual estimates of the severity of coronary stenoses have traditionally demonstrated substantial intra- and interobserver variability. For example, a comparison of site and quality-control readings of 870 angiograms from the Coronary Artery Surgery Study [21] found that when one reader identified a stenosis of 50% or more in the left main coronary artery, there was a 19% chance that *no* lesion was found by the second reader. Important contributing factors to the variability of visual readings are lesion location, image quality, and expertise of the reader. The severity of the stenosis in question is also a determinant, as illustrated in this graph. Shub *et al.* [22] reported that when two angiographers read films at baseline and then again 3 months later, the interobserver (a-b) and intraobserver (a-a, b-b) variabilities were relatively small (mean differences less than 5%) for stenoses less than 20% or greater than 80%, but were higher (mean differences 8% to 14%) for stenoses between 20% and 80%. In this graph, *D* represents the mean difference in readings between the first and second estimates. Lesions were grouped into the following ranges of percent diameter stenosis: 0 to 9, 10 to 29, 30 to 49, 50 to 69, 70 to 89, and 90 to 100, as shown on the abscissa. (*Adapted from* Shub and coworkers [22]; with permission.)

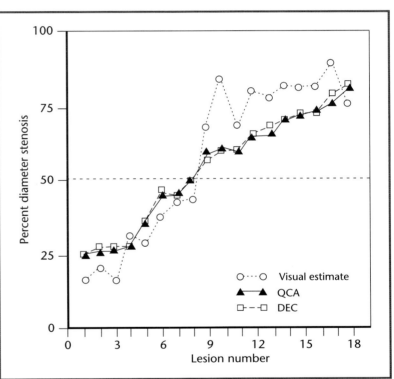

FIGURE 6-4. Visual interpretation of coronary angiography: issues of accuracy and precision. Compared with quantitative coronary angiography (QCA), visual estimates also appear to overestimate the severity of tight lesions and to underestimate the severity of mild stenoses. Shown is a study comparing measurements of percent diameter stenosis based on visual reading, digital electronic calipers (DEC), and QCA for 18 coronary lesions [23]. In severe lesions, visual analysis overestimated the percent diameter stenosis by 11% and underestimated the stenosis minimum diameter by 20% as compared with QCA. By contrast, percent diameter stenosis of mild lesions was underestimated by 5%. Separate studies have demonstrated that visual interpretation significantly overestimates initial lesion severity before balloon angioplasty and underestimates the residual stenosis postprocedure when compared with QCA measurements [24]. (*Adapted from* Scoblionko and coworkers [23]; with permission.)

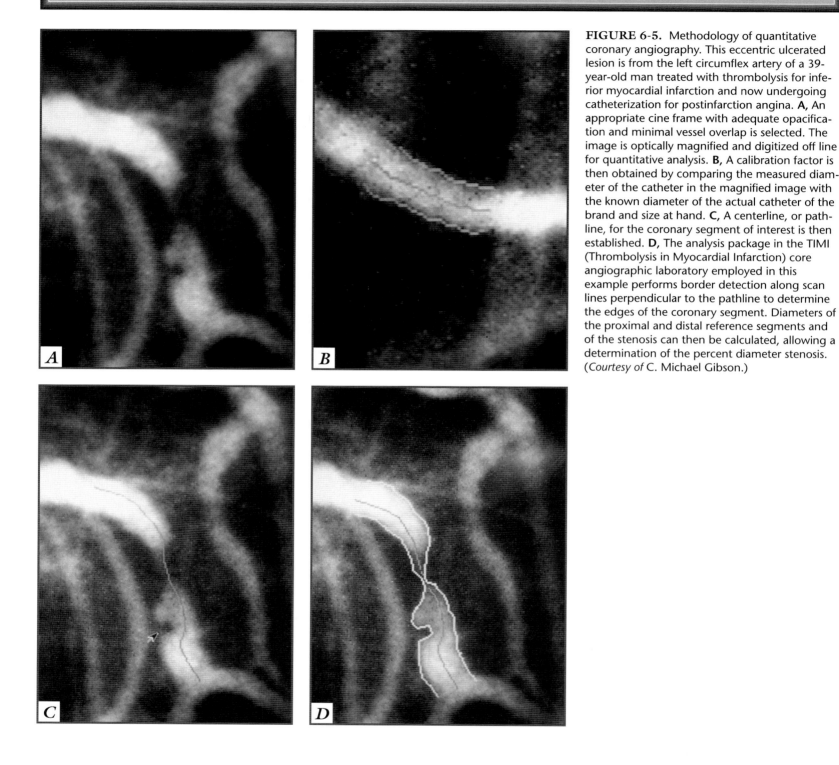

FIGURE 6-5. Methodology of quantitative coronary angiography. This eccentric ulcerated lesion is from the left circumflex artery of a 39-year-old man treated with thrombolysis for inferior myocardial infarction and now undergoing catheterization for postinfarction angina. **A,** An appropriate cine frame with adequate opacification and minimal vessel overlap is selected. The image is optically magnified and digitized off line for quantitative analysis. **B,** A calibration factor is then obtained by comparing the measured diameter of the catheter in the magnified image with the known diameter of the actual catheter of the brand and size at hand. **C,** A centerline, or pathline, for the coronary segment of interest is then established. **D,** The analysis package in the TIMI (Thrombolysis in Myocardial Infarction) core angiographic laboratory employed in this example performs border detection along scan lines perpendicular to the pathline to determine the edges of the coronary segment. Diameters of the proximal and distal reference segments and of the stenosis can then be calculated, allowing a determination of the percent diameter stenosis. (*Courtesy of* C. Michael Gibson.)

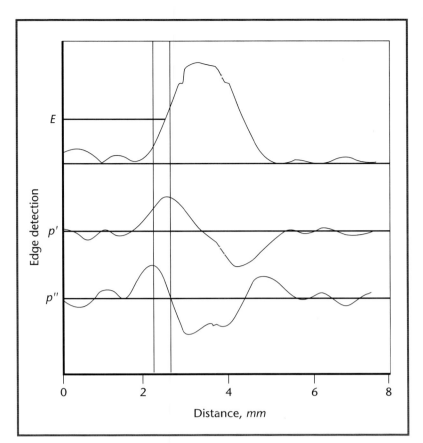

FIGURE 6-6. Edge detection algorithms. In quantitative coronary angiography, each pixel in the digitized cine image is assigned a gray scale value. Edge detection is then generally performed by analyzing the brightness profiles along scan lines perpendicular to the determined centerline of the artery. There is no uniformly accepted algorithm for this analysis; however, most systems use a weighted sum of the first and second derivatives of the brightness profile. Depicted in this example are the overall brightness profile along a scan line (p), the first derivative of the brightness profile (p'), and the second derivative of the brightness profile (p''). In this system the brightness level of the arterial edge point (E) is set at 75% of the difference between the peak of the first and second derivatives (weighted toward the first derivative). The edge points detected in this manner are then compared with neighboring edge points. Those greater than a predetermined distance from the neighboring valid edge point are discarded as spurious, and the edge at that site is linearly interpolated from the adjacent valid edge points. This type of interpolation may lead to errors in the analysis of complex angiographic lesions with overhanging edges. More recently, the gradient field transform technique [25], a technique that assesses brightness changes in all directions (not only perpendicular to the centerline), has been proposed. This allows more than one edge point to be assigned along a given scan line, thus accommodating sharp angles and overhanging edges. (*Courtesy of* Michelle T. Le Fre.)

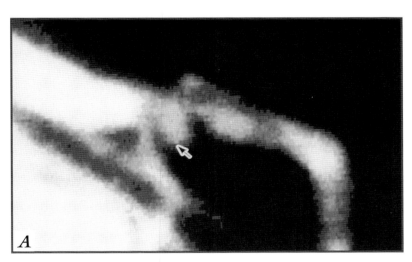

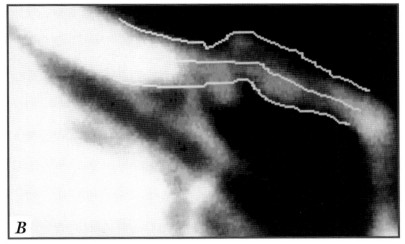

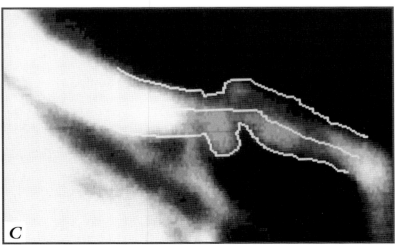

FIGURE 6-7. Limitations of edge detection algorithms. This ulcerated lesion demonstrates the difficulty automatic edge detection systems encounter in tracing sharp angulations. **A,** In the magnified and digitized image under analysis, there is an ulcerated angulated lesion (*arrow*) in the left anterior descending coronary artery just after the origin of the left circumflex coronary artery. **B,** The initial quantitative coronary analysis is unable to trace around the outpouching of the artery, and instead a relatively straight line connecting the edges proximal and distal to the outpouching is defined. **C,** The inferior edge of the artery is then manually edited to conform to the true edge of the artery. The computer algorithm subsequently redefines the edges in an iterative process based on the operator's modifications. (*Courtesy of* C. Michael Gibson.)

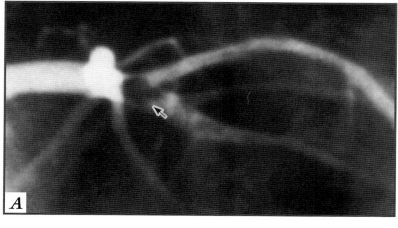

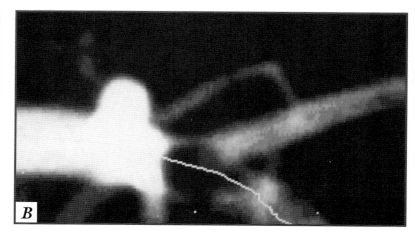

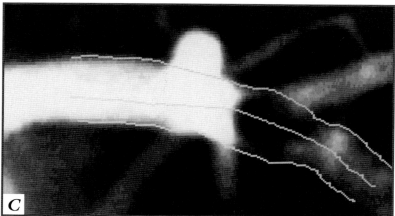

FIGURE 6-8. Assessment of thrombus with quantitative coronary angiography. This 25-year-old man with a mechanical aortic valve for congenital aortic stenosis presented with an acute anterior myocardial infarction after discontinuing warfarin against medical advice. **A,** A large globular filling defect (*arrow*) consistent with thrombus is noted at the origin of the left anterior descending coronary artery. **B,** A centerline is drawn. **C,** Although the edge-detection algorithm accurately outlines the coronary contour, there is no accounting for the intraluminal filling defect. Efforts are underway to quantify the thrombus burden by techniques such as planimetry. (*Courtesy of* C. Michael Gibson.)

CORONARY ANGIOSCOPY

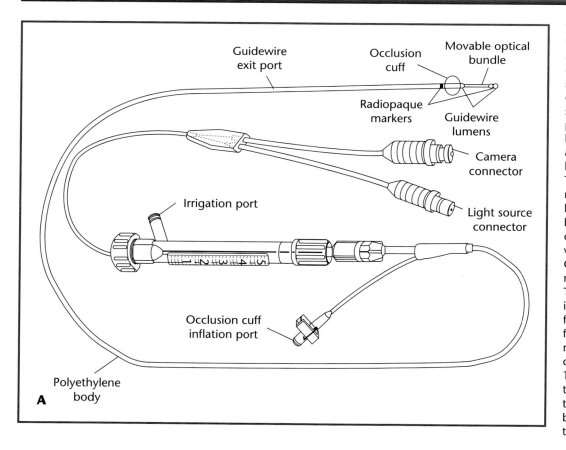

A

FIGURE 6-9. Coronary angioscopy device and technique. Coronary angioscopy was developed to allow direct visual inspection of the luminal surface of the coronary artery *in vivo*. The angioscope consists of a delivery catheter through which a fiberoptic imaging chain is transported to the coronary segment of interest. The transport catheter is equipped with a balloon at its tip to occlude antegrade blood flow into the coronary segment of interest and with a flush port through which the segment can be flushed of collateral blood to optimize imaging. The fiberoptic imaging chain is composed of illumination fibers connected to a high-intensity cold light source and an imaging bundle composed of at least 2000 optical fibers, which is connected to a closed circuit television camera, monitor, and a videotape recorder. **A,** The Baxter (Baxter Healthcare Co, Irvine, CA) angioscope is a 4.5F (1.5-mm) monorail system that accepts a 0.014-in guidewire. The fiberoptic bundle consists of a 3000-pixel fused imaging bundle surrounded by ten 120 μm light fibers, and has an objective lens at the tip with a 55° field of view and a depth of field of more than 0.5 mm. The lesion is crossed with the guidewire, the catheter is advanced proximal to the lesion, 0.5 to 1.0 mL/s of warm Ringer's lactate is infused through the flush port, the occlusion balloon is inflated, and the imaging bundle is then advanced up to 5 cm beyond the tip of the delivery catheter to visualize the segment of interest.

(Continued on next page)

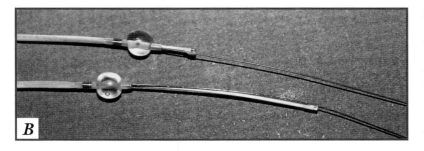

B

FIGURE 6-9. (*Continued*) **B,** The Baxter angioscope with the occlusion balloon inflated and the imaging bundle in the retracted (*top*) or extended (*bottom*) positions. Potential technical limitations of the procedure include inadequate space for the occlusive cuff for imaging extremely proximal segments, insufficient flexibility of the imaging chain to negotiate severe angulations, a restricted field of view owing to lack of steerability of the tip, limited viewing time owing to ischemia induced by balloon inflation, and insufficient flushing to clear collateral blood flow from the segment of interest. (Part A *adapted from* Ramee and coworkers [26]; part B *from* Teirstein and coworkers [27]; with permission.)

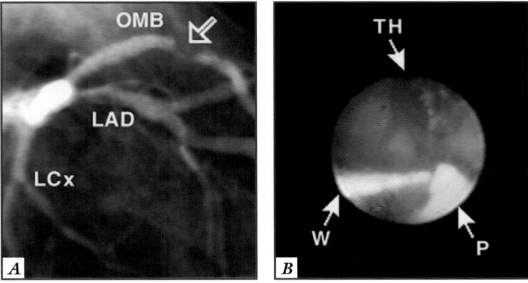

A | **B**

FIGURE 6-10. Detection of thrombus with angioscopy. This image demonstrates the disparity between angiographic and angioscopic findings in a patient with severe unstable angina. **A,** Angiogram showing a high-grade eccentric lesion (*arrow*) in the obtuse marginal branch (OMB). There is no intraluminal filling defect surrounded on three sides by contrast medium to fulfill the rigorous angiographic definition of thrombus. **B,** Angioscopy reveals a complex lesion composed of thrombus (TH) and yellow plaque (P). The guidewire (W) is also seen in the lumen. Multiple studies have demonstrated the increased sensitivity of coronary angioscopy when compared with angiography for the detection of intracoronary thrombus [1,2,27,28]. Thrombus is defined angioscopically as a protruding, intraluminal, or superficial mass that adheres to the vessel surface but that clearly is a separate structure persisting when flushed with saline. In one study of patients undergoing catheterization within 8 hours of presentation with acute infarction, both angioscopy and angiography detected thrombus in nearly all cases [2]. Thrombus was also detected by angioscopy in 14 of 15 patients with unstable angina who were studied within 48 hours of presentation. None of these 15 patients had "occlusive thrombi" by angiography, although the prevalence of filling defects was not reported. Angioscopy has also demonstrated a significantly higher prevalence of thrombus in unstable versus stable angina [28] and in patients with postinfarction angina versus those with an uncomplicated postinfarction course [29]. Using angioscopy as the reference standard, angiography has been reported to detect thrombus with a sensitivity of 21%, a specificity of 94%, and a positive predictive value of 94% [27]. The true prevalence of thrombus may be underestimated even with angioscopy because the technique is often performed upstream of the culprit lesion, missing poststenotic thrombus [30]. LAD—left anterior descending coronary artery; LCx—left circumflex artery. (*From* Ramee and White [26]; with permission.)

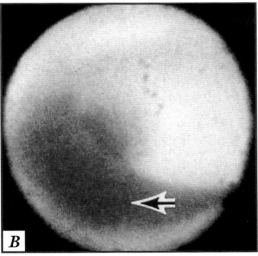

A | **B**

FIGURE 6-11. Thrombus in unstable coronary syndromes. **A,** Angiogram (left anterior oblique projection) of a 70-year-old man with angina at rest showing a severe stenosis in the proximal left anterior descending coronary artery (*arrow*). No filling defect was observed in any projection by angiography. **B,** Angioscopic image of the same stenosis reveals a crescent-shaped, partially occlusive, fresh thrombus (*arrow*). Nonocclusive red thrombi, if present, are usually identified on angioscopy. A direct relationship exists between the time elapsed since the last episode of chest pain and the likelihood of detecting a thrombus on angiography. Such thrombi have been associated with an unfavorable in-hospital clinical outcome. (*From* Sherman and coworkers [1]; with permission.)

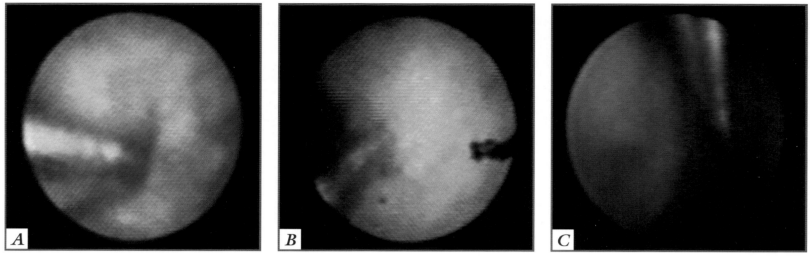

FIGURE 6-12. Thrombus color and relationship to acute coronary syndromes. Thrombus found at angioscopy can also be categorized by color as red, white, or mixed red and white. The category of white thrombus remains somewhat controversial owing to the difficulty in differentiating such a finding from flaps or intimal disruption [30]. Images from three patients with unstable angina or non–Q-wave myocardial infarction (MI) are depicted. **A,** Disrupted yellow plaque without thrombus. **B,** Predominantly white plaque with a disrupted surface and attached white thrombus. **C,** A spherical red and white thrombus protruding into the lumen. Studies to date have generally reported a higher prevalence of grayish-white thrombus in the setting of crescendo angina and more red thrombus with angina at rest or MI [2]. These findings are consistent with pathologic studies showing that whereas white thrombus is platelet-rich, red thrombus contains an abundance of fibrin mixed with erythrocytes and platelets [2]. Comparison of the histologic composition of white and red thrombi identified in angioscopic studies, however, has not been performed. Therefore, it is possible that differences in thrombus color in these settings may relate to other factors such as disparate ages of the thrombi or the more frequent presence of vessel occlusion in patients studied after having an MI. (*From* Waxman and coworkers [30]; with permission.)

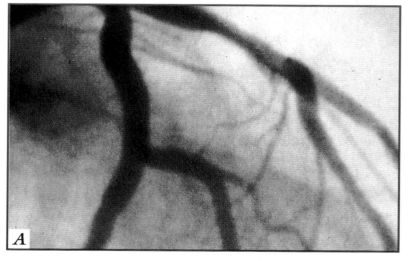

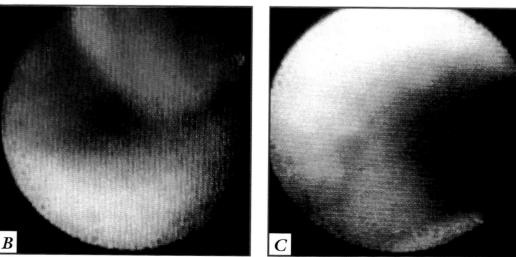

FIGURE 6-13. Angioscopy at the site of coronary spasm. **A,** Coronary artery spasm in the proximal portion of the left anterior descending coronary artery is documented angiographically. **B,** Angioscopy demonstrates that spasm is accompanied by intimal hemorrhage at the 2 o'clock position. **C,** Intracoronary thrombus between the 5 and 8 o'clock positions. (*From* Etsuda and coworkers [31]; with permission.)

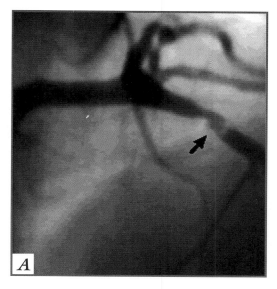

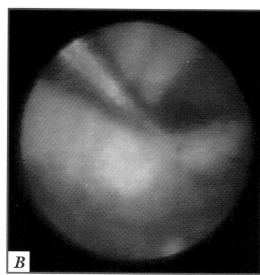

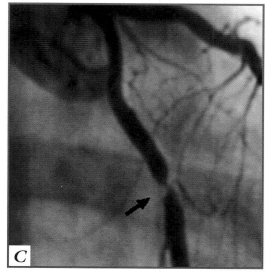

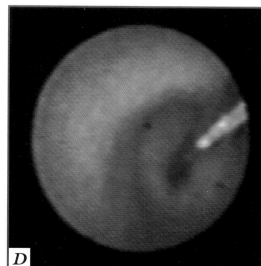

FIGURE 6-14. Relationship of angioscopic appearance of the lesion to plaque composition. **A,** Coronary angiogram of a patient with angina at rest demonstrating an eccentric ulcerated lesion (*arrow*) in the mid left anterior descending coronary artery with an intraluminal filling defect consistent with thrombus. **B,** Corresponding angioscopic image showing a disrupted yellow plaque with red and white thrombus. **C,** Coronary angiogram of another lesion (*arrow*) in the circumflex artery of a patient with angina at rest. **D,** Angioscopically, this lesion is a smooth white plaque without evidence of thrombus. Atherectomy specimens have been obtained and analyzed after angioscopic evaluation of the target lesion to establish a histomorphologic basis for the interpretation of the angioscopic findings. In one study, whereas yellow lesions predominated in patients with unstable angina (89%), a relatively equal distribution of yellow (57%) and gray-white (43%) plaque was noted in those with stable angina [32]. The prevalence of yellow lesions increased from 40% among patients with stable angina with no prior myocardial infarction (MI), to 69% in those with stable angina and an MI more than 3 months before, to 91% in those with an MI within 3 months. Histologic analysis of the atherectomy specimens demonstrated that gray-white lesions correlated with fibrous plaque, mostly without degeneration. By contrast, gray-yellow lesions represented degenerated plaque in most cases and deep yellow or yellow-red lesions were associated with either atheroma or degenerated plaque. In addition, the surface area of the gray-yellow and deep yellow lesions was frequently ruptured. These data suggest that yellow color is an important marker of plaque instability. It has been speculated that yellow color reflects the presence of a lipid pool covered only by a very thin fibrous or endothelial cap, which is vulnerable to rupture. (*From* Nesto and coworkers [33]; with permission.)

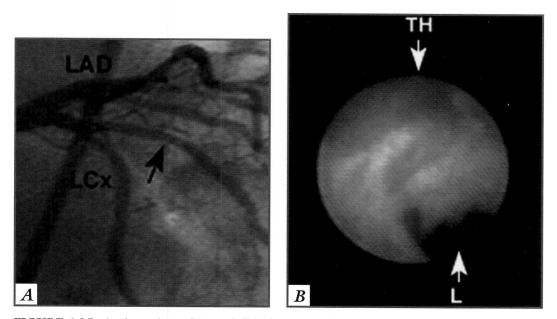

culprit lesion might reveal important morphologic details with superior power over angiography to predict clinical outcome in patients undergoing percutaneous coronary intervention. In one study involving 60 patients, the prognostic information from angiography, intravascular ultrasound (IVUS) imaging, and angioscopy was compared. Multivariable predictors of recurrent ischemia at 1 year postintervention were plaque rupture on the preprocedure angioscopy and angioscopic visualization of thrombus after angioplasty [34]. Other variables from either quantitative coronary angiography or IVUS imaging did not predict outcome. Other investigators have reported that angioscopic evidence of yellow color, plaque disruption, and thrombus at the target site before percutaneous coronary intervention conveys an eightfold increase in the risk of ischemic complications within the first 24 hours postprocedure [30]. Angioscopic evidence of a protruding thrombus pre- or postangioplasty has also been found to predict restenosis, whereas angioscopic evidence of dissection postprocedure has not [35]. LAD—left anterior descending coronary artery; LCx—left circumflex artery. (*From* Ramee and coworkers [26]; with permission.)

FIGURE 6-15. Angioscopic predictors of clinical outcome after percutaneous coronary intervention. **A,** Angiogram of a patient with recurrent unstable angina after percutaneous coronary angioplasty of the obtuse marginal branch (*arrow*) showing a widely patent vessel without evidence of intraluminal pathology. **B,** Angioscopy of the same lesion, however, shows yellow and white plaque, thrombus (TH), and the lumen (L). Angioscopists have speculated that direct endoluminal inspection of the

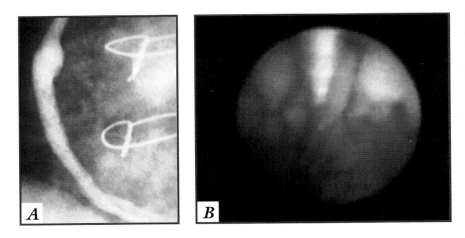

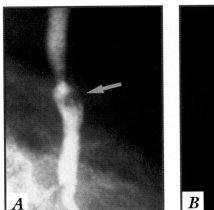

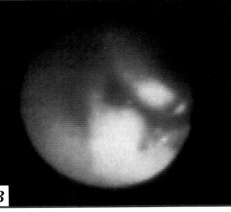

FIGURE 6-16. Angioscopy after stent placement. **A,** Angiography after stent deployment demonstrating a smooth lumen without evidence of thrombus. **B,** Angioscopy clearly demonstrating red material (mural thrombus) overlying stent struts and adherent to the luminal wall at the 12 o'clock to 4 o'clock position. The guidewire is seen at the 12 o'clock position. (*From* Teirstein and coworkers [27]; with permission.)

FIGURE 6-17. Angioscopy of an intraluminal filling defect. Not all intraluminal filling defects seen on angiography represent thrombi. **A,** Angiography of a saphenous vein graft demonstrating a globular intraluminal filling defect (*arrow*) consistent with thrombus. Angioscopy does not reveal thrombus at the site of the filling defect; however, evidence exists of a ruptured venous valve at that site (**B**). (*Courtesy of* Paul S. Teirstein.)

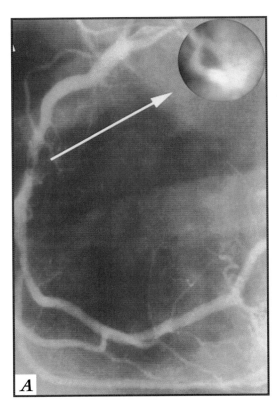

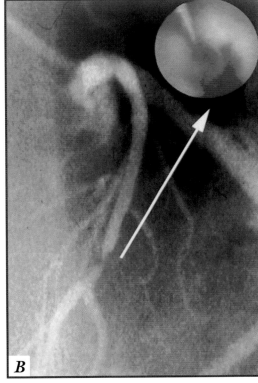

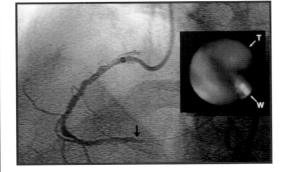

FIGURE 6-19. Angioscopy of abrupt vessel closure. This left anterior oblique angiogram shows abrupt closure of the distal right coronary artery (*arrow*). There is TIMI (Thrombolysis in Myocardial Infarction Study Group) 0 flow past the site, even with the angioplasty guidewire across the lesion. Angioscopy at the site of occlusion (*inset*) shows intraluminal thrombus (T) at the 12 o'clock to 2 o'clock position with the guidewire (W) at the 4 o'clock position. In one study [36], angioscopy performed in 17 cases of abrupt vessel closure demonstrated that dissection was responsible in 14 patients (82%), and intracoronary thrombus was the primary mechanism in three patients (18%). Using angioscopy as the reference standard, angiography correctly identified the specific cause of closure in only five of 17 patients ($P < 0.001$), four of 14 patients (29%) with deep dissections, and one of three patients (33%) with occlusive thrombi. (*From* White and coworkers [36]; with permission.)

FIGURE 6-18. Angiographic versus angioscopic evaluation of lesions. **A,** Left anterior oblique angiogram demonstrating a filling defect in the mid right coronary artery, consistent with thrombus. Angioscopy at this site (*arrow and inset*) shows the guidewire at the 11 o'clock position and white tissue at the lesion, representing ruptured plaque. No thrombus is apparent. **B,** Left anterior oblique-cranial angiogram demonstrating a focal concentric stenosis in the mid left anterior descending artery. Angioscopy of the lesion (*arrow and inset*) shows a red thrombus at the 4 o'clock to 6 o'clock position, which was not suspected based on the angiogram. (*Courtesy of* Christopher A. White.)

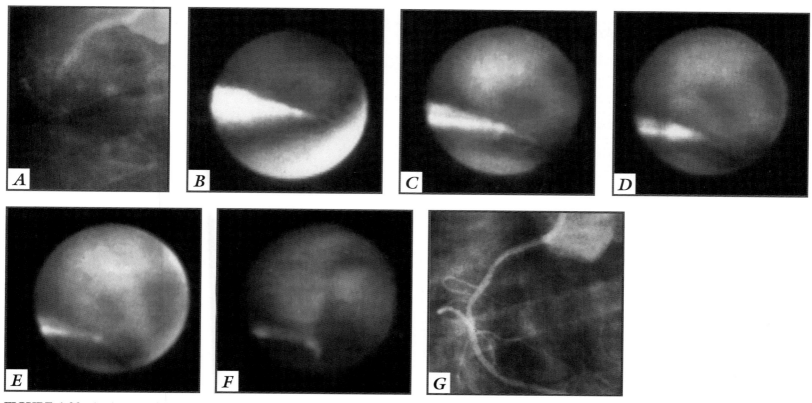

FIGURE 6-20. Angioscopy during intracoronary thrombolysis. **A,** Occluded right coronary artery. **B** to **E,** Angioscopy after initial reperfusion is achieved with ballon angioplasty shows evidence of mural red thrombus at the 12 o'clock to 3 o'clock position in addition to the guidewire seen at the 7 o'clock to 9 o'clock position. Each image demonstrates the thrombus at the same point in time but imaged at different angles and with different gains. **F,** Twenty minutes after administration of intracoronary urokinase, 250,000 U, thrombus is no longer detectable by angioscopy. **G,** A subsequent angiogram demonstrating a widely patent vessel. (*Courtesy of* Paul S. Teirstein.)

INTRAVASCULAR ULTRASOUND IMAGING

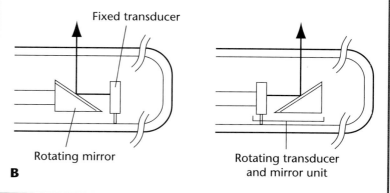

FIGURE 6-21. Three types of intravascular ultrasound (IVUS) catheters. IVUS catheters used for imaging coronary arteries now range from 2.9F to 3.5F (diameters of approximately 1 mm) and have ultrasound frequencies of 20 to 30 MHz. The two types of transducer design are the mechanically rotated devices and multiple array. Both designs result in an ultrasound beam that sweeps around the catheter to provide a 360° tomographic image perpendicular to the catheter tip. **A,** Rotating transducer design in which the ultrasound crystal rotates within an outer sheath. The sheath is inserted over a guidewire into the most distal area to be examined, and the guidewire is withdrawn into a more proximal chamber in the sheath. The transducer can be advanced or withdrawn within the stationary sheath to image the artery without any guidewire artefact. **B,** Rotating mirror designs in which a mirror rotates to reflect an ultrasound beam from a transducer. This design increases the distance the ultrasound must travel between the transducer and the arterial wall, and theoretically helps to reduce some of the ultrasound artefact that occurs within the first few tenths of a millimeter from the transducer (called the *ringdown artefact*). However, the addition of a mirror increases the length of the rigid tip and can reduce catheter handling characteristics.

(*Continued on next page*)

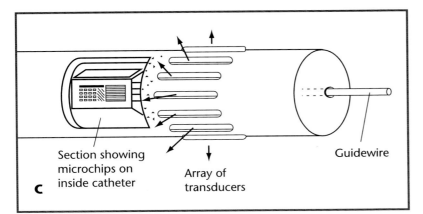

FIGURE 6-21. (*Continued*) C, Multiple array design in which multiple transducer elements surround the outside of the catheter tip. The catheter has built-in microcomputer chips to sequentially activate the transducers and amplify the signals. The computer software integrates the signals from each transducer element to construct an image of the artery. The new multiple array catheters have a more flexible design, do not require retraction of the guidewire, and have an image frame rate that is the same as that of mechanical transducer designs (30 frames/s). The difference in image quality between the catheters is generally small, and all types of designs are used successfully in clinical practice and research.

NORMAL MORPHOLOGY OF THE CORONARY ARTERY SHOWN ON INTRAVASCULAR ULTRASOUND IMAGING

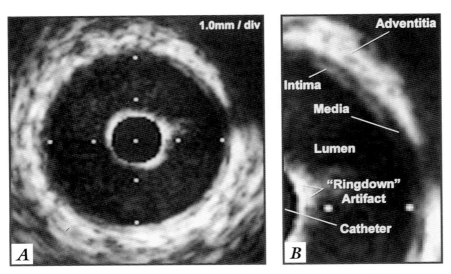

FIGURE 6-22. Normal artery showing trilaminar appearance (**A**) and with an arc from the 12 o'clock to 4 o'clock positions enlarged and labeled in **B**. The intravascular ultrasound (IVUS) image is constructed from the reflection of ultrasound from different layers and structures that have differences in acoustic impedance. The normal coronary artery can exhibit a three-layer or monolayer ultrasound appearance. The ultrasound catheter is represented by a black void in the center of the picture. This figure shows a normal trilaminar appearance of the arterial wall with a leading intimal edge, hypoechogenic media, and echoreflective adventitia in the predominantly muscular coronary arteries. The lumen of the artery is hypoechogenic, and in real time, often has a moving speckled appearance from flowing blood that is accentuated with microbubbles generated with injections of angiographic contrast or other agents. An intimal leading edge is visualized when the mismatch in acoustic impedence between the lumen and intima is large enough to become a good reflector of ultrasound. In this case, the artery will have a trilaminar appearance. However, the thickness of the normal intima measured from ultrasound reflects the axial resolution of the ultrasound system as well as the true histologic thickness of this structure. A 30-MHz transducer has an axial resolution of approximately 100 μm, and will identify all echoreflective structures less than 100 μm thick as a line 100 μm thick. Thus normal intima that appears to be 100 μm thick on ultrasound may be thinner than this on histologic examination. Studies have shown that the trilaminar appearance is more common in arteries that have a thicker intima on histology [37], and this may reflect changes in the acoustic properties of thicker intima. Intra-arterial contrast agents have also been used to help identify the lumen-wall interface [38]. However, as ultrasound technology improves, the role of these agents may be restricted to imaging complex structures, such as identification of the extent of dissection in the arterial wall. The ringdown artefact in this image appears as a flare around the catheter void. (*Adapted from* Nissen and coworkers [39]; with permission.)

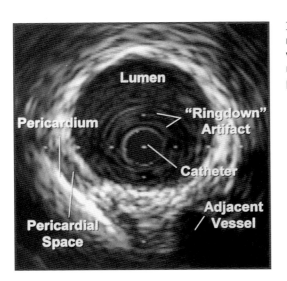

FIGURE 6-23. Normal artery showing monolayer appearance. A normal coronary artery can also have a monolayer appearance on intravascular ultrasound imaging, especially in younger individuals. The arterial wall has a monolayer appearance where the intima is not visualized. The ringdown artefact from this rotating transducer catheter appears in this image as rings close to the edge of the catheter void. The pericardial space increases in systole and virtually disappears in diastole. Scale is 1.0 mm/division.

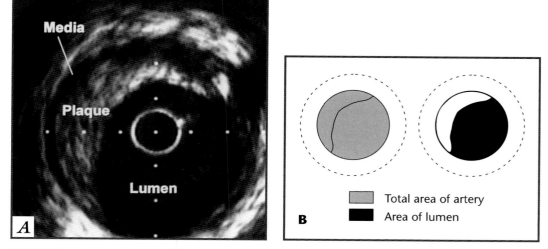

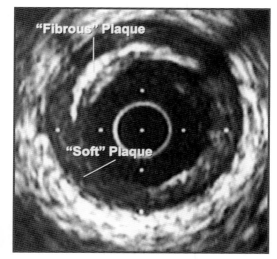
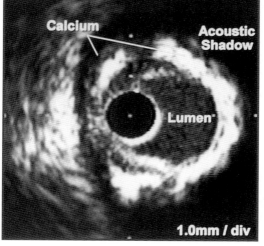
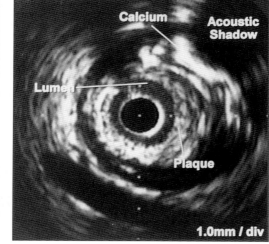

FIGURE 6-24. Eccentric "soft" sonolucent plaque. **A,** Intravascular ultrasound (IVUS) image in which the hypoechogenic media forms a dark border that divides the adventitia from the eccentric plaque and intima. The plaque and intima are not differentiated by IVUS imaging, and the outer edge of the adventitia is not clearly identified because this is associated with perivascular tissue that has similar echoreflective properties. **B,** The most common measurements of atherosclerotic arteries include the total area, lumen area, and plaque or intimal area, which is the difference between the total and lumen areas. The total area is bounded by the media-adventitia interface and corresponds to the external elastic lamina that is closely related to the total artery area on histologic specimens. The plaque or intimal area represents intima and structures within atherosclerotic plaques. *In vitro* studies demonstrate that these areas are highly correlated with similar areas obtained at histologic examination [40–43]. IVUS imaging may yield slightly larger total artery and lumen areas [42,44]. However, this may be a result of tissue shrinkage during histologic preparation of artery specimens. When phantom vessels are studied, there is high agreement of IVUS-derived areas with the known areas, although eccentric placement of the catheter and nonuniform rotational distortions may affect the accuracy of IVUS measurements. Scale is 1.0 mm/division. (*Courtesy of* Steven E. Nissen.)

FIGURE 6-25. Concentric mixed fibrous and soft plaque. Soft plaques have a grayer appearance than do fibrous plaques, which appear whiter and more speckled. Although there is controversy over their exact interpretation, the variations in appearance reflect some difference in plaque composition. Histologic studies suggest that whereas the more echogenic fibrous plaques have a higher proportion of fibrous tissue, the soft plaques have a higher content of the more hypoechogenic lipids [40,43]. In more homogenous plaques, the plaque appearance can be altered by changing the ultrasound gain settings. Scale is 1.0 mm/division. (*From* Topol and Nissen [45]; with permission.)

FIGURE 6-26. Superficial calcium. Calcium within a plaque is very echogenic, appears white, and is distinguished from fibrous plaque because calcium reflects virtually all the ultrasound, resulting in a dark acoustic shadow that prevents imaging more distant structures. Compared with angiography, intravascular ultrasound (IVUS) imaging is a very sensitive method of identifying calcium within the arterial wall. In one study, IVUS imaging identified calcium in 73% of atherosclerotic lesions analyzed compared with 38% of the same lesions analyzed by angiography [46]. A rim of superficial calcium surrounds most of the artery lumen, leaving a narrow acoustic window between the 8 o'clock and 11 o'clock positions. (*Courtesy of* Steven E. Nissen.)

FIGURE 6-27. Deep calcium. Mixed soft and fibrous plaques are visualized, with a deep layer of calcium between the 1 o'clock and 2 o'clock positions. (*Courtesy of* Steven E. Nissen.)

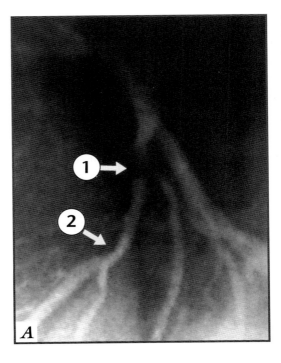

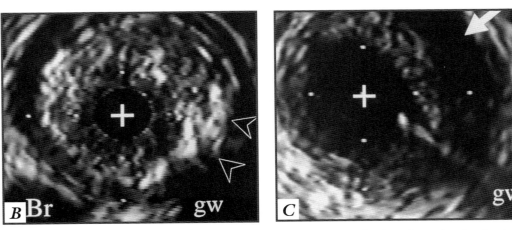

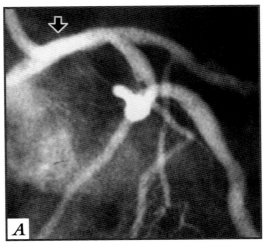

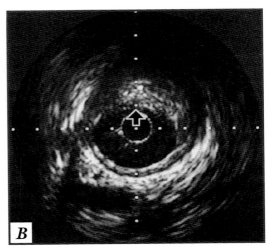

FIGURE 6-28. Lipid pool. Lipid is hypoechogenic, and occasionally lipid pools can be visualized with intravascular ultrasound (IVUS) imaging. **A,** A coronary angiogram demonstrating a 95% stenosis in the left anterior descending artery (*1*) and a 50% stenosis in the middle portion of the vessel (*2*). **B,** IVUS imaging of the proximal lesion showing a concentric fibrous plaque with calcium deposits (*arrowheads*) at the 4 o'clock to 5 o'clock positions. *Dagger* denotes the catheter void. **C,** The more distal lesion shows concentric soft plaque with a large echolucent area that is indistinguishable from the media and represents a necrotic lipid pool (*arrow*). Br—diagonal branch; gw—guidewire artefact. Scale is 1.0 mm/division. (*From* Kimura and coworkers [47]; with permission.)

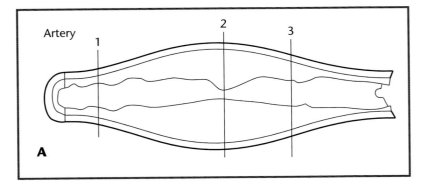

FIGURE 6-29 Left main disease. The diffuse nature of atherosclerosis often is not detected by angiography. Angiography visualizes the arterial lumen and relies on comparisons to reference segments that may also be diseased. In contrast, intravascular ultrasound (IVUS) imaging visualizes the arterial wall and the lumen and is a more sensitive method of identifying atherosclerosis. In this example, coronary angiography (**A**) shows a normal-appearing left main coronary artery (*arrow*). However, IVUS imaging (**B**) reveals substantial disease, with an eccentric plaque from the 9 o'clock to 3 o'clock positions that reduces the lumen by 50% (*arrow*). (*From* Topol and Nissen [45]; with permission.)

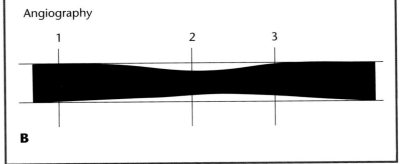

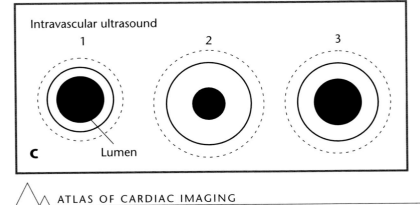

FIGURE 6-30. Compensatory enlargement. Compensatory enlargement was first described by Glagov *et al.* [7]. It refers to the gradual enlargement of the total arterial diameter at sites of atherosclerosis to accommodate the growing plaque, thereby reducing the narrowing of the lumen. The enlarging artery is shown at a focal stenosis within a coronary artery that has atheroma. **A** has mild intimal thickening that appears normal on angiography (**B**), but is identified by intravascular ultrasound (IVUS) **C.** *Section 3* has moderate intimal thickening that is detectable by IVUS, but a normal angiographic appearance is maintained due to compensatory enlargement at this site. *Section 2* has severe atheroma that encroaches on the lumen sufficiently to be detectable by angiography. Compensatory enlargement is overwhelmed when the plaque approaches approximately 30% of the arterial area, and from this point, further plaque growth decreases the arterial lumen [48].

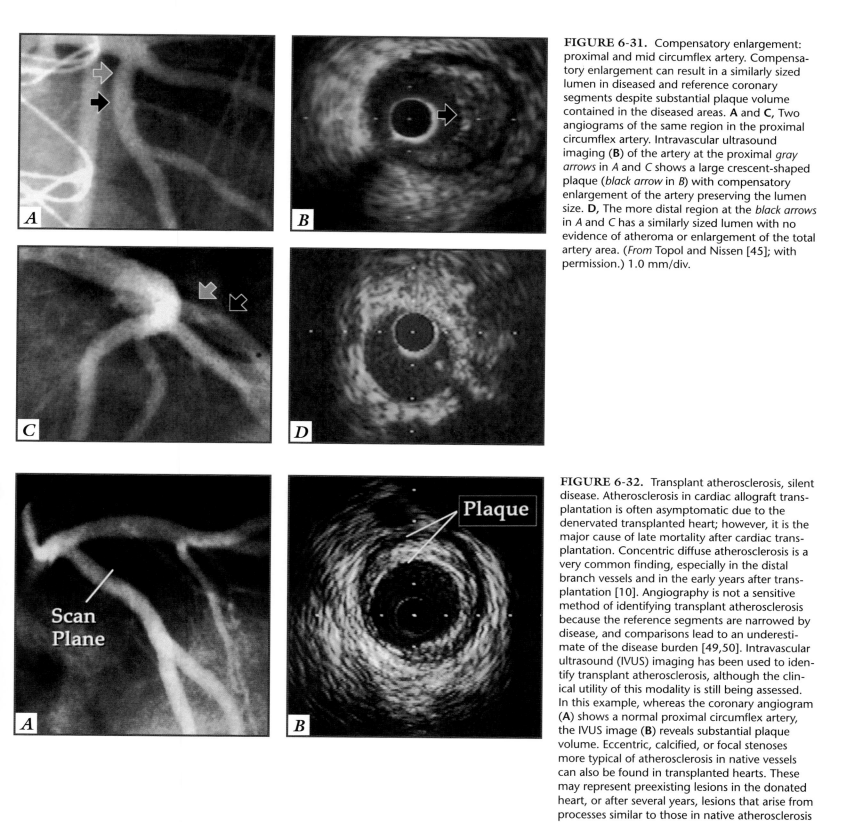

FIGURE 6-31. Compensatory enlargement: proximal and mid circumflex artery. Compensatory enlargement can result in a similarly sized lumen in diseased and reference coronary segments despite substantial plaque volume contained in the diseased areas. **A** and **C,** Two angiograms of the same region in the proximal circumflex artery. Intravascular ultrasound imaging (**B**) of the artery at the proximal *gray arrows* in *A* and *C* shows a large crescent-shaped plaque (*black arrow* in *B*) with compensatory enlargement of the artery preserving the lumen size. **D,** The more distal region at the *black arrows* in *A* and *C* has a similarly sized lumen with no evidence of atheroma or enlargement of the total artery area. (*From* Topol and Nissen [45]; with permission.) 1.0 mm/div.

FIGURE 6-32. Transplant atherosclerosis, silent disease. Atherosclerosis in cardiac allograft transplantation is often asymptomatic due to the denervated transplanted heart; however, it is the major cause of late mortality after cardiac transplantation. Concentric diffuse atherosclerosis is a very common finding, especially in the distal branch vessels and in the early years after transplantation [10]. Angiography is not a sensitive method of identifying transplant atherosclerosis because the reference segments are narrowed by disease, and comparisons lead to an underestimate of the disease burden [49,50]. Intravascular ultrasound (IVUS) imaging has been used to identify transplant atherosclerosis, although the clinical utility of this modality is still being assessed. In this example, whereas the coronary angiogram (**A**) shows a normal proximal circumflex artery, the IVUS image (**B**) reveals substantial plaque volume. Eccentric, calcified, or focal stenoses more typical of atherosclerosis in native vessels can also be found in transplanted hearts. These may represent preexisting lesions in the donated heart, or after several years, lesions that arise from processes similar to those in native atherosclerosis [11]. (*Courtesy of* Alan C. Yeung.)

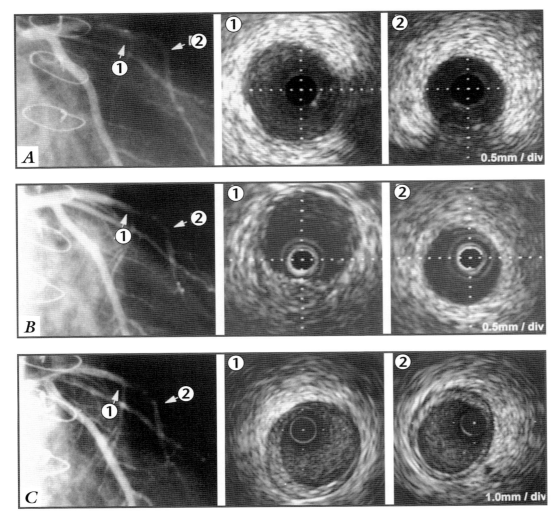

FIGURE 6-33. Transplant atherosclerosis, serial survey. Intravascular ultrasound (IVUS) imaging has helped to characterize the rapid progression of atherosclerosis in the coronary arteries of some transplant recipients. In this example, angiography and IVUS imaging of *sites 1* and *2* of the left anterior descending coronary artery are compared in a patient who had cardiac catheterization 3 weeks after transplantation (**A**), and then at year 1 (**B**) and year 2 (**C**) after transplantation. At each examination, coronary angiography revealed no evidence of atherosclerosis. IVUS imaging showed no intimal thickening at the baseline, but did show substantial growth of atherosclerosis in matched segments from year 1 to year 2 after transplantation.

USE OF INTRAVASCULAR ULTRASOUND IMAGING IN CORONARY ARTERY INTERVENTIONS

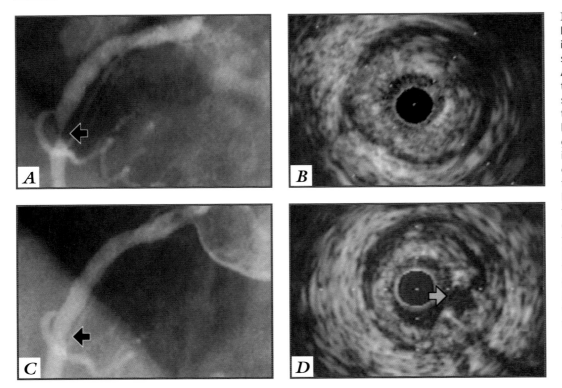

FIGURE 6-34. Balloon angioplasty. Intravascular ultrasound (IVUS) has provided important insights into the mechanisms for the success and failure of coronary interventions. **A,** Angiogram showing a tight stenosis (*arrow*) of the right coronary artery. **B,** IVUS imaging of this site shows a predominantly fibrous lesion, with the IVUS catheter nearly occluding the narrowed lumen. **C,** After balloon angioplasty, the angiogram shows an excellent result (*arrow*). **D,** IVUS imaging, however, reveals a more modest increase in lumen size resulting from a fracture in the plaque (*arrow*). Studies using IVUS imaging have revealed that balloon angioplasty increases the lumen area mainly by stretching the artery wall (increasing total artery area), and by cracking, tearing, or causing slight compression of plaque [12,13]. Most of the smaller dissections and fractures are not apparent on angiography, and the eccentric nature of many of these changes can lead to overestimates of the increase in lumen size with angiography. (*From* Topol and Nissen [45]; with permission.)

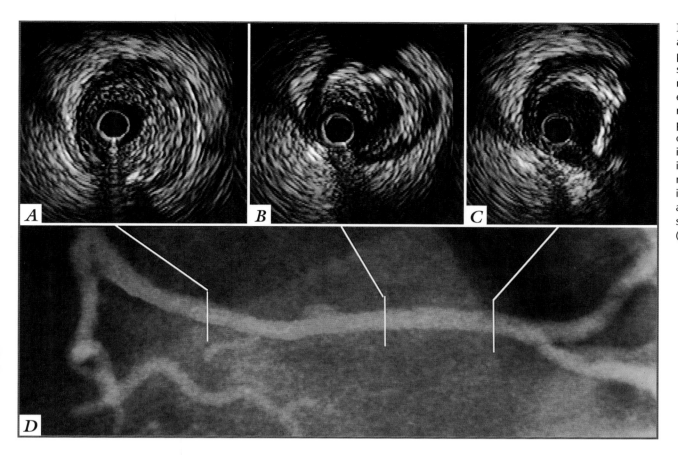

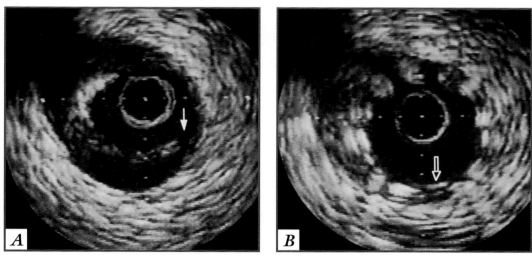

FIGURE 6-35. Balloon angioplasty. Balloon angioplasty of the middle segment of this obtuse marginal branch yields an excellent angiographic result compared with the proximal and distal sections of this artery (**A**). However, intravascular ultrasound imaging reveals diffuse moderately severe disease in this artery (**B** and **C**) and a crack in the plaque at the site of angioplasty (**D**). (*Courtesy of* Alan C. Yeung.)

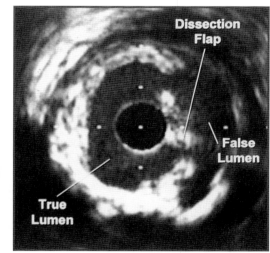

FIGURE 6-36. Dissection flap. Severe dissections are often identified on angiography; however, smaller ones are usually missed. Because it is a more sensitive tool for identifying dissection, intravascular ultrasound (IVUS) imaging has helped in understanding the risks of acute complications associated with disruptions of the artery wall, In this example, a large dissection flap is identified by IVUS imaging. Dissected flaps can be underestimated or missed in smaller arteries when the ultrasound catheter "props" the flap up against the artery wall. Scale is 1.0 mm/division. (*Courtesy of* Steven E. Nissen.).

FIGURE 6-37. Intracoronary stenting of a dissected flap. Intravascular ultrasound imaging has been critical in the improvement of coronary stenting techniques. **A**, A large dissection from the 4 o'clock to 12 o'clock positions. *Arrow* indicates the edge of the true lumen. **B**, An intracoronary stent that is appropriately deployed and tacks the flap against the artery wall. The *arrow* points to an echogenic metal strut of the stent. Scale is 1.0 mm/division. (*Courtesy of* Alan C. Yeung.).

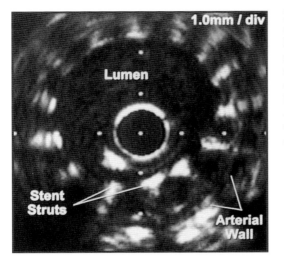

FIGURE 6-38. Poorly deployed stent. Coronary stents were initially deployed at pressures that were commonly used in balloon angioplasty (4 to 8 atm). Although angiography generally showed an excellent lumen with no residual stenosis, intravascular ultrasound (IVUS) imaging revealed that many of the stents deployed in this fashion were not fully expanded [15,16]. In this example, the echogenic stent struts abut the arterial wall in the top half of the artery but are not apposed to the wall from the 4 o'clock to 7 o'clock positions. Poor stent deployment is a principle risk factor for acute stent thrombosis. IVUS imaging studies have shown that high-pressure balloon dilation (typically from 12 to 20 atm) of slotted tube stents is required to expand these devices properly. This practice has revolutionized coronary stenting by reducing thrombotic complications and the need for aggressive anticoagulation. (*Courtesy of* Steven E. Nissen.)

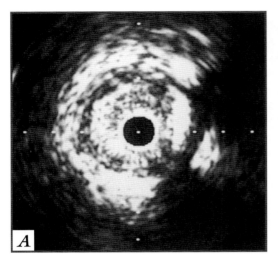
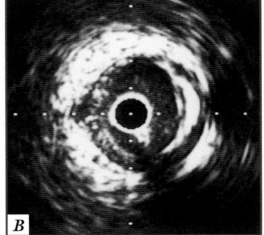

FIGURE 6-39. Directional coronary atherectomy (DCA). DCA is differentiated from balloon angioplasty by its ability to remove atheroma and thereby debulk coronary stenoses. However, it is not particularly effective at removing calcified plaque. Intravascular ultrasound (IVUS) imaging can identify suitable target lesions for DCA, and it can locate branch vessels and other landmarks that help direct the cutting window to the correct side of the vessel, although this is not an easy task. Compared with angiography, IVUS imaging also provides a superior assessment of the success of DCA. **A,** Concentric fibrous plaque surrounds the ultrasound catheter, which is occluding the lumen of the vessel. Calcium is present between the 2 o'clock and 4 o'clock positions. **B,** After DCA, plaque has been removed from much of the segment; however, most of the calcium remains. (*From* Nissen and coworkers [39]; with permission.)

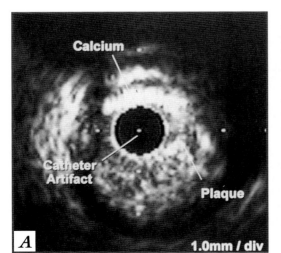
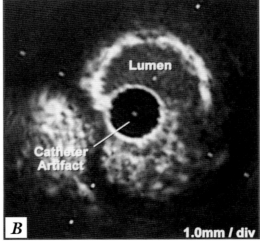

FIGURE 6-40. Rotational atherectomy (ROTA). ROTA uses a diamond-studded burr rotating at high speed to grind off atheroma. Unlike directional coronary atherectomy, this device preferentially removes superficial calcium. For this reason, intravascular ultrasound (IVUS) imaging can help in the choice of atherectomy devices. **A,** Superficial calcium is present between the 11 o'clock and 1 o'clock positions. **B,** IVUS imaging after RCA shows that most of the plaque removed was from the area with calcium. (*Courtesy of* Steven E. Nissen.)

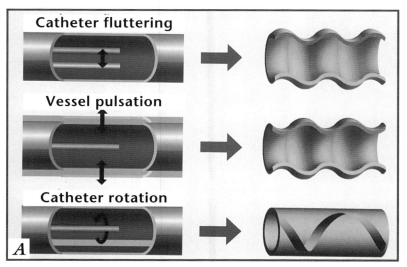

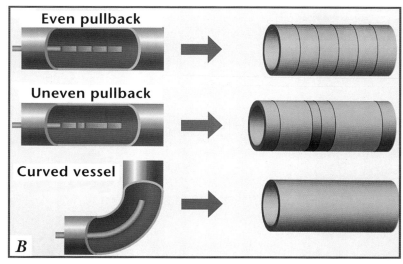

FIGURE 6-41. Errors in two- and three-dimensional reconstruction. Two- and three-dimensional reconstruction is currently being developed to help identify the spatial relationships between structures identified on different cross-sectional images acquired by intravascular ultrasound catheters. Using a constant pullback rate on the ultrasound catheter, sequential ultrasound slices can be compiled using a computer program that assumes a fixed distance between slices in relation to the speed of pullback and the time between slices. However, catheter and artery motion not taken into account during computer reconstruction lead to errors in the subsequent two- and three-dimensional image. **A,** Three-dimensional error by catheter movements and vessel pulsation. Catheter fluttering, artery pulsation, and rotation of the catheter during pullback can cause artefacts in the reconstructed image. The effect of artery pulsation can be reduced by gating image acqui- sition to the R-wave on the electrocardiogram [51]; however, this increases acquisition time. **B,** Three-dimensional error during catheter pullback. An uneven pullback leads to erroneous assumptions on the length of various segments, which can be reduced by using mechanical pullback devices with a constant pullback speed [51]. However, even these devices do not guarantee a constant pullback speed at the transducer in the catheter tip. Because the catheter is used as the reference point by the computer program, curves in vessels appear as straight segments on two-and three-dimensional recon- struction. These drawbacks limit the applicability of reconstruction tech- niques but illustrate the potential for combining cross-sectional ultrasound images to yield greater qualitative and quantitative information on artery morphology. (*Courtesy of* Alan C. Yeung.)

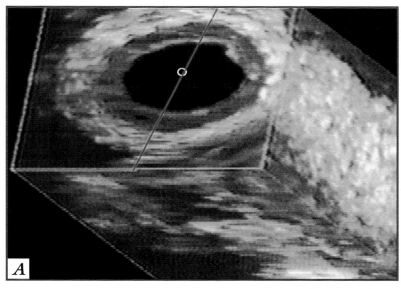

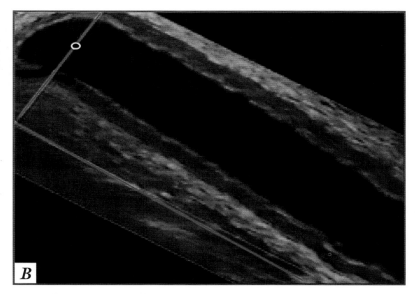

FIGURE 6-42. Longitudinal reconstruction. **A,** Sequential ultrasound slices have been "stacked" on top of each other to create a three-dimen- sional artery. **B,** A computer algorithm is able to slice the artery in a selected longitudinal view. The diffuse atheromatous plaque is evident throughout this reconstructed image. (*Courtesy of* Alan C. Yeung.)

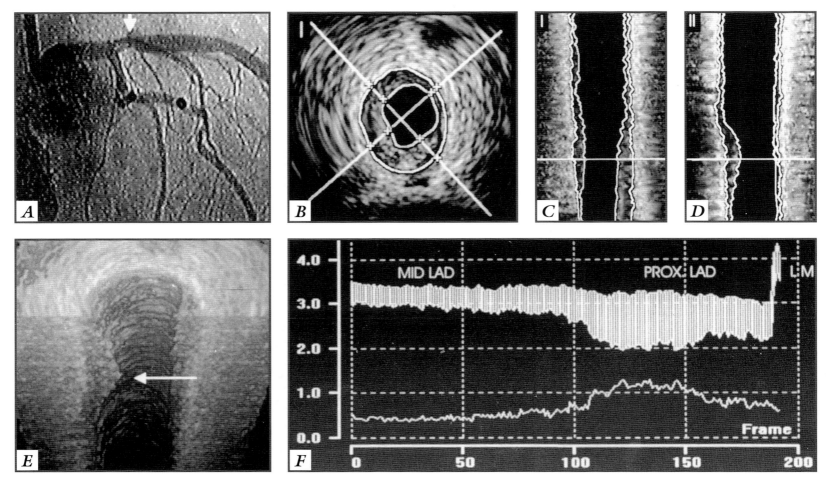

FIGURE 6-43. Computerized assessment of luminal and plaque areas. Recent advances in computer software have resulted in the development of algorithms that can help computers identify the luminal and media-adventitia interfaces and help quantify the plaque volume in three-dimensional reconstructed images [51–53]. **A,** An angiogram with an *arrow* at the proximal segment of the left anterior descending coronary artery (LAD) that is visualized by ultrasound. **B,** A representative two-dimensional intravascular ultrasound image with two perpendicular lines used to generate the longitudinal images in **C** and **D**. The longitudinal images help the automated contour detection program identify the center and range of the boundary-searching process used to identify the lumen interface and media-adventitia interface in the sequential two-dimensional cross-

sectional images. The operator can make corrections to the longitudinal contours before to the final automated contour detection of the cross-sectional images. **E,** A three-dimensional view of half of the vessel with an *arrow* identifying a focal stenosis. **F,** An *upper line* indicating the total area of the artery along the segment analyzed, a *middle line* indicating the lumen area, and the *hatched area* indicating the plaque volume. The *left-hand axis* refers to diameter (in mm), and the *horizontal* axis refers to cross-sectional frame. The *lower line* indicates the plaque area along the artery segment and quantifies the focal stenosis in the proximal LAD. LM—left main artery; MID LAD—mid-left anterior descending coronary artery; PROX LAD—proximal left anterior descending coronary artery. (*Adapted from* von Birgelen and coworkers [52]; with permission.)

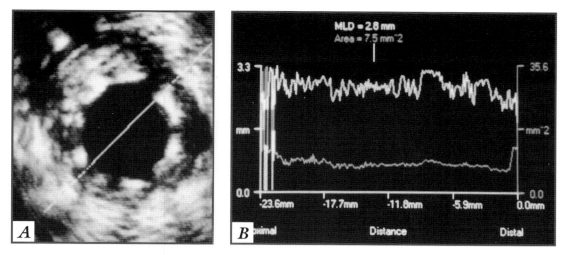

FIGURE 6-44. Use of reconstruction in the assessment of stent deployment. Reconstructed ultrasound images are used to assess an optimally deployed Palmaz-Schatz stent (Johnson & Johnson, Warren, NJ) in an eccentric coronary atherosclerotic plaque. Using computer algorithms similar to those used in the previous example, the cross-sectional ultrasound images (**A**) are used to create a reconstructed longitudinal image of the stent (**C**). **B**, Graph showing the lumen diameter along the stent (*upper line* and *left axis*), which yields a minimal lumen diameter (MLD) of 2.8 mm. The lumen area is represented by the *lower line* and *right axis*. (*From* von Birgelen and coworkers [54]; with permission.)

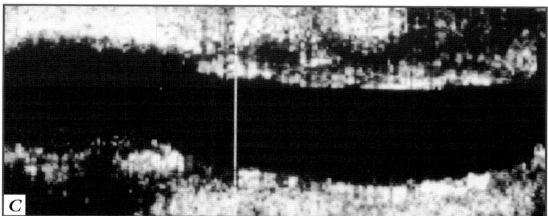

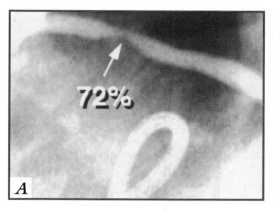

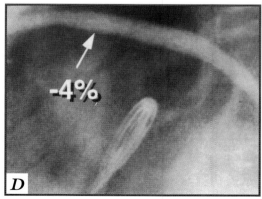

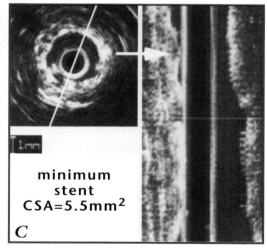

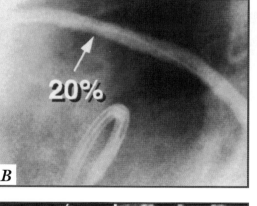

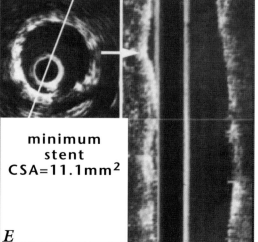

FIGURE 6-45. Use in stent deployment. Longitudinal reconstructed images can help identify regions in which stents are underdeployed. **A,** A focal stenosis is treated with an intracoronary stent (Palmaz-Schatz stent; Johnson & Johnson, Warren, NJ). **B,** Minimal evidence of residual stenosis on angiography. **C,** A cross-sectional intravascular ultrasound image at a narrowed segment of the stent that was identified from a two-dimensional longitudinal reconstructed image. High-pressure postdeployment balloon inflation improves the angiographic result slightly (**D**); however, it leads to marked improvement in the ultrasound images (**E**) CSA—cross-sectional area. (*Courtesy of* Gary S. Mintz.)

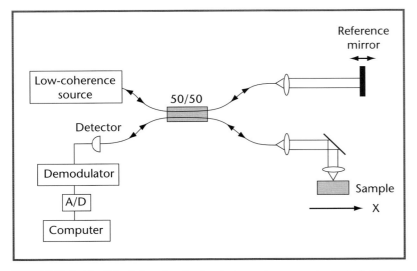

single-mode fiberoptic cable. Light is then split evenly at a 50/50 optical fiber splitter, with one fiber directing light to the sample tissue, and the other fiber directing it to a moving reference mirror whose position is precisely controlled electronically. The reflected light intensity from structures within the tissue is measured by recombining its signal with that returning from the reference mirror (whose distance is accurately known). Interference occurs only when the two paths are matched within the coherence length of the light source, allowing precise measurement of depth on a micron scale. The magnitude of optical interference is a measurement of the intensity of optical backscatter or reflection from the tissue. Tomographic images can thus be obtained with OCT in a manner similar to radar by measuring the intensity of backscattering light from within the tissue plotted as a function of depth and transverse position. Images are displayed either in gray scale or false color in order to differentiate tissue microstructure. OCT was initially used to image transparent tissues of the eye owing to limited penetration of only a few millimeters in tissue that is not transparent. However, imaging penetration depth can be enhanced by using longer wavelength light in the near-infrared range (1300 nm with a 50-nm bandwidth). OCT imaging of *in vitro* human aortic plaques with this methodology has been demonstrated to achieve an axial resolution of 16 ± 1 μm, superior to *in vivo* magnetic resonance imaging (> 100 μm) or *in vivo* high-frequency intravascular ultrasound imaging (> 100 μm) at 20 to 30 MHz. A/D—analog/digital. (*From* Brezinski and coworkers [55]; with permission).

FIGURE 6-46. Principles of optical coherence tomography (OCT). OCT has been proposed as a method of imaging the internal microstructure of atherosclerotic plaques with high resolution. OCT uses infrared light in a technique analogous to the use of acoustical waves in B-mode ultrasound imaging. Light generated from a low-coherence diode is coupled into a

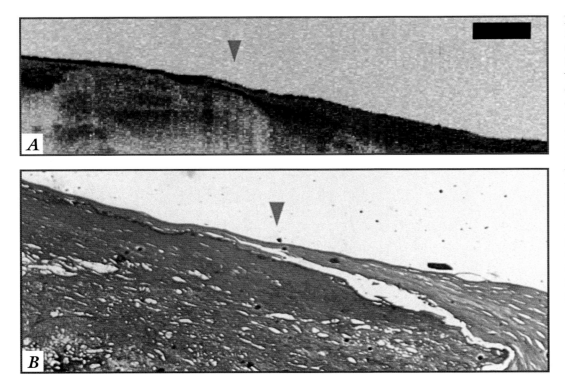

FIGURE 6-47. Calcified atherosclerotic plaque. Shown are an *in vitro* optical coherence tomography (OCT) image and histologic section of human abdominal aortic atherosclerotic plaque from a fresh autopsy specimen. **A,** The OCT image demonstrating a small intimal layer (*arrowhead*), covering a large atherosclerotic plaque (*left*). The plaque is heavily calcified with relatively low lipid content. Although intravascular ultrasound imaging cannot penetrate heavily calcified tissue, infrared light is less strongly reflected from calcified tissues. Thus, OCT imaging is possible even within structures containing calcium. OCT allows high-resolution delineation of microstructural details, such as thickness of the intimal cap, which may be important features of unstable coronary plaques. **B,** The corresponding histology of the plaque stained with hematoxylin and eosin. The *bar* represents 500 μm; *arrowhead* indicates the small intimal layer. (*From* Brezinski and coworkers [55]; with permission.)

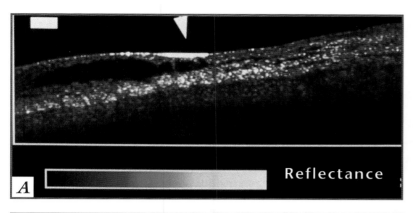

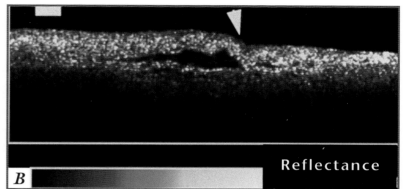

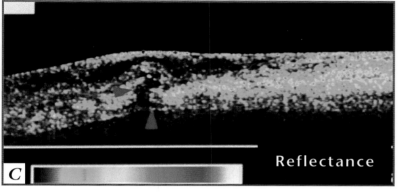

FIGURE 6-48. Atherosclerotic plaque with lipid core. All of these optical coherence tomography (OCT) images were obtained *in vitro* from fresh autopsy specimens of human abdominal aorta. **A,** An *in vitro* OCT image of a thin-walled atherosclerotic plaque. The small plaque has a lipid-filled core (*dark area* within walls) separated from the lumen by a small intimal cap (*arrowhead*). The thin cap and the lipid-rich core may predispose such plaques to rupture. **B,** A thicker-walled (*arrowhead*) atherosclerotic plaque with a smaller lipid core. **C,** A small plaque with a complicated internal structure. The low backscattering areas (*dark areas*) within the wall correspond to lipid that extends in both longitudinal and axial directions. The *arrowheads* identify a small penetration into deeper intima followed by tracking at the intima-media border. Structural changes within plaques are believed to play an important role in atherosclerosis and the progression of myocardial infarction. The color table has been changed in this image to delineate deeper structures more effectively. The *bars* represent 500 µm. (*From* Brezinski and coworkers [55]; with permission.)

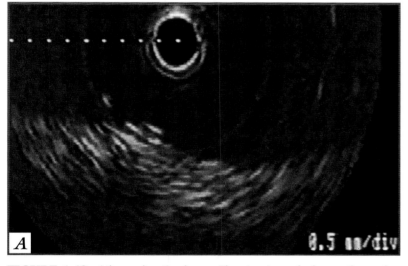

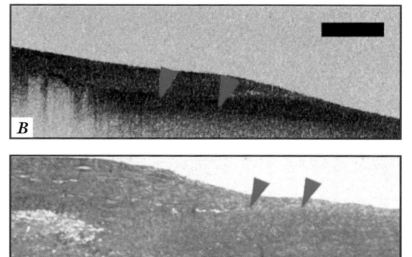

FIGURE 6-49. Atherosclerotic plaque. The structure of a large atherosclerotic plaque in a fresh autopsy specimen of human abdominal aorta is imaged with intravascular ultrasound (IVUS) imaging and optical coherence tomography (OCT). **A,** The IVUS image. **B,** The OCT image demonstrating a large plaque to the left with a well-demarcated layer of smooth muscle cell proliferation (*arrowheads*) running through the intima of the adjacent arterial wall. **C,** Histology of the plaque, with *arrowheads* at the same site as in *B*. (*From* Brezinski and coworkers [56]; with permission.)

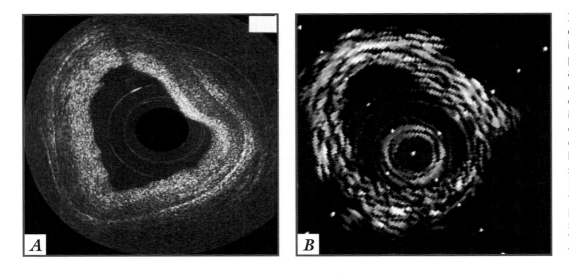

FIGURE 6-50. Coronary imaging with optical coherence tomography (OCT). *In vitro* OCT imaging of human coronary arteries has been performed using a prototype catheter-based approach. **A,** An image of an *in vitro* human coronary artery generated with a recently developed OCT catheter. The prototype OCT catheter is 2.9F and contains no transducer within the catheter frame. The adventitia and media are well differentiated, in addition to moderate intimal hyperplasia. **B,** A 3.2F, 20-MHz intravascular ultrasound transducer (Cardiovascular Instrument Systems, Sunnyvale, CA) was used to image the same arterial segment. The data in *B* were processed and displayed with the Insight III ultrasound system (Cardiovascular Instrument Systems). The *bar* in *A* and the *gratings* in *B* are 1 mm. (From Tearney and coworkers [57]; with permission.)

REFERENCES

1. Sherman CT, Litvack F, Grundfest, *et al.*: Coronary angioscopy in patients with unstable angina pectoris. *N Engl J Med* 1986, 315:913–919.

2. Mizuno K, Satomura K, Miyamoto A, *et al.*: Angioscopic evaluation of coronary-artery thrombi in acute coronary artery syndromes. *N Engl J Med* 1992, 326:287–291.

3. Brown BG, Lin JT, Schefer SM, *et al.*: Niacin or lovastatin, combined with colestipol regress coronary atherosclerosis and prevent clinical events in men with elevated apolipoprotein B. *N Engl J Med* 1990, 323:1289–1298.

4. Kinlay S, Selwyn AP, Delagrange D, *et al.*: Biological mechanisms for the clinical success of lipid-lowering in coronary artery disease and the use of surrogate end-points. *Curr Opin Lipidol* 1996, 7:389–397.

5. Treasure CB, Klein JL, Weintraub WS, *et al.*: Beneficial effects of cholesterol-lowering therapy on the coronary endothelium in patients with coronary artery disease. *N Engl J Med* 1995, 332:481–487.

6. Anderson TJ, Meredith IT, Yeung AC, *et al.*: The effect of cholesterol-lowering and antioxidant therapy on endothelium-dependent coronary vasomotion. *N Engl J Med* 1995, 332:488–493.

7. Glagov S, Weisenberg E, Zarins CK, *et al.*: Compensatory enlargement of human atherosclerotic coronary arteries. *N Engl J Med* 1987, 316:1371–1375.

8. Mintz GS, Popma JJ, Pichard AD, *et al.*: Arterial remodeling after coronary angioplasty: a serial intravascular ultrasound study. *Circulation* 1996, 94:35–43.

9. Lim TT, Liang DH, Botas J, *et al.*: Role of compensatory enlargement and shrinkage in transplant coronary artery disease: serial intravascular ultrasound study. *Circulation* 1997, 95:855–859.

10. Johnson DE, Gao SZ, Schroeder JS, *et al.*: The spectrum of coronary artery pathologic findings in human cardiac allografts. *J Heart Transplant* 1989, 8:349–359.

11. Rickenbacher PR, Pinto FJ, Chenzbraun A, *et al.*: Incidence and severity of transplant coronary artery disease early and up to 15 years after transplantation as detected by intravascular ultrasound. *J Am Coll Cardiol* 1995, 25:171–177.

12. Di Mario C, Gil R, Camenzind E, *et al.*: Quantitative assessment with intracoronary ultrasound of the mechanisms of restenosis after percutaneous transluminal coronary angioplasty and directional coronary atherectomy. *Am J Cardiol* 1995, 75:772–777.

13. Baptista J, Di Mario C, Ozaki Y, *et al.*: Impact of plaque morphology and composition on the mechanisms of lumen enlargement using intracoronary ultrasound and quantitative angiography after balloon angioplasty. *Am J Cardiol* 1996, 77:115–121.

14. Kovach JA, Mintz GS, Pichard AD, *et al.*: Sequential intravascular ultrasound characterization of the mechanisms of rotational atherectomy and adjunct balloon angioplasty. *J Am Coll Cardiol* 1993, 22:1024–1032.

15. Görge G, Haude M, Ge J, *et al.*: Intravascular ultrasound after low and high inflation pressure coronary artery stent implantation. *J Am Coll Cardiol* 1995, 26:725–730.

16. Moussa I, Di Mario C, Di Francesco L, *et al.*: Subacute stent thrombosis and the anticoagulation controversy: changes in drug therapy, operator technique, and the impact of intravascular ultrasound. *Am J Cardiol* 1996, 78:13–17.

17. Schömig A, Neumann FJ, Kastrati A, *et al.*: A randomized comparison of antiplatelet and anticoagulant therapy after the placement of coronary-artery stents. *N Engl J Med* 1996, 334:1084–1089.

18. Nakamura S, Hall P, Gaglione A, *et al.*: High pressure assisted coronary stents implantation accomplished without intravascular ultrasound guidance and subsequent anticoagulation. *J Am Coll Cardiol* 1997, 29:21–27.

19. Powers ER: Coronary angiography. In *Atlas of Heart Diseases: Chronic Ischemic Heart Disease.* Edited by Braunwald EB, Beller GA. Philadelphia: Current Medicine; 1995.

20. Johnson DE, Alderman EL, Schroeder JS, *et al.*: Transplant coronary artery disease: histopathologic correlations with angiographic morphology. *J Am Coll Cardiol* 1991, 17:449–457.

21. Fisher LD, Judkins MP, Lesperance J, *et al.*: Reproducibility of coronary arteriographic reading in the coronary artery surgery study. *Cathet Cardiovasc Diagn* 1982, 8:565–575.

22. Shub C, Vlietstra RE, Smith HC, *et al.*: The unpredictable progression of symptomatic coronary artery disease: a serial clinical-angiographic analysis. *Mayo Clin Proc* 1981, 56:155–160.

23. Scoblionko DP, Brown BG, Mitten S, *et al.*: A new digital electronic caliper for measurement of coronary arterial stenosis: comparison with visual estimates and computer-assisted measurements. *Am J Cardiol* 1984, 53:689–693.

24. Fleming RM, Kirkeeide RL, Smalling RW, Gould KL: Patterns in visual interpretation of coronary arteriograms as detected by quantitative coronary arteriography. *J Am Coll Cardiol* 1991, 18:945–951.

25. van der Zwet PM, Reiber JH: A new approach for the quantification of complex lesion morphology: the gradient field transform; basic principles and validation results. *J Am Coll Cardiol* 1994, 24:216–224.

26. Ramee SR, White CJ: Percutaneous coronary angioscopy. In *Textbook of Interventional Cardiology.* Edited by Topol EJ. Philadelphia: WB Saunders; 1994:1122–1135.

27. Teirstein PS, Schatz RA, DeNardo SJ, *et al.*: Angioscopic versus angiographic detection of thrombus during coronary interventional procedures. *Am J Cardiol* 1995, 75:1083–1087.

28. White CJ, Ramee SR, *et al.*: Coronary thrombi increase PTCA risk. Angioscopy as a clinical tool. *Circulation* 1996, 93:253–258.

29. Tabata H, Mizuno K, Arakawa K, *et al.*: Angioscopic identification of coronary thrombus in patients with postinfarction angina. *J Am Coll Cardiol* 1995, 25:1282–1285.

30. Waxman S, Sassower M, Mittelman MA, *et al.*: Angioscopic predictors of early adverse outcome after coronary angioplasty in patients with unstable angina and non-Q wave myocardial infarction. *Circulation* 1996, 93:2106–2113.

31. Etsuda H, Mizuno K, Arakawa K, *et al*.: Angioscopy in variant angina: coronary artery spasm and intimal injury. *Lancet* 1993, 342:1322–1324.

32. Thieme T, Wernecke KD, Meyer R, *et al*.: Angioscopic evaluation of atherosclerotic plaques: validation by histomorphologic analysis and association with stable and unstable coronary syndromes. *J Am Coll Cardiol* 1996, 28:1–6.

33. Nesto RW, Waxman S, Mittleman MA, *et al*.: Angioscopy of culprit coronary lesions in unstable angina: correlation of clinical presentation with plaque morphology. *Am J Cardiol* 1997, in press.

34. Feld S, Ganim M, Carell ES, *et al*.: Comparison of angioscopy, intravascular ultrasound imaging and quantitative coronary angiography in predicting clinical outcome after coronary intervention in high risk patients. *J Am Coll Cardiol* 1996, 28:97–105.

35. Bauters C, Lablanche JM, McFadden EP, *et al*.: Relation of coronary angioscopic findings at coronary angioplasty to angiographic restenosis. *Circulation* 1995, 92:2473–2479.

36. White CJ, Ramee SR, Collins TJ, *et al* : Coronary angioscopy of abrupt occlusion after angioplasty. *J Am Coll Cardiol* 1995, 25:1681–1684.

37. Fitzgerald PJ, St Goar FG, Connolly AJ, *et al*.: Intravascular ultrasound imaging of coronary arteries is three layers the norm? *Circulation* 1992, 86: 154–158.

38. Hausmann D, Krishnankutty S, Mullen WL, *et al*.: Contrast-enhanced intravascular ultrasound: validation of a new technique for delineation of the vessel wall boundary. *J Am Coll Cardiol* 1994, 23:981–987.

39. Nissen SE, Tuzcu EM, De Franco AC: Coronary intravascular ultrasound: diagnostic and interventional applications. In *Textbook of Interventional Cardiology*, update 14. Edited by Topol EJ. Philadelphia: WB Saunders; 1994:215–219.

40. Di Mario C, The SHK, Madretsma S, *et al*.: Detection and characterization of vascular lesions by intravascular ultrasound: An in vitro study correlated with histology. *J Am Soc Echocardiogr* 1992, 5:135–146.

41. Nishimura RA, Edwards WD, Warnes CA, *et al*.: Intravascular ultrasound imaging: in vitro validation and pathologic correlation. *J Am Coll Cardiol* 1990, 16:145–154.

42. von Birgelen C, van der Lugt A, Nicosia A, *et al*.: Computerized assessment of coronary lumen and atherosclerotic plaque dimensions in three-dimensional intravascular ultrasound correlated with histomorphometry. *Am J Cardiol* 1996, 78:1202–1209.

43. Potkin BN, Bartorelli AL, Gessert JM, *et al*.: Coronary artery imaging with intravascular high-frequency ultrasound. *Circulation* 1990, 81:1575–1585.

44. Anderson MH, Simpson IA, Katritsis D, *et al*.: Intravascular ultrasound imaging of the coronary arteries: an in vitro evaluation of measurement of area of the lumen and atheroma characterization. *Br Heart J* 1992, 68:276–281.

45. Topol EJ, Nissen SE: Our preoccupation with coronary luminology: the dissociation between clinical angiographic findings in ischemic heart disease. *Circulation* 1995, 92:2333–2342.

46. Mintz GS, Popma JJ, Pichard AD, *et al*.: Patterns of calcification in coronary artery disease: a statistical analysis of intravascular ultrasound and coronary angiography in 1155 lesions. *Circulation* 1995, 91:1959–1965.

47. Kimura BJ, Russo RJ, Penny WF: Images in cardiovascular medicine. Plaque types. *Circulation* 1996, 94:3382.

48. Hermiller JB, Tenaglia AN, Kisslo KB, *et al*.: In vivo validation of compensatory enlargement of atherosclerotic coronary arteries. *Am J Cardiol* 1993, 71:665–668.

49. St Goar FG, Pinto FJ, Alderman EL, *et al*.: Intracoronary ultrasound in cardiac transplant recipients. In vivo evidence of "angiographically silent" intimal thickening. *Circulation* 1992, 85:979–987.

50. Pflugfelder PW, Boughner DR, Rudas L, Kostuk WJ: Enhanced detection of cardiac allograft arterial disease with intracoronary ultrasonographic imaging. *Am Heart J* 1993, 125:1583–1591.

51. Di Mario C, von Birgelen C, Prati F, *et al*.: Three dimensional reconstruction of cross sectional intracoronary ultrasound: clinical or research tool? *Br Heart J* 1995, 73(suppl 2):26–32..

52. von Birgelen C, Di Mario C, Serruys PW: Structural and functional characterization of an intermediated stenosis with intracoronary ultrasound and doppler: a case of "reverse Glagovian modeling." *Am Heart J* 1996, 132:694–696.

53. von Birgelen C, Slager CJ, Di Mario C, *et al*.: Volumetric intracoronary ultrasound: a new maximum confidence approach for the quantitative assessment of progression-regression of atherosclerosis? *Atherosclerosis* 1995, 118(suppl):103–113.

54. von Birgelen C, Kutryk MJB, Gil R, *et al*.: Quantification of the minimal luminal cross-sectional area after coronary stenting by two- and three-dimensional intravascular ultrasound versus edge detection and videodensitometry. *Am J Cardiol* 1996, 78:520–525.

55. Brezinski ME, Tearney GJ, Bouma BE, *et al*.: Optical coherence tomography for optical biopsy. Properties and demonstration of vascular pathology. *Circulation* 1996, 93:1206–1213.

56. Brezinski ME, Tearney GJ, Weissman NJ, *et al*.: Assessing atherosclerotic plaque morphology: comparison of optical coherence tomography and high frequency intravascular ultrasound. *Br Heart J* 1997, 77:397–403.

57. Tearney GJ, Brezinski ME, Boppart SA, *et al*.: Catheter-based optical imaging of a human coronary artery. *Circulation* 1996, 94:3013.

CHAPTER 7

Computed Tomography Imaging of the Heart

George G. Hartnell

Computed tomographic (CT) scanning has been widely available for more than 20 years but has had relatively little impact on cardiac diagnosis. This is due mainly to the long acquisition times that most CT scanners require to generate images. Conventional CT scanners acquire images by rotating an x-ray tube and a variable number of x-ray detectors around the patient, a process that may take several seconds. Even with the fastest new spiral CT (SCT) scanners, image acquisition still takes at least half a second, during which time the heart can move considerably. Conventional CT images of the heart, therefore, are affected by motion blurring. Because there is less motion in the aorta and other adjacent structures, conventional CT scanning is more useful for evaluating the aorta and the adjacent great veins. It was only with the development of Ultrafast CT (UFCT; Imatron, South San Francisco, CA) scanning using electron beam technology (EBT) that realistic routine CT investigation of the heart itself became possible [1,2].

Conventional CT scan is widely available, and the general principles are widely known. Briefly, an x-ray tube and multiple detectors are rotated on a gantry around the patient. The tube-detector gantry rotates a predetermined angle between each data acquisition. A pulse of x-rays is produced, and transmitted x-rays are received by the detector array. The output from the detector array is converted into digital data. The gantry rotates a number of times to produce all the information required to generate an image, which usually takes several seconds. The digital data is processed by computer using variations of a back-projection algorithm to produce a single two-dimensional image. Although conventional CT can show some cardiac abnormalities, its main use in this context is the investigation of adjacent abnormalities of the aorta and mediastinum.

Spiral computed tomography scan is a development of conventional CT in which the tube-detector gantry continuously rotates as the patient is moved slowly (typically 5 to 15 mm/s) through the scanner aperture. X-rays are generated and data acquired continuously, allowing faster imaging, and hence, reducing motion blurring for cardiac imaging. Movement of the patient causes data to be acquired along a spiral trajectory, producing a three-dimensional data set. The data set allows reconstruction of three-dimensional images of vessels with sufficiently high contrast, usually after contrast enhancement, a technique called *CT angiography* (CTA). This technique is especially useful for aortic imaging and visualizing other major arteries and is fast enough to show intracardiac abnormalities [3]. Cardiac motion during SCT image acquisition, however, is too great to allow CTA of coronary arteries. Such imaging also requires electrocardiographic (ECG) gating, which is difficult to achieve with SCT. Much faster ECG-gated image acquisition is required for this and for some other cardiac applications [1,2], which is provided by UFCT.

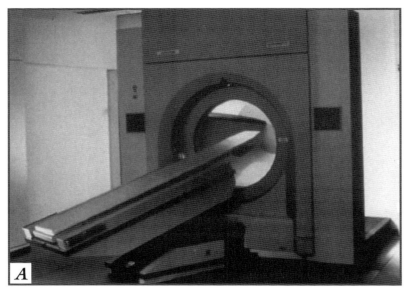

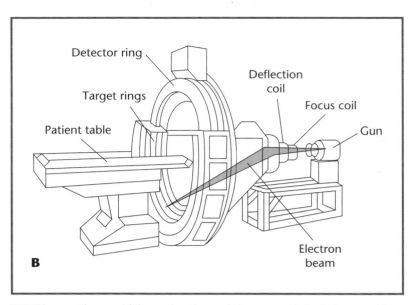

FIGURE 7-1. A, Ultrafast CT (UFCT; Imatron, South San Francisco, CA) scanner. Electron beam UFCT scanner uses an electron gun to produce a stream of electrons that are deflected onto tungsten target rings by a changing magnetic field. Bombardment of the tungsten rings generates x-rays that are detected by a semicircular x-ray detector array. **B,** Diagrammatic representation of the UFCT scanner. There are no moving parts in this system except for the examination couch, which moves the patient through the machine. The advantage of no moving parts is that image acquisition time can be extremely short (as few as 50 ms). Image acquisition can be triggered by the patient's electrocardiogram and can effectively freeze cardiac motion. This makes it possible to image the heart and to see even very small structures, such as the coronary arteries, without significant motion blurring. Therefore, UFCT provides a possible method for examining many aspects of cardiac disease. Newer versions can also perform spiral CT (called *continuous volume scanning*, or CVS). In either mode, UFCT can be used for three-dimensional image acquisition and reconstruction.

UFCT has not been widely used so far, and there are relatively few machines (less than 100) available around the world.

The only commercial UFCT scanner at this time is manufactured by Imatron and is distributed in the United States as the Evolution Scanner by Siemens Medical Systems (Iselin, NJ). This scanner is well suited for cardiac imaging, but has a slightly poorer performance for general-purpose CT imaging when compared with some other CT scanners designed for noncardiac imaging (*ie*, for neurologic imaging). In addition, the machine is rather expensive and has a restricted aperture for patient examination (limited by the cone formed by the electron gun). For this reason, the number of UFCT scanners available for clinical and research work is limited, which has restricted the development of some applications. However, recent commercial alliances and the promotion of this device in the Far East have increased the installed base of machines, which has resulted in an acceleration in the clinical and research development of UFCT for cardiac and related diagnoses. (*Courtesy of* Siemens Medical Systems, Iselin, NJ.)

Anatomy

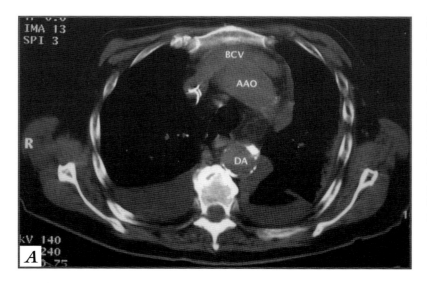
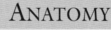

FIGURE 7-2. The great vessels and major cardiac chambers are usually easy to identify on computed tomography (CT), even without contrast opacification. Identification of intracardiac structures requires contrast injection, unless these structures are either of high (calcific) or low (fatty) radiographic attenuation. The relative prominence of areas of different attenuation can be modified electronically and optimized for viewing different attenuation areas. **A,** The descending aorta (DA) usually runs caudally just to the left of the spine. In this patient the DA is calcified, indicated by peripheral high attenuation (*white area*). There is a pacing wire (high-attenuation star-shaped artefact in the brachiocephalic vein [BCV] running anterior to the ascending aorta [AAO]). Very high attenuation objects (usually metal implants) cause perturbations in image reconstruction that can produce this sort of artefact. The high attenuation of undiluted contrast in the superior vena cava can also produce artefacts that may obscure or mimic pathology in the aorta.

(*Continued on next page*)

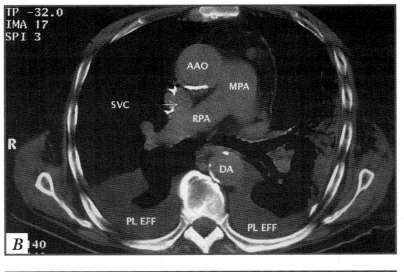

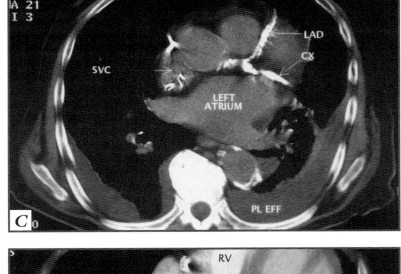

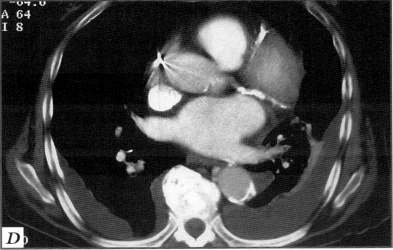

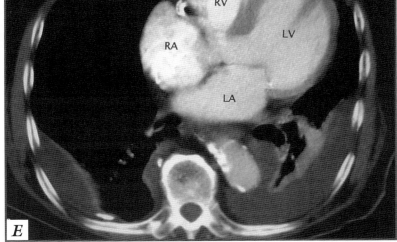

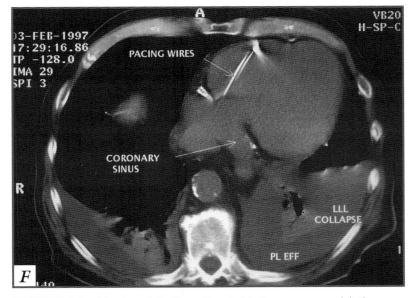

anterior to AAO and MPA. This may give the appearance of a widened mediastinum on a chest radiograph, even when the other mediastinal structures are of normal size.

C, The coronary arteries can be seen particularly well when they are heavily calcified, as in this case in which calcified left anterior descending (LAD) and circumflex (CX) coronary arteries are indicated. The SVC in this patient is still visible at the level of the left atrium (LA), which is shown receiving the pulmonary veins. This image was acquired approximately 3 cm caudal to B.

D, Image acquired approximately 30 seconds after the intravenous injection of conventional iodinated contrast medium at the same level as in C. Note the marked change in attenuation of the intracardiac structures. Contrast opacification is required to delineate most intracardiac structures. This image shows the aorta, right ventricular outflow tract, LA, and thicknesses of their walls (*see* part E).

E, Intracardiac anatomy is only well shown after contrast administration, as in this image approximately 2 cm caudal to D. Note that with contrast opacification and rapid exposure using fast spiral CT, the tricuspid and mitral valve leaflets can be seen. An apparent defect in the intraventricular septum between the right ventricle (RV) and the left ventricle (LV) is due to the thinness of the intraventricular septum at this level and its oblique passage through the imaging plane.

F, On this most caudal image, acquired without contrast medium, the coronary sinus (*arrow*) is shown running into the inferior vena cava. Pacing wires are shown passing toward their attachment on the free wall of the RV. This patient has bilateral lobar collapse (particularly left lower lobe [LLL] collapse, as indicated) and bilateral pleural effusions. LA–left atrium; RA—right atrium.

FIGURE 7-2. (*Continued*) **B,** On a slice that is 2 cm more caudal, the superior vena cava (SVC) runs in the angle between the AAO and the right pulmonary artery (RPA). The RPA runs horizontally along the plane of the image from the main pulmonary artery (MPA). The left pulmonary artery is more vertically oriented and, therefore, is only seen over a short length. Incidental findings include bilateral pleural effusions (Pl Eff) and lobar collapse (*see* part E). Mediastinal fat is seen as an area of low attenuation

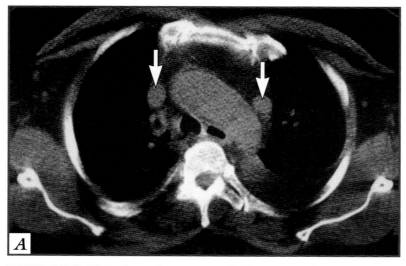

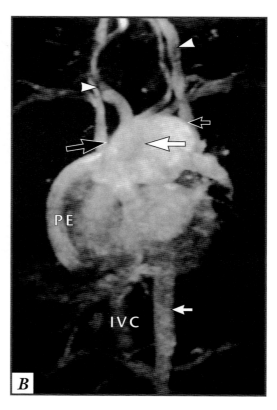

FIGURE 7-3. Bilateral superior vena cava (SVC). Congenital systemic venous abnormalities are not uncommon. **A,** Unenhanced computed tomography image showing the left SVC (*left arrow*) and the right SVC (*right arrow*) on either side of the aortic arch. **B,** Three-dimensional maximum intensity projection reconstruction from coronal unenhanced magnetic resonance angiography showing the right SVC (*long black arrow*) and the left SVC (*short black arrow*), with no bridging brachiocephalic vein. *Arrowheads* indicate common carotid arteries; *long white arrow* indicates aortic arch; *short white arrow* indicates abdominal aorta. IVC—inferior vena cava; PE—pericardial effusion.

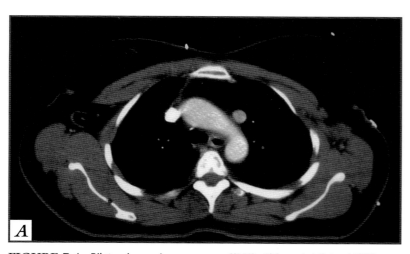

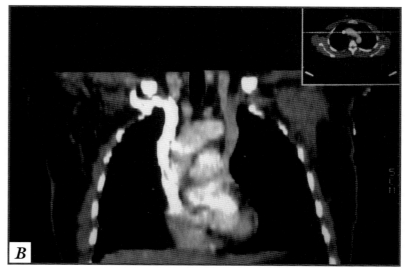

FIGURE 7-4. Bilateral superior vena cava (SVC). Although bilateral SVC anomalies can be diagnosed on unenhanced computed tomography scan, communication between the two, if present, may only be shown if contrast medium is injected. **A,** Contrast medium was injected via the patient's right arm and shows enhancement of the right SVC but no enhancement of the left SVC imaged at the level of the aortic arch. **B,** Two-dimensional coronal reconstruction, in the position indicated, shows the right SVC entering the right atrium separately from the left SVC, which drains into the coronary sinus.

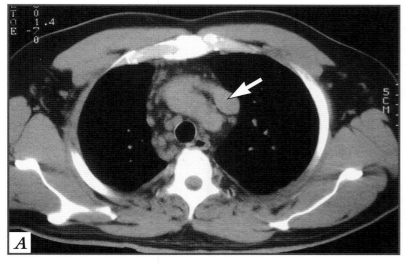

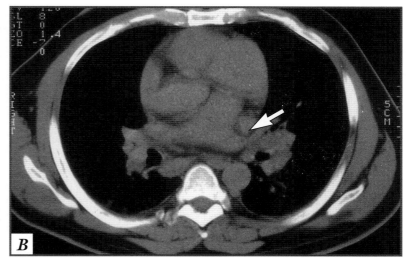

FIGURE 7-5. Left superior vena cava (SVC; *arrows*). **A,** In patients with a left SVC anomaly and no right SVC anomaly, the right brachiocephalic vein enters the left SVC at the level of the apex of the aortic arch. **B,** More caudally, the SVC runs anterior to one of the pulmonary veins before inserting into the coronary sinus. Note that in *A,* the numerous vessels seen in the mediastinum represent anomalous small veins that eventually drain into the SVC. No right SVC and no right azygous system are seen in the conventional positions. This abnormality was first noted during a difficult Swan-Ganz catheter insertion, when the catheter repeatedly passed to the left of the midline before entering the heart.

CARDIAC CALCIFICATION

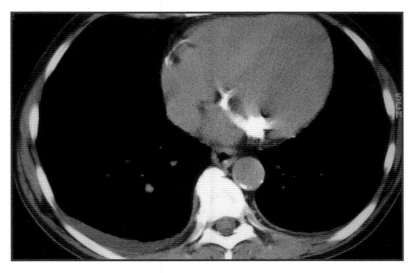

FIGURE 7-6. Mitral annulus calcification. Mitral annulus calcification is shown on this unenhanced Ultrafast CT (UFCT; Imatron, South San Francisco, CA) scan at the level of the mitral valve. Very heavy calcification is shown as a dense white mass in the region of the mitral annulus, on both its septal and posterior aspects. Mitral annulus calcification is a common incidental finding on conventional computed tomography (CT) scan and UFCT in the elderly. Calcification in the mitral valve leaflets (well shown by UFCT but blurred on conventional CT) may occur with mitral annulus calcification but is more commonly a feature of rheumatic mitral stenosis. Occasionally, tumors in the same position may also calcify to some degree, but these are extremely uncommon.

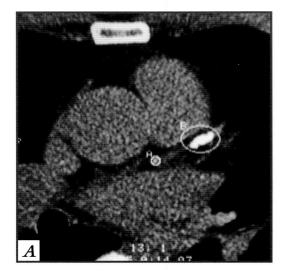

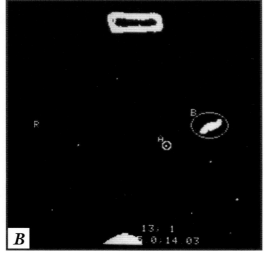

FIGURE 7-7. Coronary artery calcification. One of the unique applications of Ultrafast CT (UFCT; Imatron, South San Francisco, CA) to coronary imaging is the detection and reliable quantification of coronary artery wall calcification [4,5]. **A** and **C,** On conventional (soft tissue) window UFCT scan, coronary calcification is bright white, with regular soft tissue (*ie,* myocardium) being gray. These images are used to identify areas of coronary calcification (*circled*), in this case the left anterior descending and distal left main coronary arteries (**A** and **B**) and right coronary artery (**C** and **D**).

(*Continued on next page*)

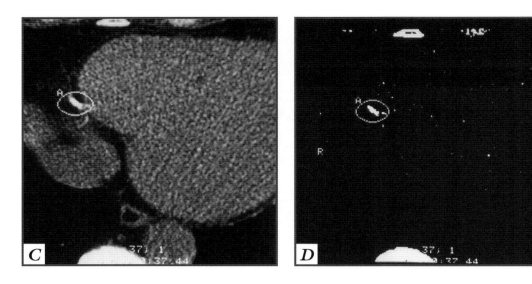

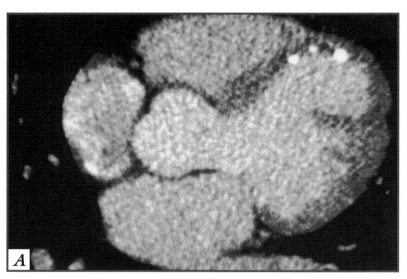

FIGURE 7-7. (*Continued*) **B** and **D,** These calcifications are highlighted by changing the display parameters so that the window is narrow (conventionally one Hounsfield unit [HU]) and set at a level that highlights calcification only (conventionally 130 HU). Multiple regions of interest (ROIs) are traced manually around coronary calcifications, as shown in these examples. The UFCT scanner automatically measures the attenuation of these areas, determines the area of calcification within each ROI, expressed as a number of pixels, and from this calculates a coronary calcification score. The total calcification score can be combined with other demographic information to give an estimate of the probability of underlying significant coronary artery disease.

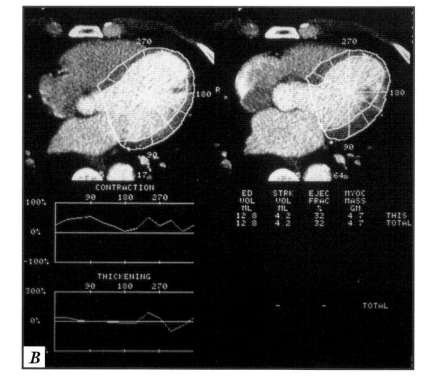

FIGURE 7-8. Left ventricular aneurysm. This patient has a history of possible, but unproven, myocardial infarction. **A,** This Ultrafast CT (UFCT; Imatron, South San Francisco, CA) image demonstrates calcification in a thin-walled left ventricular (LV) apex that did not move on cine computed tomography angiography (CTA). This represents a moderately sized apical infarction with myocardial thinning but without frank aneurysm formation after left anterior descending coronary artery occlusion. Only 50 mL of intravenous contrast medium was required for this cine study of LV function. With cine UFCT, multiple images are acquired during a single heartbeat at a rate of 17 scans/s. **B,** Using a semi-automated edge detection program to trace the endocardial surface at end-diastole and end-systole, ejection fractions can be calculated and abnormalities of regional wall motion quantified.

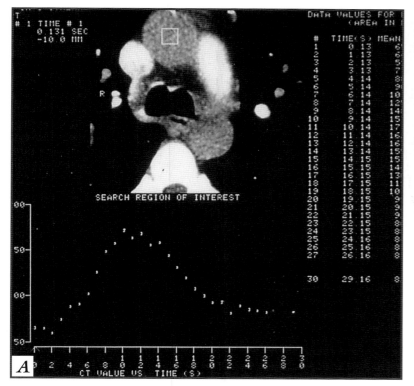

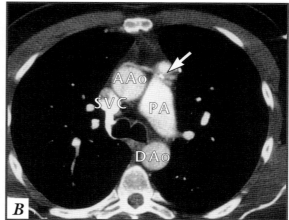

FIGURE 7-9. Coronary artery bypass graft (CABG). Definition of coronary artery and CABG anatomy is dependent on a tight, well-timed bolus of contrast medium arriving in the heart and the ascending aorta (AAo) [6]. Timing is determined by injecting a small volume of contrast (typically 16 mL at 4 mL/s) into a peripheral or central vein. Images are acquired at the same level using cine mode (1 image per R-R interval) through the AAo. **A,** Time density curve is constructed and time to the peak of contrast enhancement is estimated. The peak contrast enhancement indicates that the delay should be applied to starting the image acquisition for coronary or CABG computed tomography angiography (CTA). After an appropriately timed contrast injection (typically 120 mL), multilevel Ultrafast CT (UFCT; Imatron, South San Francisco, CA) is performed (typically 40 X 3 mm sections with 1 mm overlap between each section). For coronary or CABG CTA, an image is acquired for each cardiac cycle (usually after 80% of the R-R interval). **B,** This axial UFCT image shows excellent contrast opacification of the AAo and two saphenous vein bypass grafts arising from the anterior part of the AAo. Accuracy for UFCT detection of CABG patency is 92% to 96% [7]. *Arrow* indicates left internal mammary artery graft. DAo—descending aorta; PA—pulmonary artery; SVC—superior vena cava.

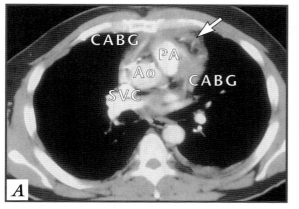

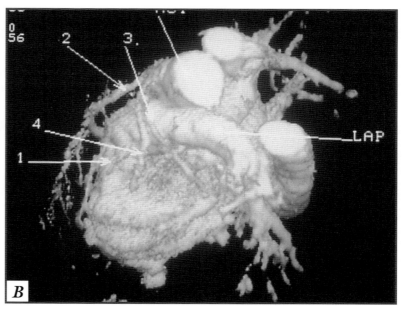

FIGURE 7-10. Coronary artery bypass graft (CABG). **A,** Axial spiral computed tomography angiography (CTA) image of patient with patent saphenous vein bypass grafts. Spiral CTA is more susceptible to motional blurring than is Ultrafast CT (UFCT; Imatron, South San Francisco, CA), but despite this can still provide good images of patent CABGs, with accuracies of 92% to 96% [8]. A good contrast bolus is required (typically 100 to 120 mL) to provide adequate opacification, as determined by a timing bolus. This image demonstrates three patent CABGs: two saphenous vein bypass grafts and one left internal mammary artery (LIMA) graft (*arrow*). Spiral CTA can provide good-quality three-dimensional data that can be reformatted using a variety of three-dimensional reconstruction techniques to demonstrate bypass graft patency. **B,** In this surface-shaded rendering from the same patient as in *A,* there are patent LIMA (1), right coronary artery (2), left-sided coronary artery (3 and 4) and saphenous vein bypass grafts. Although graft patency is well demonstrated using spiral CTA, the lack of electrocardiographic gating still produces sufficient blurring to make these scans unreliable for assessing intragraft stenoses or for assessing the distal anastomosis. AOT—ascending aorta; LAP—left pulmonary artery; PA—pulmonary artery; SVC—superior vena cava.

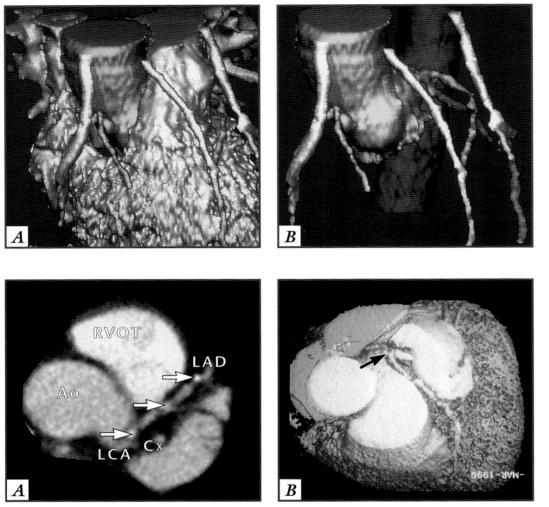

FIGURE 7-11. Color-coded (*not shown*) coronary artery bypass graft (CABG). The potential utility of Ultrafast CT (UFCT; Imatron, South San Francisco, CA) for noninvasive coronary angiography is increasing as postprocessing techniques become more sophisticated. In this work from Beijing, surface-shaded rendering and color coding have been used to highlight the CABGs. **A,** Surface-shaded reconstruction showing the position of the CABGs on the surface of the heart. **B,** The same data with the underlying heart edited away, leaving only the CABGs. Three CABGs (one to the left anterior descending coronary artery, one to the right coronary artery, and a jump graft to the circumflex artery and a diagonal artery) are shown against the native vessels. With UFCT, CABG can often be followed all the way to the distal anastomosis. (*Courtesy of* Imatron and Dai Ru Ping.)

FIGURE 7-12. Coronary artery disease on computed tomography angiography (CTA). One of the most active areas of Ultrafast CT (UFCT; Imatron, South San Francisco, CA) research is the development of intravenous coronary angiography. Although not yet a clinical tool and not intended to be a replacement for conventional coronary angiography, UFCT shows potential for imaging the proximal coronary arteries with reasonable accuracy. **A,** Thin slice projection constructed from several axial contrast-enhanced UFCT images, demonstrating the origin of the left main coronary artery and the length of the left anterior descending coronary artery (LAD). There is irregular narrowing of the LAD with several areas of calcification (*arrows*). The calcifications make it difficult to see the true luminal diameter of the associated vessel, one of the limitations of UFCT for noninvasive coronary angiography. **B,** Surface-shaded rendering three-dimensional image showing the origin of the LAD (*arrow*) and the left main coronary artery well. The circumflex artery (Cx) is obscured by the pulmonary artery. A stenosis in the LAD seen on the source images is also shown. Ao—aorta; LCA—left main coronary artery; RVOT—right ventricular outflow tract.

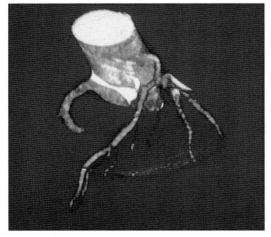

FIGURE 7-13. Three-dimensional coronary computed tomography angiography (CTA). New image processing software makes it possible to edit out many structures that surround the coronary arteries that can obstruct a clear view of coronary anatomy. In this three-dimensional surface-shaded rendering from a normal volunteer with coronary CTA, most of the heart and great vessels has been edited out of the raw data. The image shows only the coronary arteries arising from the aortic root.

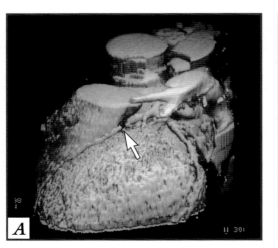
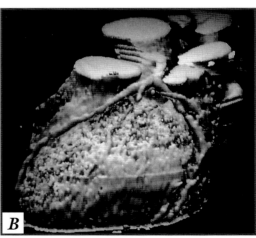

FIGURE 7-14. Three-dimensional coronary computed tomographic angiography (CTA). Pre– and post–percutaneous transluminal coronary angioplasty (PTCA). Intravenous coronary angiography by Ultrafast CT (UFCT; Imatron, South San Francisco, CA) can show the full length of the major coronary arteries, although the definition of smaller, more distal, or branch vessels is unreliable. **A,** Stenoses of the proximal major coronary artery are well shown by CTA, as in this example of a proximal left anterior descending coronary artery (LAD) stenosis (*arrow*) represented on a surface-shaded three-dimensional rendering. With this sort of lesion, it should be possible to use UFCT to reliably follow the results of PTCA, as is the case here [9]. **B,** Post-PTCA image showing that the stenosis seen on UFCT before PTCA has disappeared and there is a widely patent LAD at this level. (*From* Moshage and coworkers [9]; with permission.)

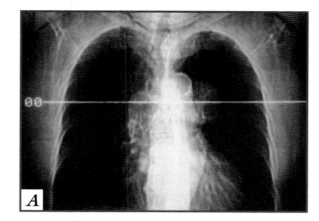

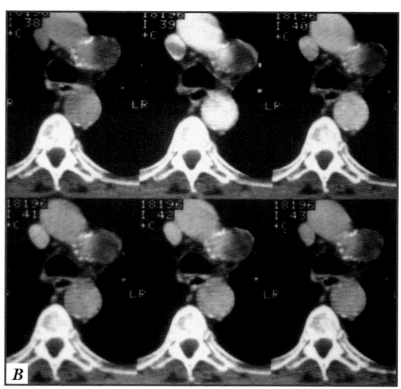

FIGURE 7-15. Saccular aortic aneurysm. Some aortic aneurysms can be relatively small and largely thrombosed. In this situation it may be difficult, particularly on an unenhanced scan, to differentiate them from tumors or other masses adherent to the aortic arch that may be suggested by the chest radiograph. **A,** On this scout image, an equivalent image to the chest radiograph is provided by computed tomography (CT) scan showing a mass adjacent to the aortic arch. In this situation, a dynamic study with contrast injection and multiple acquisitions at the same level (*horizontal line*) may clarify the anatomy. In this patient a partly calcified mass is seen adjacent to the ascending aorta. **B,** Dynamic scan (6 images illustrated) showing contrast enhancement opacifying the base of the aneurysm, indicating that this is a saccular aneurysm of the aortic arch rather than an adherent tumor.

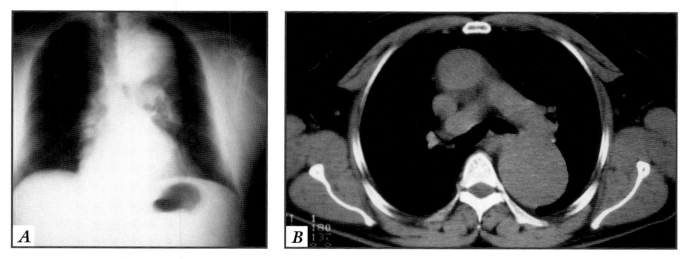

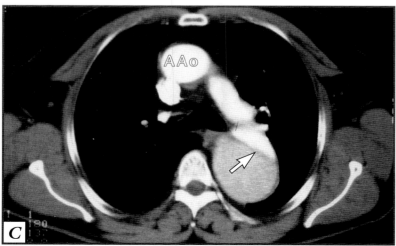

FIGURE 7-16. Type B aortic dissection. Aortic dissection is a relatively uncommon but important indication for computed tomography (CT) scan of the aorta [10]. **A,** Chest radiography may suggest the diagnosis of aortic dissection; however, confident diagnosis requires some form of cross-sectional imaging. **B,** Unenhanced CT scan may show dilatation of the aorta but does not provide adequate information about the internal aortic anatomy. Contrast enhancement is essential for any suspected aortic dissection. **C,** Image after injection of contrast medium at the same level as in *B,* showing dense opacification of the true lumen and faint opacification of the false lumen. The dissection flap in the descending aorta is well shown (*arrow*). Pulsatility artefact in the ascending aorta (AAo) should not be mistaken for a flap in the AAo.

Spiral acquisition allows rapid imaging of the whole of the chest and three-dimensional image reconstruction. The next version of the Ultrafast CT (UFCT; Imatron, South San Francisco, CA), which is now available, has a much larger area of coverage in conventional and spiral modes.

(Continued on next page)

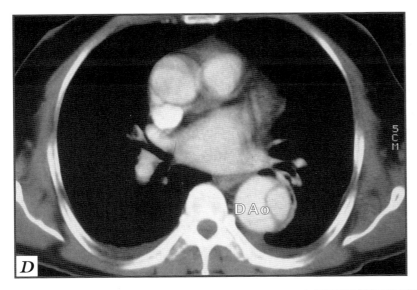

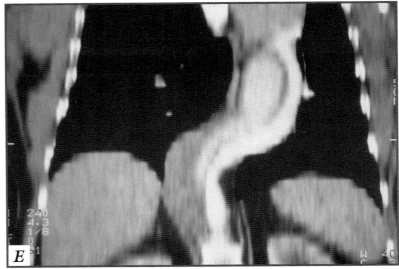

FIGURE 7-16. (*Continued*) **D,** Image from spiral CT acquisition 3 cm below image in *C,* showing the opacification of true and false lumens in the descending aorta (DAo) at the level of the left atrium with pulsatility artefact but no dissection flap in the AAo. **E,** Two-dimensional coronal reformatted image from the three-dimensional data set shows the curved path of the dissection flap and the partially thrombosed lower part of the false lumen. The dissection flap arises distal to the left subclavian artery origin (Type A or III) and runs caudally in the DAo, with equal opacification of true and false lumen. **F,** Surface-shaded three-dimensional reconstruction from the same data sets shows some pulsatility artefact in the AAo, the origin of the dissection from the upper part of the descending thoracic aorta, and the false lumen spiraling around the true lumen. **G,** Correlative digital subtraction aortogram shows the same basic proximal anatomy; however, contrast medium fails to fully opacify the lower part of the false lumen.

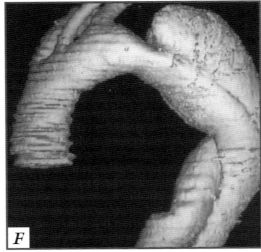

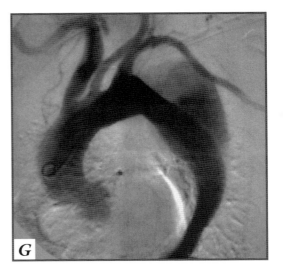

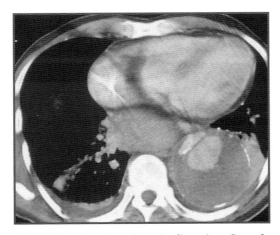

FIGURE 7-17. Type B aortic dissection. One of the advantages of computed tomography (CT) scan compared with conventional aortography is its capability of showing the full size of the aorta. Aortography can only show the patent lumen. In this patient with a partly thrombosed Type A (III) dissection, well shown by contrast-enhanced spiral CT, the full diameter of the aorta would be underestimated by aortography, and the dissection flap would not be profiled in the conventional 60° left anterior oblique view used for most standard aortography.

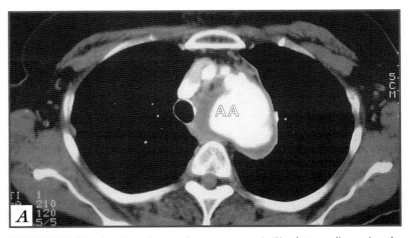

FIGURE 7-18. Aortic arch saccular aneurysm. **A,** Single two-dimensional computed tomography (CT) image through the aortic arch shows a large saccular aneurysm (AA) arising from the distal aortic arch immediately beyond the origin of the left subclavian artery, causing displacement of the trachea to the right.

(Continued on next page)

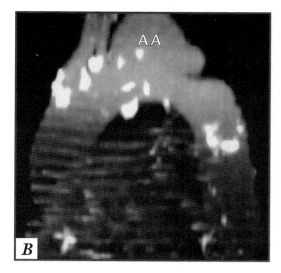

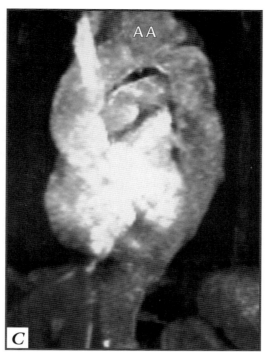

FIGURE 7-18. (*Continued*) **B,** Three-dimensional maximum intensity projection (MIP) reconstruction of the CT angiography images is affected by pulsatility artefact in the ascending aorta but clearly shows the saccular aneurysm (AA) arising from the apex of the aortic arch. Note the displacement of the subclavian artery and the other major aortic arch branches. Also on this reconstruction, areas of calcification appear as white areas superimposed on the gray of the opacified aortic lumen. **C,** The same patient underwent magnetic resonance angiography (MRA) using multiple oblique sagittal breath-hold imaging, without the need for contrast agent. These were reconstructed using MIP to produce a similar image, although with a larger field of view. MRA and CTA produce similar images, but only CT shows the distribution of calcification.

CONGENITAL AORTIC ARCH ANOMALIES

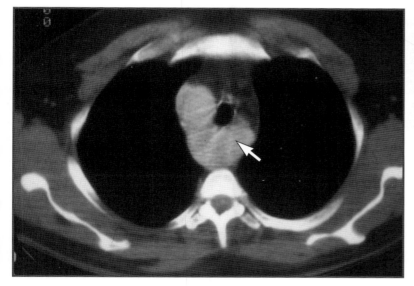

FIGURE 7-19. Right aortic arch. Computed tomography (CT) scan is an important method for diagnosing congenital aortic arch anomalies. This axial image shows a right aortic arch with anomalous origin of the left subclavian artery (*arrow*) from the distal aortic arch and passing posterior to the trachea. This is the normal arrangement in patients with a right aortic arch without congenital heart disease, a mirror image of an anomalous right subclavian artery, *ie*, the first branches are the common carotid arteries followed by the right subclavian artery and then most distally by the left subclavian artery. As shown in this image, there may be dilatation of the origin of the anomalous subclavian artery, representing a remnant of the diverticulum of Kommerell.

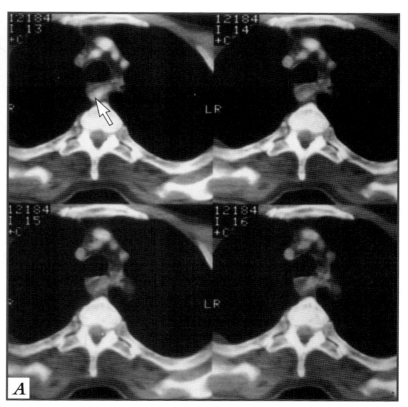

FIGURE 7-20. Aberrant right subclavian artery. A normal-sized aberrant subclavian artery may be difficult to show convincingly on unenhanced computed tomography (CT) scan. **A,** Sequence of four images acquired at the same level during contrast enhancement showing an anomalous right subclavian artery (*arrow*) posterior to the trachea.

(Continued on next page)

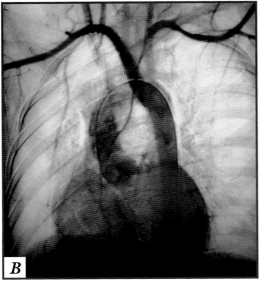

FIGURE 7-20. *(Continued)* **B,** Conventional arch aortogram (photographic subtraction) showing delayed filling of the anomalous right subclavian artery.

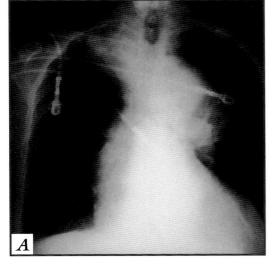

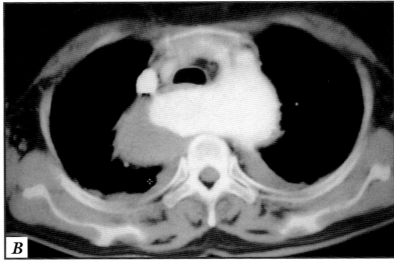

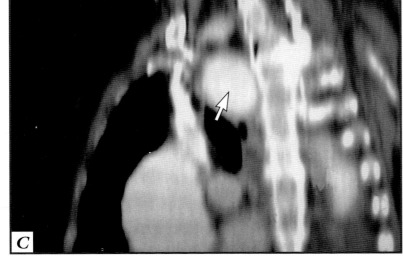

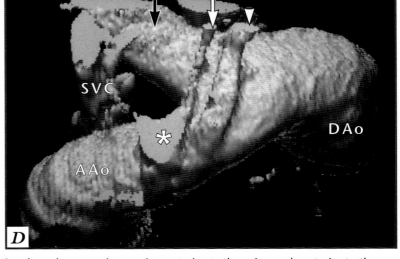

FIGURE 7-21. Aneurysm of an aberrant right subclavian artery. **A,** Chest radiograph showing a large tortuous structure extending from the aortic arch in a patient with dysphagia. **B,** Axial contrast-enhanced spiral computed tomography (SCT) image at the level of the aortic arch showing a large vascular structure, an aneurysmal anomalous right subclavian artery, arising from the aortic arch and passing posterior to the esophagus and the trachea. There is luminal thrombus in its lateral aspect. **C,** Two-dimensional sagittal image reconstructed from the SCT data showing the anomalous artery *(arrow)* in a lateral perspective passing anterior to the spine and posterior to the trachea. **D,** Surface-rendered three-dimensional reconstruction showing more clearly the anomalous right subclavian artery *(black arrow)* arising from the distal part of the aortic arch. Note the position relative to the origin of the left common carotid artery *(white arrow)* and left subclavian artery *(arrowhead)*. *Asterisk* indicates stump of brachiocephalic artery (removed for clarity). AAo—ascending aorta; DAo—descending aorta; SVC—superior vena cava.

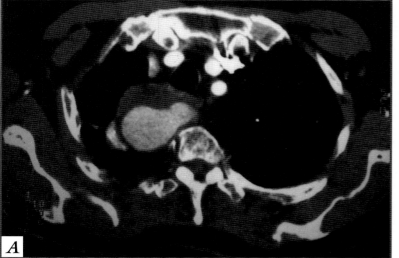

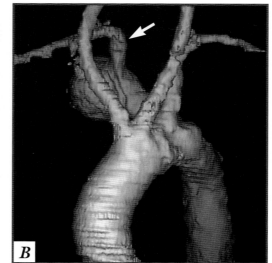

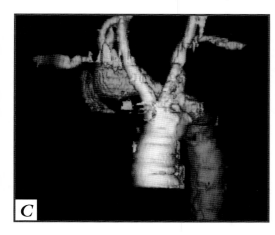

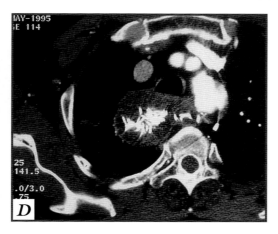

FIGURE 7-22. Saccular aneurysm of an aberrant right subclavian artery. This patient presented with a large superior mediastinal mass on chest radiography. **A,** Enhanced spiral computed tomography (SCT) scan (axial slice) showing a large round mass with contrast enhancement in its center. **B,** Surface-shaded rendering three-dimensional reconstruction showing this to be a saccular aneurysm of an anomalous right subclavian artery (*arrow*). **C,** After surgical bypass the aneurysm is still filled, as shown on this surface-rendered image. There has been a right common carotid to right subclavian bypass; however, the contrast medium still opacifies the aneurysm through a small defect at the surgical closure site from the distal arch of the aorta. This was treated by coil embolization. **D,** Postcontrast axial CT images after embolization at a level similar to that in *A* showing the high-attenuation steel coils in the aneurysm but no contrast enhancement in the aneurysm. The patient remains well more than 1 year following embolization.

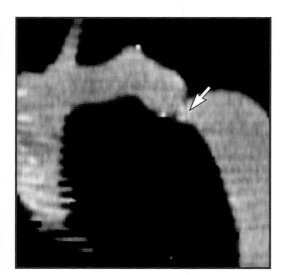

FIGURE 7-23. Coarctation of the aorta. There is limited value to Ultrafast CT (UFCT; Imatron, South San Francisco, CA) in the evaluation of patients with congenital heart disease and associated problems related to the need to give intravenous contrast medium and the use of radiation. Although intracardiac conditions can be demonstrated by UFCT, these are usually well shown by echocardiography, with additional imaging by magnetic resonance imaging (MRI) if needed. MRI better assesses congenital aortic conditions such as coarctation in adults, and echocardiography, with or without MRI, better assesses children. However, there are patients who cannot undergo MRI in whom echocardiography is adequate. The maximum intensity projection reconstruction shows coarctation (*arrow*) involving the distal aortic arch.

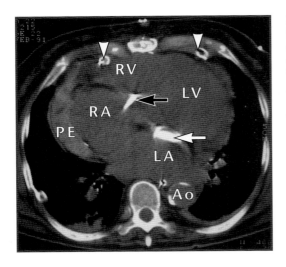

FIGURE 7-24. Postoperative pericardial effusion (PE). Computed tomography (CT) scan is valuable for evaluating postoperative complications, particularly in patients in whom acoustic access for echocardiography is limited due to surgical wounds, hyperinflation in patients on ventilators, and lack of mobility. An unenhanced CT demonstrates an unsuspected PE adjacent to the right atrium (RA). The patient has a mitral valve prosthesis (*white arrow*), bilateral chest drains (*arrowheads*), bibasilar atelectasis, and bilateral pleural effusions. There is a large left atrium (LA) and artefacts from the Swan-Ganz catheter (*black arrow*) passing through the RA and tricuspid valve. Ao—aorta; LV—left ventricle; RV—right ventricle.

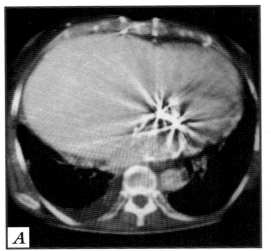

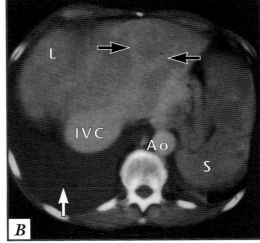

FIGURE 7-25. Mitral valve disease with congestive heart failure (CHF). Patients with long-standing rheumatic heart disease may be examined incidentally by computed tomography (CT), although their normal cardiac evaluation examination would initially be by echocardiography. **A,** Extensive "streaking" or beam-hardening artefact is produced by the metal in this MV prosthesis. In this patient, chronic rheumatic MV disease has caused right heart failure, with a huge right atrium that extends out to the right chest wall. **B,** A more caudal image in the same patient showing that the inferior vena cava (IVC) is displaced laterally and the hepatic veins are dilated (*black arrows*) due to CHF. There is also a large right pleural effusion. *White arrow* indicates ascites. Ao—aorta; L—liver; S—spleen.

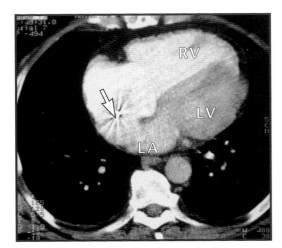

FIGURE 7-26. Right ventricular (RV) dysplasia. This contrast-enhanced computed tomography angiography (CTA) scan demonstrates a dilated poorly contracting RV in a patient with an RV dysplasia [11]. The anterior RV wall adjacent to the contrast-enhanced cavity is of low attenuation, indicating some fatty infiltration; however, it is so thin that it is difficult to see. There is artefact from the pacing wire (*arrow*) in the right atrium. Contrast medium passes through the RV slowly, hence the poor opacification of the left ventricle (LV). There is displacement of the interatrial septum toward the left atrium (LA), indicating high right atrial pressure.

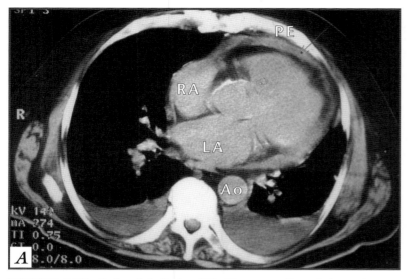

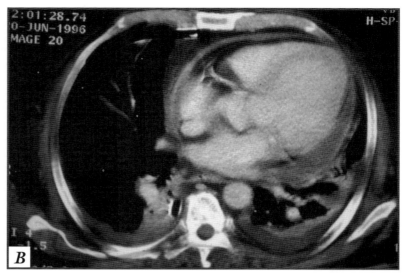

FIGURE 7-27. Pericardial effusion (PE). PEs are usually well shown by echocardiography. However, they are often a finding on conventional computed tomography (CT) scan or Ultrafast CT (UFCT; Imatron, South San Francisco, CA). As shown in Figure 7-24, CT may show loculated pericardial fluid that cannot be shown by echocardiography. **A,** On unenhanced scans, a PE often has attenuation similar to soft tissue and therefore has the same density as do myocardium and blood pool. PE is usually visible as a layer of abnormal thickening separated from the heart by a line of low-attenuation epicardial fat, as shown in this example. Sometimes the epicardial fat is very thin; however, it still should be visible.

B, If there is doubt whether there is a PE or if there is no epicardial fat, intravenous contrast medium will enhance the myocardium but not the pericardial fluid. The attenuation of the myocardium will increase, as shown in this patient with lymphoma invading the pericardium, whereas the attenuation of the pericardial fluid (here mostly loculated posteriorly) is unchanged, enhancing the difference between the two. Although CT is not recommended as the first line method for detecting PEs, it frequently shows underlying conditions such as tumor, which may lead to pericardial effusion. In addition, in patients who are poor subjects for echocardiography, CT will show PEs, including effusions loculated in areas difficult to examine by echocardiography. Ao—aorta; LA—left atrium; RA—right atrium.

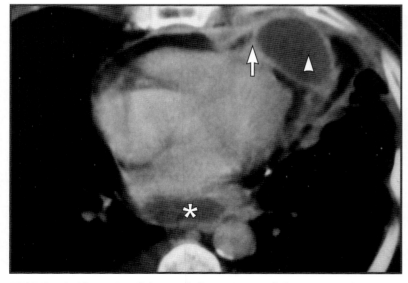

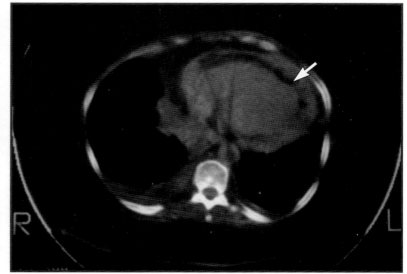

FIGURE 7-28. Pericardial mesothelioma. Pericardial tumors can have a variety of appearances, most of which are not characteristic. In this contrast-enhanced computed tomography (CT) scan in a patient with pericardial mesothelioma (*arrow*), irregular thickening of the pericardium is shown along with a well-defined loculated pericardial effusion (*arrowhead*) close to the apex of the heart. There is a smaller pericardial effusion (*asterisk*) behind the left atrium. Tumor attenuation is increased by contrast medium injection, and the fluid in the loculated pericardial effusion remains of low attenuation.

FIGURE 7-29. Pericardial metastasis. Diffuse pericardial thickening with areas of irregular thickening and other areas of normal-thickness pericardium raises the possibility, in the appropriate clinical context, of pericardial malignancy, especially metastases. This unenhanced computed tomography scan shows extensive pericardial thickening (*arrow*) owing to direct invasion by small cell carcinoma of the lung.

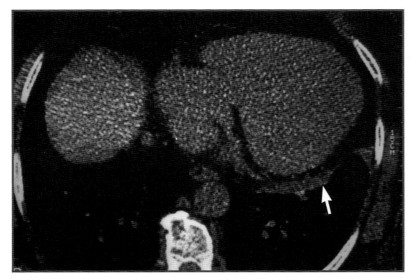

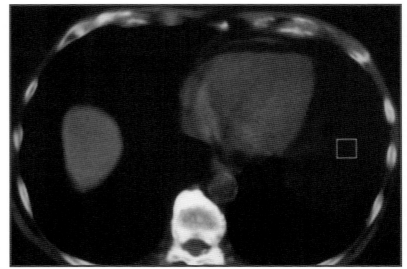

FIGURE 7-30. Pericardial thickening. Ultrafast CT (UFCT; Imatron, South San Francisco, CA) is probably the most accurate method for measuring the thickness of the pericardium *in vivo*. Spiral computed tomography (CT) scan is also relatively accurate, although it includes some blurring of the pericardium because of the longer exposure time. Magnetic resonance imaging is also appropriate but tends to have a slightly larger range of normal thicknesses. In this patient, unenhanced UFCT shows focal pericardial thickening posteriorly (*arrow*). The pericardium is seen as an area of soft tissue attenuation separated from the posterior part of the left ventricle by a rim of low-attenuation epicardial fat. Diffuse pericardial thickening is more common with hemodynamically significant pericardial constriction.

FIGURE 7-31. Pericardial lipoma. The attenuation coefficients of different types of tissue sometimes give useful information about tissue type. High attenuation usually indicates calcification (*ie,* attenuation over 100 Hounsfield units [HU] on unenhanced scans). Low attenuation (below 0 HU and usually in the region of -100 HU) indicates the presence of fat. This is useful in evaluating pericardial or epicardial masses. Epicardial fat pads are common. Larger masses with low attenuation and a homogeneous internal structure, as shown in this unenhanced computed tomography (CT) scan, represent pericardial lipomas. As long as there is uniform low attenuation throughout these tumors, a confident pathologic diagnosis can be made. Irregular attenuation should raise concern that the mass might represent a liposarcoma.

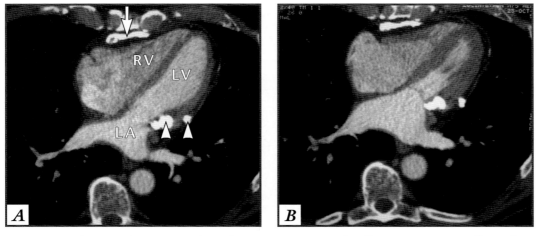

FIGURE 7-32. Constrictive pericarditis. Chronic constrictive pericarditis may not necessarily produce changes over the entire pericardium. Characteristically, there is pericardial thickening, often with calcification, concentrated on the atrioventricular (AV) sulci. Because computed tomography (CT) scan not only shows thickening of pericardium but also shows calcium very well, this is possibly the best technique for fully evaluating the pericardium in constrictive pericarditis. **A,** Although the rest of the pericardium is of normal thickness, there is extensive pericardial calcification in this patient in the AV grooves. On the diastolic image there is an impression on the anterior surface of the right ventricle (RV), indicating some restriction of right heart filling. **B,** On the systolic image, the left ventricle (LV) contracts to a very small volume, again suggesting limited cardiac filling. Contrast-enhanced CT scan is recommended before surgical stripping to ensure that there is adequate thickness of RV myocardium under areas of pericardial thickening. With conventional CT, the normal thickness of the pericardium is up to approximately 3 mm but may be slightly less with the more precise Ultrafast CT (UFCT; Imatron, South San Francisco, CA). *Arrow* indicates calcification in the anterior AV grooves; *arrowheads* indicate those in the posterior AV grooves. LA—left atrium.

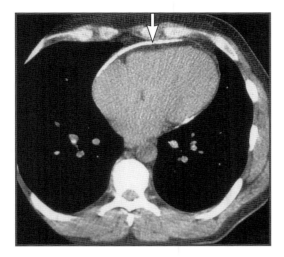

FIGURE 7-33. Pericardial calcification. There are numerous causes for pericardial calcification. In this patient, a road traffic accident many years ago caused a localized hemopericardium, which led to focal pericardial calcification with mild thickening, with a sharp transition to a normal thickness noncalcified pericardium. This contrast-enhanced Ultrafast CT (UFCT; Imatron, South San Francisco, CA) image shows focal pericardial thickening and calcification (*arrow*). There were no features of constrictive pericarditis (*ie*, no hemodynamic abnormalities or symptoms to suggest impaired cardiac filling).

CARDIAC TUMORS AND MASSES

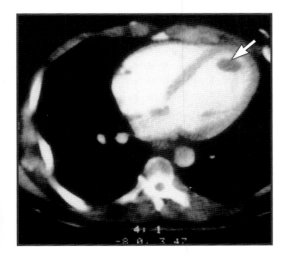

FIGURE 7-34. Left ventricular thrombus. Contrast enhanced Ultrafast CT (UFCT; Imatron, South San Francisco, CA) is useful for evaluating intracardiac tumors, cardiac tumors, and other masses. In this patient with a dilated left ventricle after myocardial infarction, there is thinning of the cardiac apex associated with an intraluminal filling defect (*arrow*) representing intraluminal thrombus. (*Courtesy of William Stanford.*)

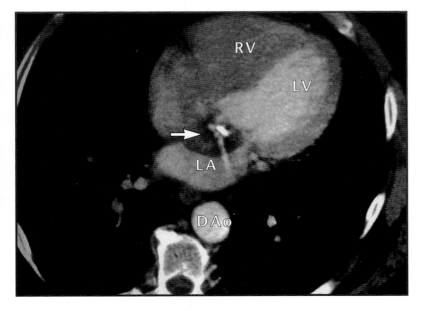

FIGURE 7-35. Left atrial myxoma. Ultrafast CT (UFCT; Imatron, South San Francisco, CA) provides very clear visualization of cardiac tumors. Contrast-enhanced UFCT showing a left atrial myxoma (*arrow*), outlined by contrast in the left atrium (LA). The myxoma arises from the interatrial septum (the most common position), does not enhance, and has a central fleck of calcification. This is a characteristic appearance. DAo—descending aorta; LA—left atrium; LV—left ventricle; RV—right ventricle.

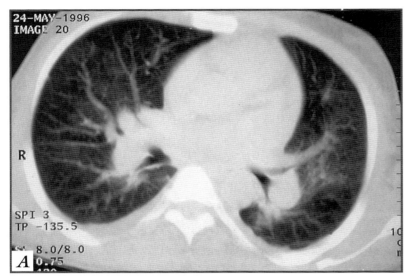

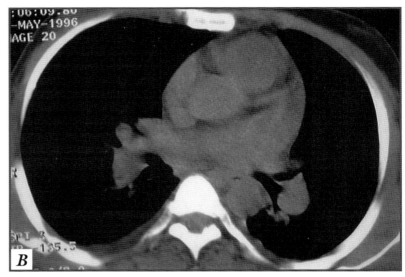

FIGURE 7-36. Pulmonary edema. **A,** Breath-hold spiral computed tomography (SCT) scan at the lung windows showing extensive ground-glass density in both lungs, with large pulmonary vessels. **B,** The pulmonary changes are not visible on the soft tissue window image generated from the same data; however, the large pulmonary arteries are still visible. In patients with interstitial or alveolar lung disease with an unclear cause, CT is often helpful in the diagnosis by demonstrating a characteristic distribution of changes within the lungs that may indicate heart failure as a cause. Demonstration of intracardiac abnormalities that can cause heart failure may provide a clue to the diagnosis.

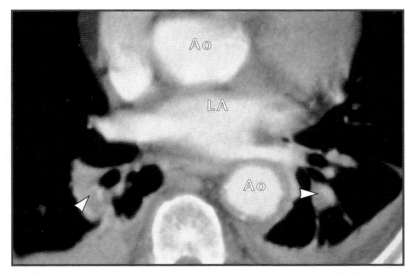

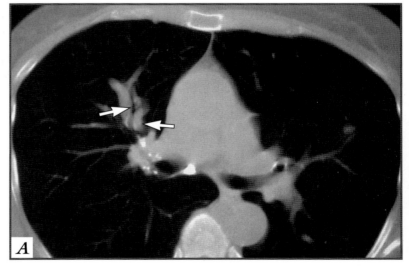

FIGURE 7-37. Pulmonary embolus. The noninvasive diagnosis of pulmonary embolus has been facilitated by computed tomographic angiography (CTA) [12]. Contrast-enhanced pulmonary computed tomography can show single or multiple pulmonary emboli (*arrowheads*) with considerable accuracy, shown here as intraluminal filling defects, as far out as the fourth order branches of the pulmonary arteries. Ao—aorta; LA—left atrium.

FIGURE 7-38. Pulmonary arteriovenous malformations (PAVMs). **A,** Unenhanced computed tomography (CT) scan is useful for detecting primary pulmonary conditions, which may have cardiac manifestations. This unenhanced axial spiral CT image shows large vessels (*arrows*) running to the anterior part of the right lower lobe.

(*Continued on next page*)

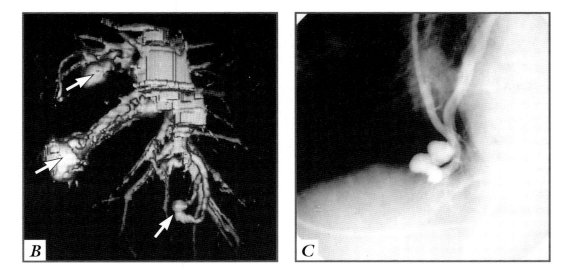

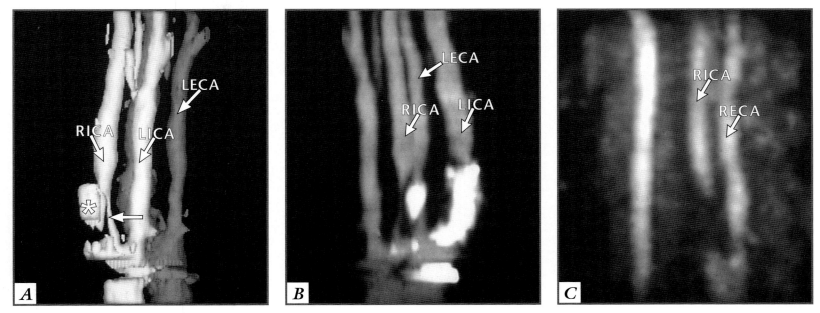

FIGURE 7-38. (*Continued*) **B,** Three-dimensional surface-shaded reconstruction demonstrating multiple PAVMs (*arrows*). This is one situation in which injected contrast medium is not required to perform three-dimensional reconstructions of vessels. **C,** Selective injection at pulmonary angiography before embolization, confirming the presence of the right anterior PAVM shown in *B*.

OTHER USES OF COMPUTED TOMOGRAPHY IMAGING IN CARDIAC DISEASE

FIGURE 7-39. Carotid artery stenosis. Computed tomography angiography (CTA) is useful for evaluating carotid artery disease in patients who cannot undergo magnetic resonance angiography (MRA) [13]. It also provides useful information concerning the relative position of stenoses and calcifications around the carotid bifurcation (although calcification may obscure contrast in the true lumen of the vessel, making accurate stenosis quantification difficult). Multiple views and different three-dimensional reconstructions may be needed to show all relevant abnormalities [14]. **A,** Surface-shaded rendering does not differentiate between the high signal from the contrast medium in the arterial lumen and calcification, but in the right orientation it may project the stenosis away from the calcification. In this patient, severe right internal carotid artery (RICA) stenosis (*long white arrow*) and mild left ICA (LICA) stenosis are shown on both the surface-shaded and maximum intensity projection (MIP) images (**B**). *Asterisk* indi-

cates calcification at the origin of the RICA. **C,** An equivalent three-dimensional time-of-flight MRA view (targeted MIP) of the right ICA showing extensive signal loss consistent with a severe stenosis, without obscuration by calcification. MRA tends to overestimate very severe stenosis; however, this is usually not clinically significant with three-dimensional MRA.

Compared with MRA, CTA requires a relatively large dose of contrast medium (this type of MRA does not require contrast dye) and shows a relatively limited craniocaudal field of view. Although CTA can cover large areas with a coarse acquisition pitch, a very fine pitch is required to achieve the spatial resolution required for carotid CTA. This reduces the craniocaudal field of view to only a few centimeters above and below the bifurcation. Another benefit of CTA is that the risks of catheter manipulation, inherent with conventional angiography, are avoided. LECA—left external carotid artery.

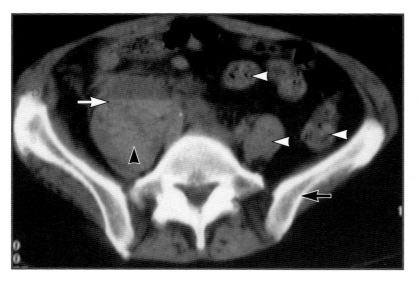

FIGURE 7-40. Retroperitoneal hematoma. It should be remembered that computed tomography (CT) has value not only in direct imaging of the heart but also in demonstrating complications of cardiac disease and investigations. This patient underwent a cardiac catheterization 1 week before this unenhanced abdominal CT scan was performed. The scan shows a large retroperitoneal hematoma (*black arrowhead*) lateral to the iliac arteries, which has a hematocrit level (*white arrow*), indicating that the blood within it has been present for some time. CT is the most appropriate method for evaluating retroperitoneal hematomas. *White arrowheads* indicate loops of bowel; *black arrow* indicates iliac wing.

REFERENCES

1. Wood AM, Hoffman KR, Lipton MJ: Cardiac function: quantification with magnetic resonance and computed tomography. *Radiol Clin North Am* 1994, 32:553–579.

2. Thompson BH, Stanford W: Evaluation of cardiac function with ultrafast computed tomography. *Radiol Clin North Am* 1994, 32:537–551.

3. Zeman RK, Silverman PM, Vieco PT, Costello P: CT angiography. *AJR Am J Roentgenol* 1995, 165:1079–1088.

4. Arad Y, Spadaro LA, Goodman K, *et al.*: Predictive value of electron beam computed tomography of the coronary arteries: 19-month follow-up of 1173 asymptomatic subjects. *Circulation* 1966, 93:1951–1953.

5. Wexler L, Brundage B, Crouse J, *et al.*: Coronary artery calcification: pathophysiology, epidemiology, imaging methods, and clinical implications. A statement for health care professionals from the American Heart Association. *Circulation* 1996, 94:1175–1192.

6. van Hoe L, Marchal G, Baert AL, *et al.*: Determination of scan delay time in spiral CT-angiography: utility of a test bolus injection. *J Comput Assist Tomogr* 1995, 19:216–220.

7. Stanford W, Brundage BH, MacMillan R, *et al.*: Sensitivity and specificity of assessing coronary bypass graft patency with ultrafast computed tomography: results of a multicenter study. *J Am Coll Cardiol* 1988, 12:1–7.

8. Tello R, Ecker C, Hartnell GG, Costello P: Spiral CT evaluation of coronary artery bypass graft patency. *J Comput Assist Tomogr* 1993, 17:253–259.

9. Moshage WEL, Achenbach S, Seese B, *et al.*: Coronary artery stenoses: three-dimensional imaging with electrocardiographically triggered, contrast-agent-enhanced, electron-beam CT. *Radiology* 1995, 196:707–714.

10. Hamada S, Takamiya M, Kimura K, *et al.*: Type A aortic dissection: evaluation with ultrafast CT. *Radiology* 1992, 183:155–158.

11. Hamada S, Takamiya M, Ohe T, Ueda H: Arrhythmogenic right ventricular dysplasia: evaluation with electron-beam CT. *Radiology* 1993, 187:723–727.

12. Teigen CL, Maus TP, Sheedy PF, *et al.*: Pulmonary embolism: diagnosis with contrast-enhanced electron-beam CT and comparison with pulmonary angiography. *Radiology* 1995, 194:313–319.

13. Cumming MJ, Morrow IM: Carotid artery stenosis: a prospective comparison of CT angiography and conventional angiography. *AJR Am J Roentgenol* 1994, 163:517–523.

14. Takahashi M, Ashtari M, Papp Z, *et al.*: CT angiography of carotid bifurcation: artefacts and pitfalls in shaded-surface display. *AJR Am J Roentgenol* 1997, 168:813–817.

CHAPTER 8

Magnetic Resonance Imaging of Coronary and Vascular Structures

Michael V. McConnell ~ Warren J. Manning
Robert R. Edelman

Magnetic resonance imaging (MRI) has become a standard medical imaging modality because it provides detailed images of the human body noninvasively with excellent tissue contrast. Flowing blood provides a form of intrinsic contrast in MRI and contributes to the ability of MRI to image vascular structures. With the high prevalence, morbidity, and mortality of cardiovascular disease, there is a clinical need for noninvasive coronary and vascular imaging.

Magnetic resonance angiography is MRI of blood vessels. The clinical value of MR angiography was initially demonstrated for imaging the aorta, which posed the fewest technical challenges owing to its large size, rapid blood flow, and limited motion. With steadily improving techniques, MR angiography has also become widley used for cerebrovascular imaging and for renal and peripheral artery imaging, as well as for imaging venous disease. Imaging the coronary arteries has been the most challenging because of their small size and substantial cardiac and respiratory motion. However, it has the potential for the greatest clinical impact. Another area of growing interest is directly imaging the vessel wall in order to detect and characterize atherosclerotic plaque.

MRI technology continues to advance rapidly, particularly as applied to the cardiovascular system. Significant improvements in hardware and software have reduced imaging times from minutes to seconds, and specialized cardiovascular MRI systems have been developed. MRI contrast agents have had a major impact on improving MR angiography image quality and are being applied to the coronary arteries. The role of MRI continues to expand as a comprehensive noninvasive cardiovascular imaging modality.

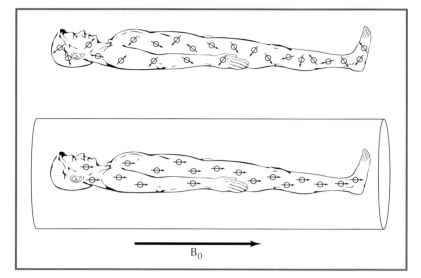

FIGURE 8-1. Basic principle of magnetic resonance. Clinical magnetic resonance imaging exploits the magnetic properties of the hydrogen atom, which is abundant in the human body primarily in water and fat. The spinning hydrogen nucleus is thus a tiny magnet. In the absence of an external magnetic field, these nuclei are randomly oriented in space (*top*). Applying an external magnetic field causes nuclei to align along the axis of the applied field (*bottom*), generating a magnetic moment (B_0) that can be measured. (*Courtesy of* Gerald G. Blackwell and Gerald M. Pohost.)

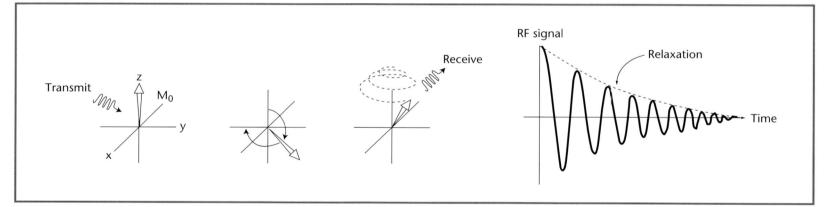

FIGURE 8-2. Radiofrequency signal. To generate a measurable signal, the nuclear spins must be perturbed. Typically, a pulse of radiofrequency (RF) energy is delivered from a transmit RF coil at the resonant frequency of the nuclei (termed the *Larmor frequency*) (**A**). This rotates the magnetization (M_0) onto the X-Y plane, where it precesses like a tipped gyroscope (**B**). This time-varying magnetic field generates a current in a receiver coil, resulting in an RF signal at the Larmor frequency (**C**). This signal decays as the magnetization returns to its equilibrium state (**D**).

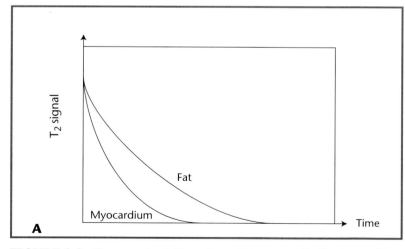

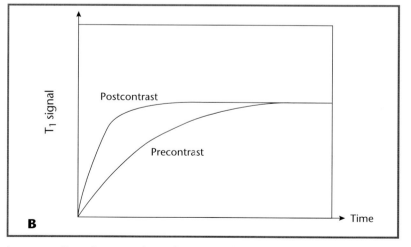

FIGURE 8-3. Tissue contrast. The return of the magnetization to equilibrium involves two major processes. These "relaxation" properties are exploited to distinguish tissue characteristics. The more rapid process is termed *transverse relaxation* (T_2) (**A**). As the magnetization rotates in the X-Y plane, individual nuclei become out of phase with each other, and the signal loses coherence. This signal loss takes longer for hydrogen nuclei in fat than in myocardium, for example, so fat appears brighter than does myocardium on a T_2-weighted image. The slower process is termed longitudinal relaxation (T_1) (**B**), which represents the time it takes to recover full magnetization along the Z axis. Magnetic resonance imaging contrast agents, for example, shorten T_1 and allow faster recovery of full magnetization for faster imaging with higher signal.

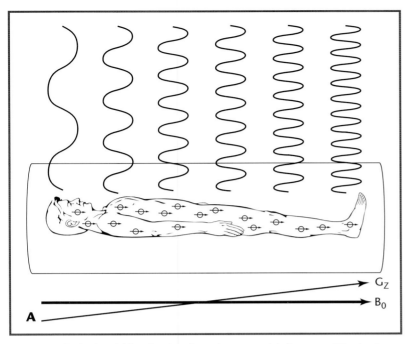

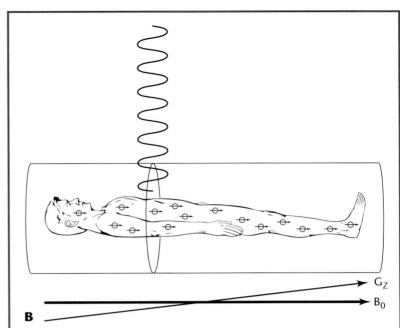

FIGURE 8-4. Spatial localization. In order to provide images of the body, the received radiofrequency (RF) signals must be localized to the part of the body from which they originated. One method is to apply a magnetic field gradient (G_z) across the body (**A**), causing the resonant frequency to be higher in nuclei from the feet compared with the head, for example. The received RF signal can then be separated into its different frequency components (by Fourier transformation), with each frequency corresponding to a different part of the body. A specific slice of the body may be imaged (**B**) by transmitting RF energy at a specific resonant frequency in the presence of a magnetic field gradient. (*Courtesy of* Gerald G. Blackwell and Gerald M. Pohost.) B_0—magnetic moment; G_z—magnetic gradient.

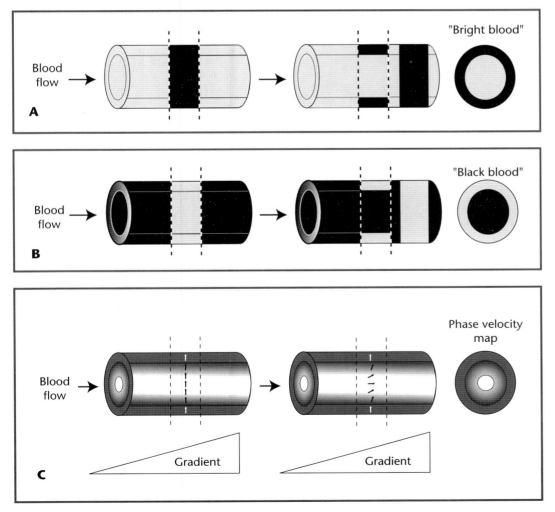

FIGURE 8-5. Vascular imaging methods. Magnetic resonance imaging is sensitive to flowing blood, which can be exploited in several different ways. **A,** The most common approach to vascular imaging is to generate an angiogram, in which flowing blood appears bright. Whereas signal from stationary structures within the imaging slice, such as the vessel wall, is "saturated" (*left*), flowing blood enters the slice with its full magnetization and thus has a high signal (*right*). This "bright-blood" technique is also termed the *time-of-flight* or *inflow* technique. **B,** The opposite approach can be used, in which flowing blood appears dark. In this technique, the desired slice is imaged to recover signal only from stationary structures (*left*). No signal is recovered from flowing blood entering the slice (*right*). This "black-blood" technique is ideal for imaging the vessel wall. **C,** A third technique, termed *phase-contrast* or *phase-velocity mapping*, allows direct quantification of blood flow velocity. The signal from spinning nuclei has both a magnitude and a phase. The nuclei (*arrows*) are initially in phase (*left*), but imaging with this technique in the presence of a magnetic field gradient induces a phase shift in moving blood that is directly proportional to velocity (*right*). The resulting phase image is thus a velocity map.

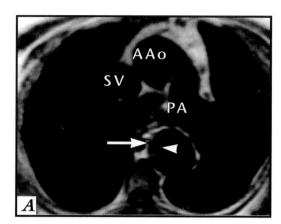

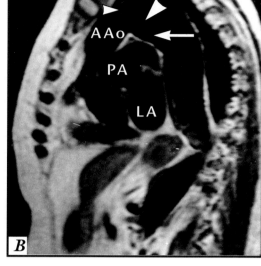

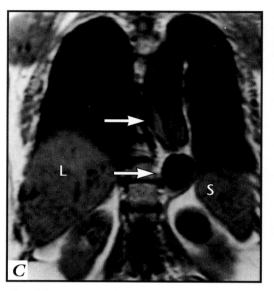

FIGURE 8-6. Magnetic resonance images of a patient with an aortic dissection from three orthogonal imaging planes [1]. **A,** Axial image showing the proximal ascending aorta (AAo), which appears intact, as well as the descending thoracic aorta, where an intimal flap (*arrowhead*) is seen separating the true lumen (*long arrow*) from the false lumen. **B,** Sagittal image showing the aortic arch and the origin of the intimal tear (*small arrowhead*) just distal to the take-off of the left subclavian artery.

The intimal flap (*large arrowhead*) is seen extending down into the abdominal aorta, separating the true lumen (*long arrow*) and false lumen. **C,** Coronal image showing the dissection flap within the descending thoracic aorta. The *long arrows* indicate the true lumen. L—liver; LA—left atrium; S—spleen; PA—pulmonary artery; SVC—superior vena cava. (*Courtesy of* Eric M. Isselbacher, Joaquin E. Cigarroa, and Kim A. Eagle.)

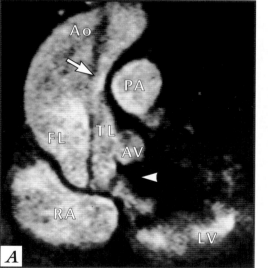

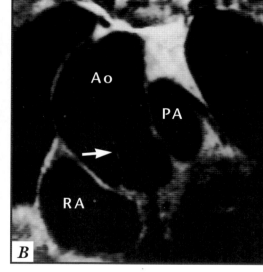

FIGURE 8-7. Magnetic resonance (MR) images of a patient with an ascending aortic dissection. **A,** The "bright blood" MR angiogram showing the ascending aorta (AAo). A dark linear structure representing the dissection flap (*arrow*) is seen extending from the level of the aortic valve (AV), which is closed in this diastolic image. There is an area of signal loss within the left ventricular (LV) outflow tract, which is caused by a jet of aortic insufficiency (*arrowhead*). **B,** The corresponding "black blood" image showing the dissection flap (*arrow*) in the AAo as a bright linear structure. FL—false lumen; PA—pulmonary artery; RA—right atrium; TL—true lumen.

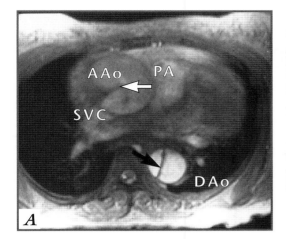

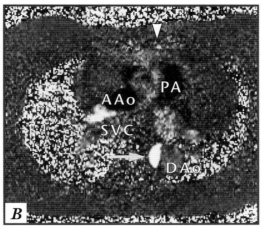

FIGURE 8-8. Phase-contrast magnetic resonance images depicting aortic flow in a patient with an ascending aortic (AAo) dissection. **A,** The magnitude image showing an enlarged AAo with a dissection flap (*white arrow*). The dissection flap (*black arrow*) is also seen in the descending thoracic aorta (DAo). **B,** The corresponding phase image depicts velocity, with blood flow toward the head appearing *black*, blood flow toward the feet appearing *white*, and no flow appearing *grey*. The true lumen is seen in the DAo as the region with high velocity (*arrow*) compared with the false lumen. Also seen are AAo and pulmonary artery (PA) flow, which appear *black*, and superior vena cava (SVC) and right internal mammary artery flow (*arrowhead*), which appear *white*.

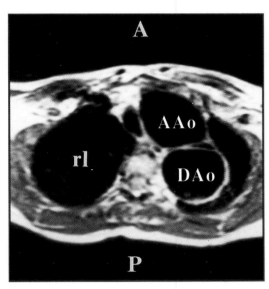

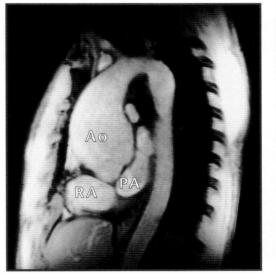

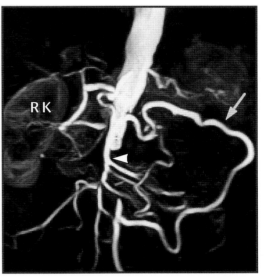

FIGURE 8-9. Magnetic resonance image of an aneurysmal aorta in a patient with Marfan syndrome. The aorta is visualized in the vicinity of the arch, and both the ascending aorta (AAo) and descending thoracic aorta (DAo) are dilated to approximately 5 to 6 cm. RL—right lung. (*Courtesy of* Carlos A. Roldan.)

FIGURE 8-10. Magnetic resonance angiogram showing an ascending aortic aneurysm. The aorta (Ao) is enlarged from the level of the aortic valve to the arch. However, the caliber appears normal beginning at the midaortic arch and extending down to the abdominal Ao. PA—pulmonary artery; RA—right atrium.

FIGURE 8-11. Magnetic resonance angiogram showing an occluded abdominal aorta. The abdominal aorta is seen to taper and then end abruptly at the level of the kidneys (*arrowhead*). The large collateral vessel (*arrow*) provides blood supply distal to the aortic occlusion. RK—right kidney.

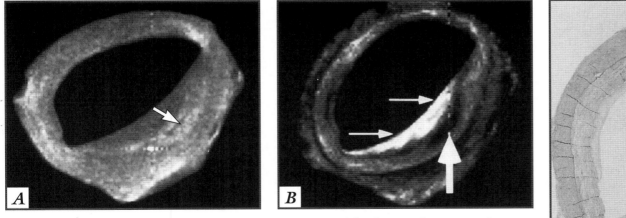

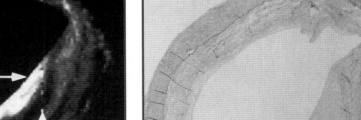

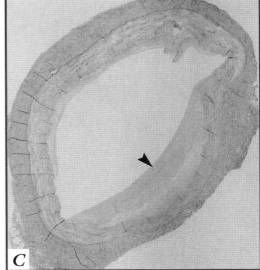

FIGURE 8-12. Human aortic plaque specimen. **A,** *In vitro* T_1-weighted magnetic resonance image showing an eccentric atherosclerotic plaque (*arrow*) with modest luminal narrowing. **B,** The matching T_2-weighted image is able to distinguish tissue characteristics within the plaque. The fibrous cap appears bright (*thin white arrows*), compared with the lipid core, which appears dark (*thick white arrow*). **C,** The matching trichrome-stained histology specimen showing the eccentric plaque (*black arrowhead*). (*From* Toussaint and coworkers [2]; with permission.)

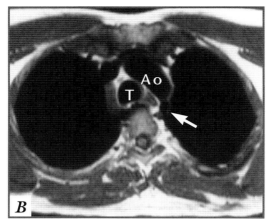

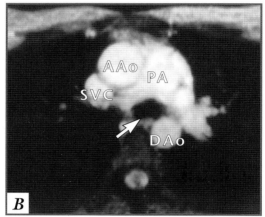

FIGURE 8-13. Magnetic resonance images of a patient with coarctation of the aorta (Ao). **A,** Sagittal image showing the aortic arch and descending thoracic aorta. There is marked narrowing at the beginning of the descending aorta (*arrow*). **B,** The axial image is at the level of the aortic arch and shows the coarctation (*arrow*) at the junction with the descending aorta. LA—left atrium; PA—pulmonary artery; RV—right ventricle; T—trachea.

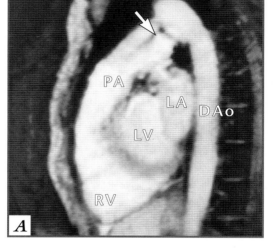

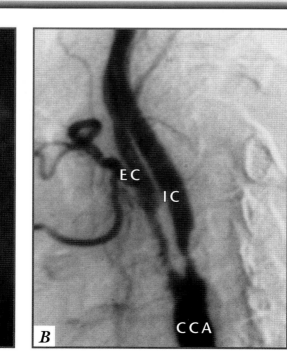

FIGURE 8-14. Matching magnetic resonance angiograms in a patient with a patent ductus arteriosus (PDA). **A,** Sagittal image showing the pulmonary artery (PA) and the descending aorta (DAo). An area of signal loss (*arrow*) is seen within the PA adjacent to the aorta, corresponding to the flow jet from the PDA. **B,** Axial image showing the ascending aorta (AAo), the DAo, and the PA at the level of its bifurcation. The flow from the DAo through the PDA causes a large area of signal loss (*arrow*) in the PA. LA—left atrium; LV—left ventricle; RV—right ventricle; SVC—superior vena cava.

CEREBROVASCULAR STRUCTURES

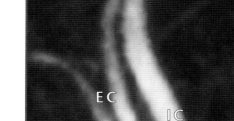

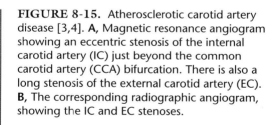

FIGURE 8-15. Atherosclerotic carotid artery disease [3,4]. **A,** Magnetic resonance angiogram showing an eccentric stenosis of the internal carotid artery (IC) just beyond the common carotid artery (CCA) bifurcation. There is also a long stenosis of the external carotid artery (EC). **B,** The corresponding radiographic angiogram, showing the IC and EC stenoses.

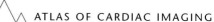

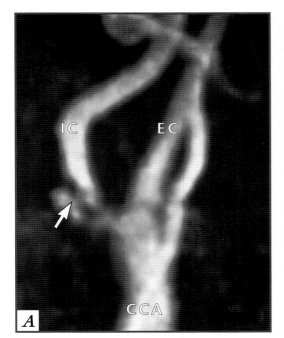

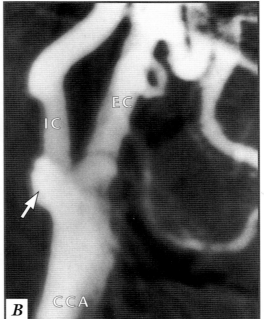

FIGURE 8-16. Carotid artery disease complicated by ulceration. **A,** Magnetic resonance angiogram of the carotid artery bifurcation showing an ulceration (*arrow*) of the internal carotid artery (IC) just after the bifurcation. **B,** The IC ulceration (*arrow*) is depicted by radiographic angiography. CCA—common carotid artery; EC—external carotid artery.

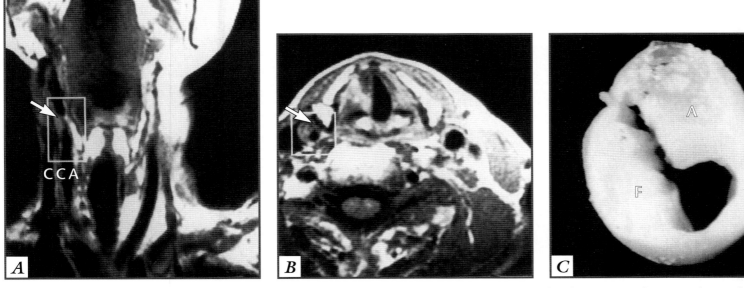

FIGURE 8-17. Carotid plaque imaging. **A,** Coronal image showing the carotid arteries extending from the neck. There is a stenosis of the right common and internal carotid arteries (*arrow*). **B,** Axial image through the right internal carotid artery stenosis showing a small lumen and a large area of atherosclerotic plaque (*arrow*). There is a relative decrease in signal intensity in the medial aspect of the plaque. **C,** Dissection microscopy of the plaque removed at carotid endarterectomy demonstrating a calcified atheromatous core (A) in the medial portion of the plaque and an overlying fibrous region (F). The tear through the plaque was caused by surgery. CCA—common carotid artery. (*From* Toussaint and coworkers [5]; with permission.)

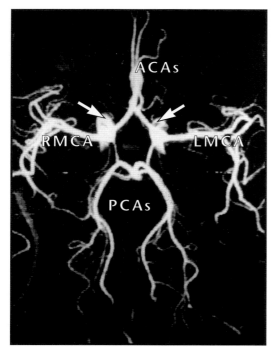

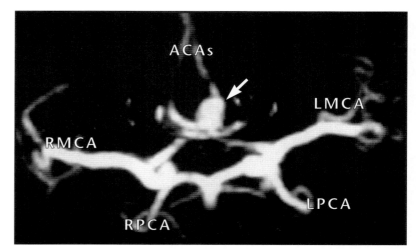

FIGURE 8-18.
Normal magnetic resonance angiogram of the cerebral vessels and the circle of Willis. The anterior, middle, and posterior cerebral arteries are seen, as well as the internal carotid arteries (*arrows*). ACAs—anterior cerebral arteries; LMCA—left middle cerebral artery; PCAs—posterior cerebral arteries; RMCA—right middle cerebral artery.

FIGURE 8-19. A magnetic resonance angiogram in a patient with a cerebral aneurysm. The anterior, middle, and posterior cerebral arteries and the circle of Willis are seen at an oblique angle. There is an aneurysm (*arrow*) of the anterior communicating cerebral artery, which is associated with an abnormal splaying of the anterior cerebral arteries (ACAs) due to bleeding from the aneurysm. LMCA—left middle cerebral artery; LPCA—left posterior cerebral artery; RMCA—right middle cerebral artery; RPCA—right posterior cerebral artery.

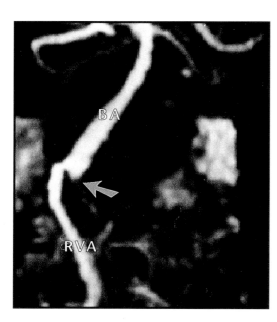

FIGURE 8-20. A magnetic resonance angiogram in a patient with a vertebrobasilar stroke [6]. The basilar (BA) and right vertebral arteries (RVA) appear intact. However, there is minimal signal in the left vertebral artery as it joins the basilar artery (*arrow*) that is consistent with occlusion, most likely from an embolic source. (*Courtesy of* Frances E. Jensen and Mark A. Creager.)

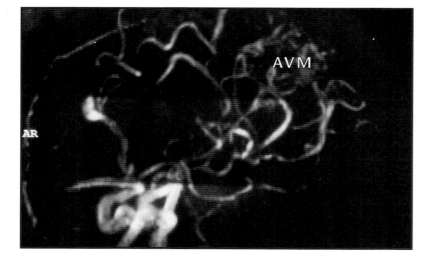

FIGURE 8-21. A sagittal magnetic resonance angiogram in a patient with an arteriovenous malformation (AVM), characterized by redundant, tortuous vessels.

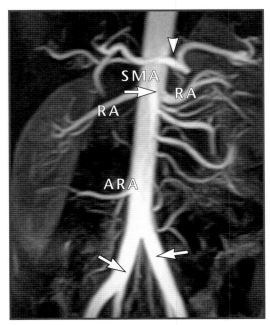

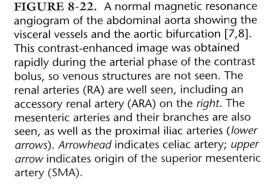

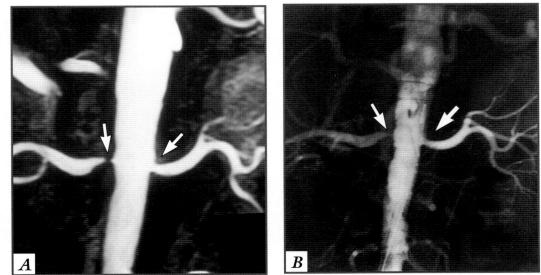

FIGURE 8-23. Renal artery stenosis [7,8]. **A,** Contrast-enhanced magnetic resonance angiogram showing a severe stenosis of the proximal right renal artery (*left arrow*) and a mild narrowing of the proximal left renal artery (*right arrow*). **B,** Matching radiographic angiogram depicting the renal artery stenoses (*arrows*).

FIGURE 8-22. A normal magnetic resonance angiogram of the abdominal aorta showing the visceral vessels and the aortic bifurcation [7,8]. This contrast-enhanced image was obtained rapidly during the arterial phase of the contrast bolus, so venous structures are not seen. The renal arteries (RA) are well seen, including an accessory renal artery (ARA) on the *right*. The mesenteric arteries and their branches are also seen, as well as the proximal iliac arteries (*lower arrows*). *Arrowhead* indicates celiac artery; *upper arrow* indicates origin of the superior mesenteric artery (SMA).

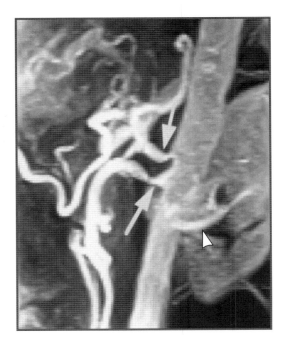

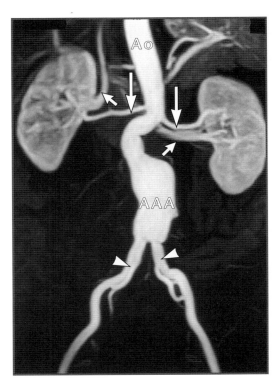

FIGURE 8-24. Contrast-enhanced magnetic resonance angiogram in a patient with mesenteric ischemia. Proximal stenoses are seen in both the celiac (*upper arrow*) and superior mesenteric (*lower arrow*) arteries. The left renal artery is also seen (*arrowhead*).

FIGURE 8-25. Contrast-enhanced magnetic resonance angiogram in a patient with an abdominal aortic aneurysm (AAA). A modest-sized aneurysm is seen originating below the renal arteries (*long arrows*) and extending to the level of the aortic bifurcation. The renal arteries and iliac arteries (*arrowheads*) are well visualized without evidence of disease. The visualization of the renal veins (*short arrows*) and renal perfusion on this study was due to later imaging after contrast injection. Ao—aorta.

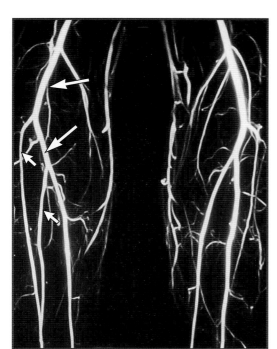

FIGURE 8-26. Normal magnetic resonance angiogram of the lower extremity arteries [9]. Contrast enhancement is used as well as subtraction of the baseline (precontrast) image to reduce background signal [9]. There are many tertiary vessels seen, even extending down to the calf vessels. The *long upper arrow* indicates the popliteal; the *short upper arrow* indicates the anterior tibial; the *long lower arrow* indicates the posterior tibial, and the *short lower arrow* indicates the peroneal.

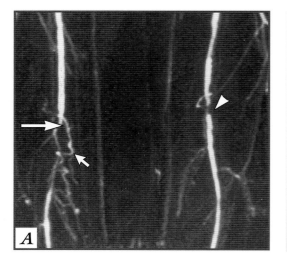

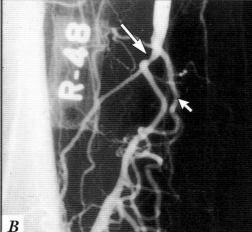

FIGURE 8-27. Lower extremity peripheral vascular disease. **A,** Magnetic resonance angiogram showing bilateral superficial femoral artery (SFA) disease. The right SFA vessel is occluded (*long arrow*) with collateral vessels (*short arrow*) reconstituting the distal vessel; the left SFA has a severe stenosis (*arrowhead*). **B,** Corresponding angiogram for the right SFA demonstrating the occluded vessel (*long arrow*) and the multiple collateral vessels (*short arrow*). (*From* Adamis and coworkers [9]; with permission.)

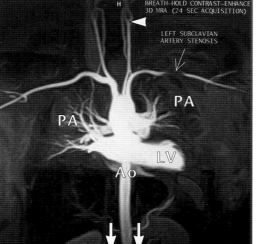

FIGURE 8-28. Contrast-enhanced magnetic resonance angiogram in a patient with upper extremity arterio-occlusive disease. A stenosis of the left subclavian artery is seen (*upper arrow*). The carotid arteries (*arrowhead*), pulmonary arteries (PAs), abdominal aorta (Ao), and renal arteries (*lower arrows*) are also seen. LV—left ventricle.

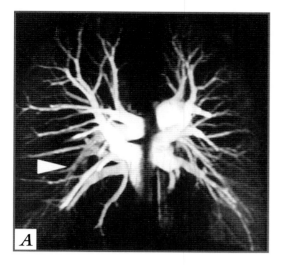

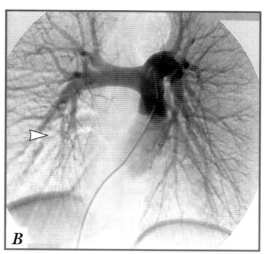

FIGURE 8-29. Pulmonary embolism (PE) [10,11]. **A,** Pulmonary magnetic resonance angiogram is obtained with contrast enhancement during breath-holding. Two separate contrast injections and breath-holds are used to separately image the right and left pulmonary arteries, which results in an artefact in the center of the image. Note the detail of the subsegmental vessels seen and the poor signal enhancement of one of the subsegmental vessels going to the right lower lobe (*arrowhead*), indicative of pulmonary embolism. **B,** Corresponding radiographic angiogram also showing the loss of vessels in the right lower lobe region (*arrowhead*) due to pulmonary embolism. (*Courtesy of* Piotr A. Wielopolski.)

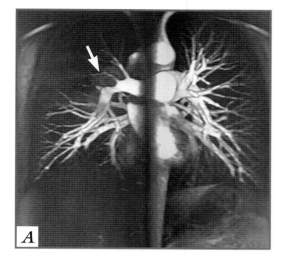

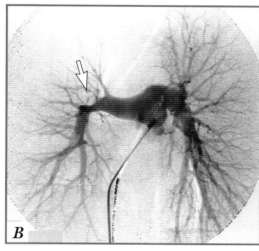

FIGURE 8-30. Tumor in the right upper lobe. **A,** Contrast-enhanced pulmonary magnetic resonance angiogram showing the normal, extensive arterial tree on the *left,* but a marked loss of pulmonary arteries in the *right* upper lobe region. **B,** The corresponding radiographic angiogram also showing the lack of pulmonary arteries to the right upper lobe. *Arrows* indicate the area of the tumor. (*Courtesy of* Piotr A. Wielopolski.)

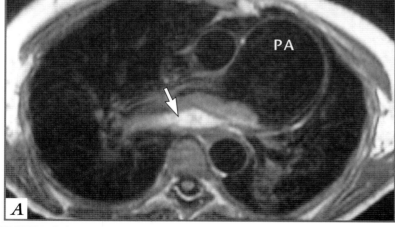

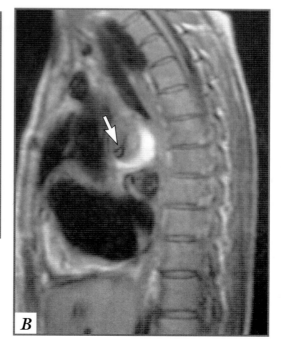

FIGURE 8-31. Magnetic resonance (MR) images of a patient with advanced pulmonary hypertension. The patient had Eisenmenger's complex, with increasing shortness of breath, right-side heart failure, and cyanosis. **A,** Axial MR image demonstrating severe enlargement of the proximal pulmonary artery (PA) with a large *in situ* thrombus seen extending into the right PA (*arrow*). **B,** Sagittal image through the right PA demonstrating an almost complete occlusion of the vessel (*arrow*). T$_2$-weighted image showing two distinct appearances of the thrombus. The *outer bright thrombus* is probably chronic in nature, with the *inner gray thrombus* likely subacute and the cause of the patient's recent symptoms. (*Courtesy of* Evan Loh.)

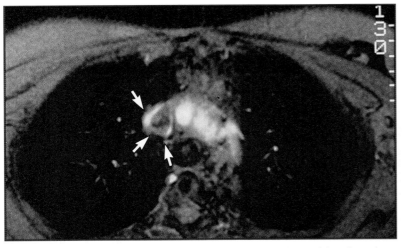

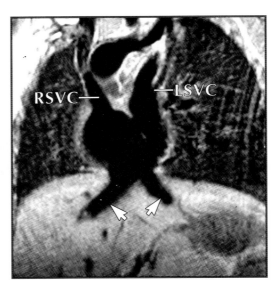

FIGURE 8-32. Magnetic resonance venogram in a patient with a thrombus (*arrows*) within the superior vena cava (SVC) [12]. On this "bright-blood" image, blood flow is only seen along the perimeter of the SVC, with a large area of signal loss corresponding to a filling defect within the center of the SVC, typical of acute venous thrombosis. (*Courtesy of* Joseph F. Polak.)

FIGURE 8-33. Magnetic resonance images showing congenitally anomalous venous anatomy. This patient has bilateral superior venae cavae as well as bilateral hepatic veins (*arrows*) draining into a common atrium. LSVC—left superior vena cava; RSVC—right superior vena cava. (*Courtesy of* Tal Geva.)

CORONARY STRUCTURES

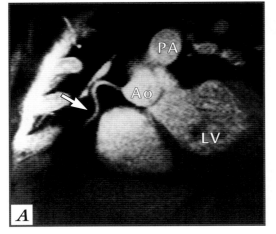

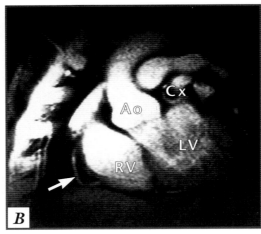

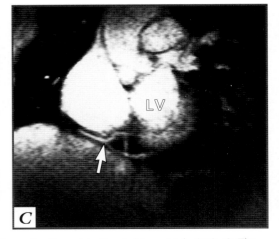

FIGURE 8-34. Coronary magnetic resonance angiograms of a normal right coronary artery (RCA). Electrocardiographic (ECG) gating timed for diastole is used during breath-holding for each image to minimize cardiac and respiratory motion. **A,** The proximal RCA (*arrow*), including shepherd's crook. Note also the left ventricle (LV) and the aortic (Ao) valve, which is closed. **B,** The mid-RCA (*arrow*) adjacent to the right ventricle (RV). **C,** The distal RCA (*arrow*), giving off posterior LV branches along the diaphragmatic surface of the heart. Cx—circumflex artery; PA—pulmonary artery. (*From* Manning and coworkers [13]; with permission.)

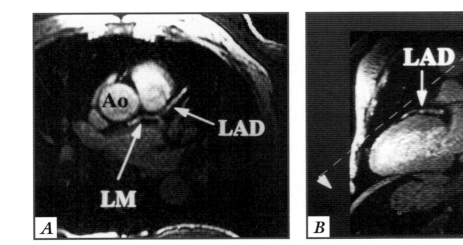

FIGURE 8-35. Breath-hold coronary magnetic resonance angiograms of a normal left coronary artery. **A,** Axial image showing the left main coronary artery (LM) bifurcating into the left circumflex and the left anterior descending coronary artery (LAD). **B,** Oblique image along the LAD showing its course along the anterior left ventricular wall. Ao—aorta.

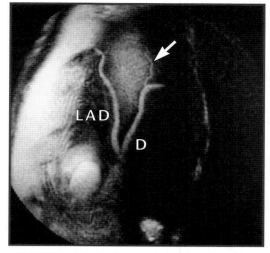

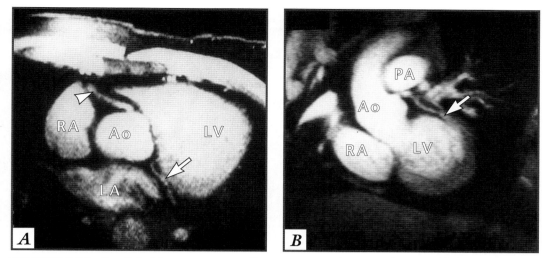

FIGURE 8-36. A high-resolution breath-hold coronary magnetic resonance angiogram of a normal left coronary artery [14]. The inplane spatial resolution is 0.8 X 0.8 mm. This oblique image showing the proximal and mid–left anterior descending artery (LAD), as well as a large diagonal branch (D), with a small tertiary branch off the diagonal (*arrow*). High resolution will be necessary to fully evaluate coronary artery disease in small distal and branch vessels. (*Courtesy of* Bob S. Hu.)

FIGURE 8-37. Breath-hold coronary magnetic resonance angiograms of a normal left circumflex artery (Cx). **A,** Axial image showing the Cx extending posteriorly in the atrioventricular (AV) groove (*arrow*). The proximal right coronary artery (RCA) extends anteriorly in the AV groove (*arrowhead*). **B,** Oblique image along the Cx showing the left main originating from the aorta (Ao) and giving off the Cx (*arrow*), which courses adjacent to the lateral left ventricular (LV) wall. LA—left atrium; LAD—left anterior descending coronary artery; PA—pulmonary artery; RA—right atrium.

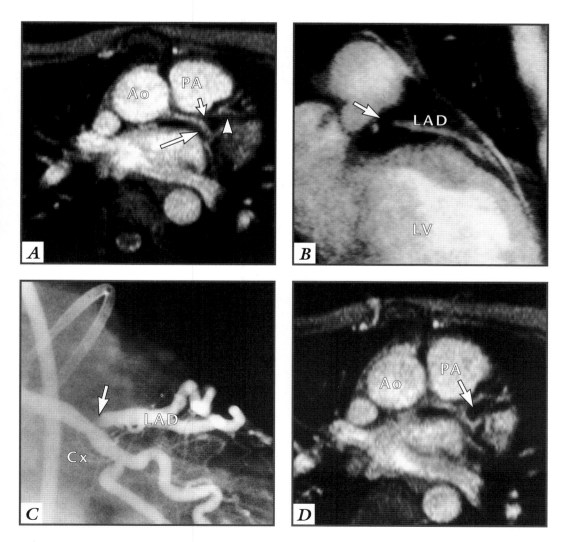

FIGURE 8-38. Magnetic resonance (MR) images from a patient with a left anterior descending coronary artery (LAD) stenosis who underwent angioplasty. **A,** Axial coronary MR angiogram showing the left main coronary artery and the bifurcation into the LAD and left circumflex artery (Cx; *large arrow*). There is signal loss in the proximal LAD just after the bifurcation (*small arrow*), indicating a significant stenosis. Distal to this stenosis, the mid-LAD and a diagonal branch (*arrowhead*) are seen. **B,** Oblique coronary MR angiogram along the LAD also showing the area of discrete signal loss due to the proximal stenosis (*arrow*). **C,** Corresponding radiographic angiogram showing the tight stenosis at the origin of the LAD (*arrow*). **D,** Axial coronary MR angiogram of the same patient after angioplasty of the LAD stenosis. Signal is now seen in the proximal LAD. Ao—aorta; PA—pulmonary artery. (Parts A and C *from* Manning and Edelman [15]; with permission.)

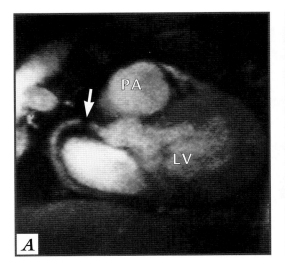

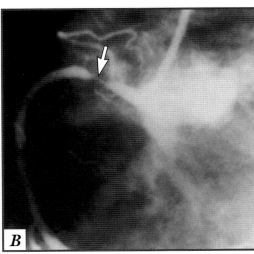

FIGURE 8-39. Proximal right coronary artery (RCA) stenosis [16]. **A,** Magnetic resonance angiogram of the entire proximal and mid-RCA produced by combining several adjacent slices into a single projection. There is an area of complete signal loss in the proximal RCA due to the stenosis (*arrow*). **B,** Corresponding radiographic angiogram demonstrating the severe proximal RCA stenosis (*arrow*). LV—left ventricle; PA—pulmonary artery.

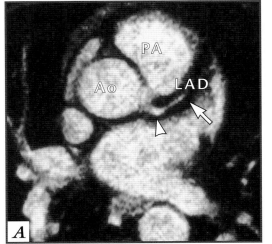

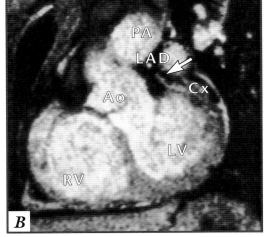

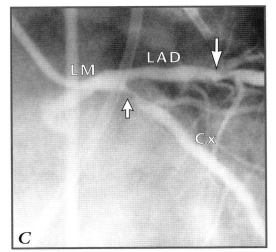

FIGURE 8-40. Magnetic resonance images from a patient with both left anterior descending and circumflex coronary artery stenoses. **A,** Axial image showing the left main (LM; *arrowhead*) and the proximal left anterior descending coronary artery (LAD). The LAD appears to end abruptly after the proximal portion (*arrow*), and the proximal circumflex (Cx) is not seen. **B,** Oblique image along the Cx showing a discrete area of signal loss in the proximal vessel (*arrow*) as it extends along the lateral left ventricular (LV) wall. The proximal LAD is seen in cross-section in this image. **C,** Corresponding radiographic angiogram showing both the LAD stenosis just beyond the proximal portion of the vessel (*large arrow*) and the Cx stenosis at its origin (*small arrow*). Ao—aorta; PA—pulmonary artery; RV—right ventricle.

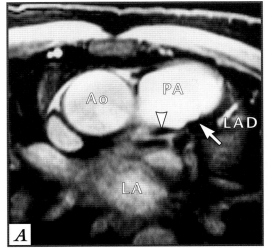

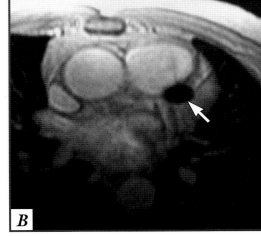

FIGURE 8-41. Coronary magnetic resonance (MR) angiograms in a patient with a coronary artery stent. Although coronary stents are not ferromagnetic and thus are not thought to be a risk for MR imaging, the metal does cause a large area of signal loss due to the induced inhomogeneity in the magnetic field. **A,** Axial coronary MR angiogram showing the left main (*arrowhead*) and left anterior descending coronary artery (LAD), with a large area of signal loss in the proximal LAD (*arrow*). As is typical, this coronary image uses a fat-suppression technique to suppress the signal from epicardial fat and increase vessel contrast. **B,** The same axial coronary MR angiogram without fat suppression. Here, the area of signal loss (*arrow*) extends well beyond the diameter of the coronary, indicating a coronary artery stent artifact and not simply a coronary artery stenosis. Ao—aorta; LA—left atrium; PA—pulmonary artery; RV—right ventricle. (*Courtesy of* André Deurinckx.)

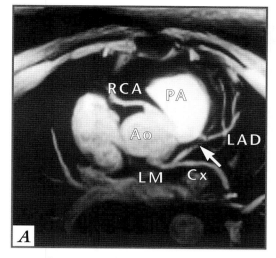 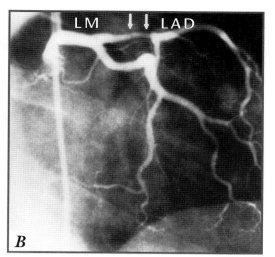

FIGURE 8-42. Coronary magnetic resonance (MR) angiogram obtained during free breathing in a patient with left anterior descending coronary artery (LAD) disease. Respiratory gating can be used instead of repetitive breath-holding [17,18]. A rapid line image (as in M-mode echocardiography) through the diaphragm is obtained during coronary imaging in order to track the motion of the diaphragm. Then, only the image data obtained at end-expiration is used to form the final image. This allows the patient to breathe freely and avoids the misregistration problem associated with trying to combine multiple separate breath-hold images. **A,** This respiratory-gated coronary MR angiogram has undergone postprocessing to combine the stack of axial images into a single projection and to segment out overlying cardiac structures. Both the left and right coronary arteries are seen, and the proximal LAD stenosis is demonstrated (*arrow*). **B,** Corresponding radiographic angiogram showing the proximal LAD stenosis (*arrows*). Ao—aorta; Cx—circumflex artery; LM—left main coronary artery; PA—pulmonary artery; RCA—right coronary artery. (*From* Haacke and coworkers [19]; with permission.)

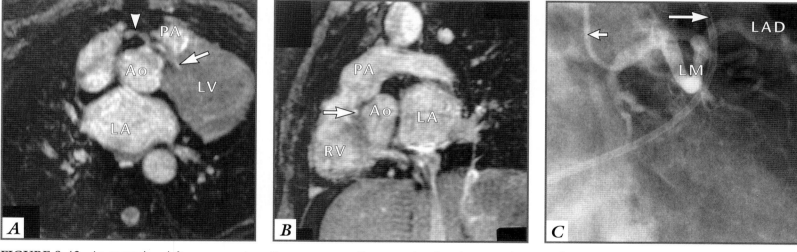

FIGURE 8-43. An anomalous left coronary artery. Coronary magnetic resonance (MR) angiography has been shown to be useful for identifying and evaluating anomalous coronary arteries and their three-dimensional path [20,21]. **A,** Axial coronary MR angiogram showing a single coronary artery originating from the right coronary cusp of the aorta (Ao). This gives rise to the right coronary artery (*arrowhead*) and the left main coronary artery (LM; *arrow*), which courses anterior to the Ao and posterior to the pulmonary artery (PA). **B,** Oblique image obtained orthogonal to the LM showing the anomalous vessel in cross section (*arrow*) between the Ao and PA. This anatomy has been associated with sudden death. **C,** Radiographic angiogram showing the LM coronary artery traversing anterior to the coronary catheter (*short arrow*) but posterior to the PA catheter (*long arrow*) before giving rise to the left anterior descending artery (LAD). LA—left atrium; LV—left ventricle; RV—right ventricle. (*From* McConnell and coworkers [20]; with permission.)

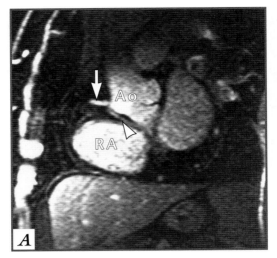

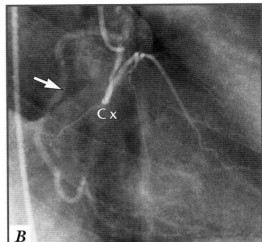

FIGURE 8-44. An anomalous left circumflex coronary artery anomaly. **A,** Coronary magnetic resonance (MR) angiogram showing two vessels originating from the right coronary cusp. In addition to a normal right coronary artery (RCA; *arrow*), a small circumflex artery (Cx; *arrowhead*) is seen coursing inferiorly and posteriorly. This anomaly is not associated with sudden death. **B,** Corresponding radiographic angiogram showing the posterior and inferior path of the anomalous Cx. The RCA is partially opacified (*arrow*). Ao—aorta; RA—right atrium. (*From* McConnell and coworkers [20]; with permission.)

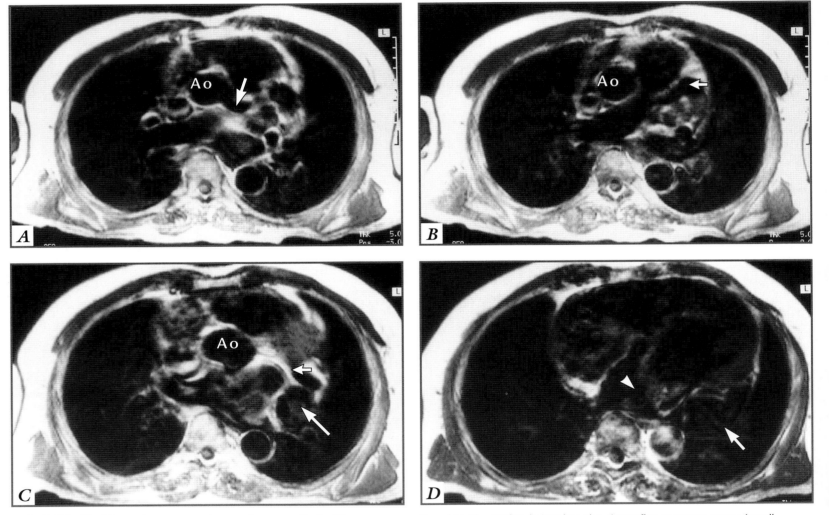

FIGURE 8-45. Magnetic resonance images from a patient with a coronary arteriovenous (AV) fistula. **A,** The increased coronary flow caused by the AV fistula results in the abnormal appearance of the coronary arteries, beginning with the markedly dilated left main coronary artery (*arrow*).

B and **C,** The AV fistula involves the circumflex coronary artery (*small arrows*), which is dilated and is connected to a large venous lake (*large arrow*). **D,** The venous lake (*arrow*) communicates with an enlarged coronary sinus (*arrowhead*). Ao—aorta.

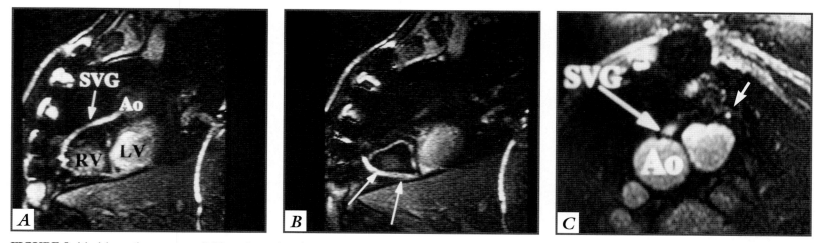

FIGURE 8-46. Magnetic resonance (MR) angiography of coronary artery bypass grafts [22]. Bypass grafts are typically larger in size and undergo less motion than do coronary arteries, which helps MR imaging. However, artefacts from metal clips, aortic markers, and sternal wires can interfere with imaging the entire graft and reliably identifying stenoses. **A** and **B**, MR angiograms showing the proximal and distal portion of a normal saphenous vein bypass graft (SVG; *arrows*) coursing from the aorta (Ao) to the posterior descending artery anterior to the right ventricle (RV). **C**, MR angiogram from a patient with an occluded saphenous vein graft (SVG). There is signal loss at the origin of the SVG due to a metal aortic marker and then the vessel ends abruptly, indicating a proximal occlusion. The bright signal of the left internal mammary artery graft (*arrow*) seen in cross-section indicates patency. LV—left ventricle.

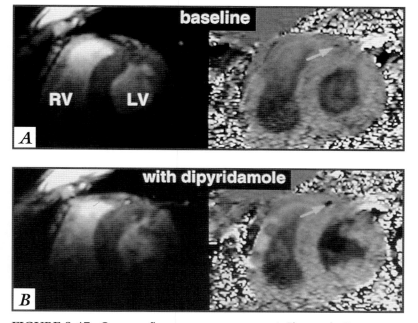
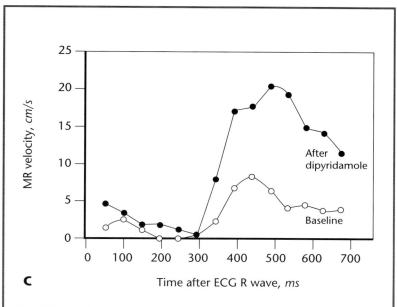

FIGURE 8-47. Coronary flow reserve measurement. Phase-velocity mapping can be applied to the measurement of coronary flow [23]. **A**, Short-axis magnitude (*left*) and phase (*right*) magnetic resonance (MR) images showing the left anterior descending coronary artery (LAD; *arrow*) in cross section. Flow is seen within the LAD on the phase image at rest. **B**, With infusion of dipyridamole, increased flow within the LAD is seen (*arrow*).

C, Coronary flow over the cardiac cycle can be measured by obtaining phase-velocity images at multiple time points. Coronary flow reserve can be calculated from the ratio of hyperemic flow to rest flow and is reduced in the presence of a flow-limiting coronary stenosis. LV—left ventricle; RV—right ventricle. (*Courtesy of* Hajime Sakuma.)

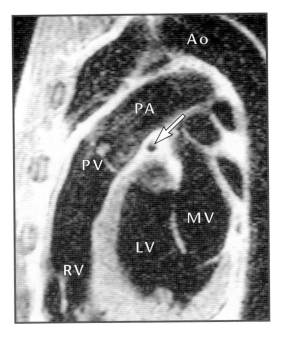

FIGURE 8-48. Imaging the coronary wall. Magnetic resonance (MR) image obtained during breath-holding using a "black-blood" technique to null the signal from blood. The left main coronary artery (LM) is seen in this normal subject (*arrow*). This technique has the potential to directly image coronary atherosclerosis. Note the pulmonic valve (PV) and mitral valve (MV) leaflets. Ao—aorta; LV—left ventricle; PA—pulmonary artery; RV—right ventricle.

REFERENCES

1. Nienaber CA, von Kodolitsch Y, Nicolas V, *et al.*: The diagnosis of thoracic aortic dissection by noninvasive imaging procedures. *N Engl J Med* 1993, 328:1–9.

2. Toussaint JF, Southern JF, Fuster V, Kantor HL: T2-weighted contrast for NMR characterization of human atherosclerosis. *Arterioscler Thromb Vasc Biol* 1995, 15:1533–1542.

3. Polack JF, Bajakian RL, Oleary DH, *et al.*: Detection of internal carotid artery stenosis: comparison of MR angiography, color Doppler sonography, and arteriography. *Radiology* 1992, 182:35–40.

4. Mattle HP, Kent KC, Edelman RR, *et al.*: Evaluation of the extracranial carotid arteries: correlation of magnetic resonance angiography, duplex ultrasonography, and conventional angiography. *J Vasc Surg* 1991, 13:838–845.

5. Toussaint JF, LaMuraglia GM, Southern JF, *et al.*: Magnetic resonance images lipid, fibrous, calcified, hemorrhagic, and thrombotic components of human atherosclerosis in vivo. *Circulation* 1996, 94:932–938.

6. Warach S, Li W, Ronthal M, *et al.*: Acute cerebral ischemia: evaluation with dynamic contrast-enhanced MR imaging and MR angiography. *Radiology* 1992, 182:41–47.

7. Prince MR, Narasimham DL, Stanley JC, *et al.*: Breath-hold gadolinium-enhanced MR angiography of the abdominal aorta and its major branches. *Radiology* 1995, 197:785–792.

8. Holland GA, Dougherty L, Carpenter JP, *et al.*: Breath-hold ultrafast three-dimensional gadolinium-enhanced MR angiography of the aorta and the renal and other visceral abdominal arteries. *AJR Am J Roentgenol* 1996, 166:971–981.

9. Adamis MK, Li W, Wielopolski PA, *et al.*: Dynamic contrast-enhanced subtraction MR angiography of the lower extremities: initial evaluation with a multi-section two-dimensional time-of-flight sequence. *Radiology* 1995, 196:689–695.

10. Meaney JF, Weg JG, Chenevert TL, *et al.*: Diagnosis of pulmonary embolism with magnetic resonance angiography. *N Engl J Med* 1997, 336:1422–1427.

11. Wielopolski PA, Haacke EM, Adler LP. Three-dimensional MR imaging of the pulmonary vasculature: preliminary experience. *Radiology* 1992, 183:465–472.

12. Erdman WA, Jayson HT, Redman HC, *et al.*: Deep venous thrombosis of extremities: role of MR imaging in the diagnosis. *Radiology* 1990, 174:425–431.

13. Manning WJ, Li W, Boyle NG, Edelman RR: Fat-suppressed breath-hold magnetic resonance coronary angiography. *Circulation* 1993, 87:94–104.

14. Meyer CH, Hu BS, Nishimura DG, Macovski A: Fast spiral coronary artery imaging. *Magn Reson Med* 1992, 28:202–213.

15. Manning WJ, Edelman RR: MR coronary angiography. *Magn Reson Q* 1993, 9:131–151.

16. Manning WJ, Li W, Edelman RR: A preliminary report comparing magnetic resonance coronary angiography with conventional angiography. *N Engl J Med* 1993, 328:828–832.

17. Wang Y, Rossman PJ, Grimm RC, *et al.*: Navigator-echo-based real-time respiratory gating and triggering for reduction of respiration effects in three-dimensional coronary MR angiography. *Radiology* 1996, 198:55–60.

18. McConnell MV, Khasgiwala VC, Savord BJ, *et al.*: Comparison of respiratory suppression methods and navigator locations for MR coronary angiography. *Am J Roentgenol* 1997, 168:1369–1375.

19. Haacke EM, Li D, Kaushikkar S: Cardiac MR imaging: principles and techniques. *Top Magn Reson Imaging* 1995, 7:200–217.

20. McConnell MV, Ganz P, Selwyn AP, *et al.*: Identification of anomalous coronary arteries and their anatomic course by magnetic resonance coronary angiography. *Circulation* 1995, 92:3158–3162.

21. Post JC, van Rossum AC, Bronzaer JGF, *et al.*: Magnetic resonance angiography of anomalous coronary arteries: a new gold standard for delineating the proximal course? *Circulation* 1995, 92:3158–3162.

22. Aurigemma GP, Reicheck N, Axel L, *et al.*: Noninvasive determination of coronary artery bypass graft patency by cine magnetic resonance imaging. *Circulation* 1989, 80:1595–1602.

23. Sakuma H, Blake LM, Amidon TM, *et al.*: Coronary flow reserve: noninvasive measurement in humans with breath-hold velocity-encoded cine MR imaging. *Radiology* 1996, 198:745–750.

9

Magnetic Resonance Imaging of Cardiac Structures

Christopher M. Kramer

Magnetic resonance imaging (MRI) is becoming increasingly useful as applied to the cardiovascular system. A thorough assessment of the structure of the cardiac chambers in congenital and acquired disease, myocardial function and perfusion, valvular function, and spectroscopic evaluation of cardiac energetics can be performed by MRI. Applications of cardiac MRI are expanding rapidly as clinicians and investigators bring to bear newer technologic advances in magnetic resonance hardware and software.

Since the early 1980s, investigators have known of the power of MRI to accurately assess the structure of the heart [1–4]. Distinguishing blood pool from cardiac structures is facilitated because of signal reduction from blood flow with spin-echo techniques and bright blood signal using gradient-echo or cine techniques. The volume and muscle mass of the left and right ventricles and the size of the left and right atrium and aorta can be readily obtained. Newer rapid imaging techniques allow evaluation of cardiac structure in one or a few breath-holds. Wall thickening and ejection fraction are easily evaluated using cine MRI techniques [5,6]. With automated analytic techniques, quantitation of left ventricular mass and volumes is

becoming simplified [7]. Newer methods for evaluation of intramyocardial function include myocardial tagging [8–12] and phase-velocity techniques [13].

To evaluate intracardiac shunts, cine MRI can demonstrate flow between chambers, and phase-velocity methods can estimate relative pulmonary and systemic blood flows. Other acquired and congenital diseases of the heart such as cardiomyopathies, both dilated and hypertrophic; myocardial infarction; intracardiac masses; right ventricular dysplasia; and pericardial diseases can be fully assessed by both spin-echo and gradient-echo imaging. The function of all the cardiac valves, including prostheses, can be evaluated by MRI.

Gadolinium-based contrast agents can be infused to assess myocardial perfusion in the setting of myocardial ischemia or acute or chronic myocardial infarction. The newest application of contrast MRI is in the evaluation of viability after myocardial infarction. Magnetic resonance spectroscopy is a specialized technology that when properly applied can assess the energy metabolism of the heart in normal and diseased states. MRI offers the potential for comprehensive imaging of the cardiovascular systems.

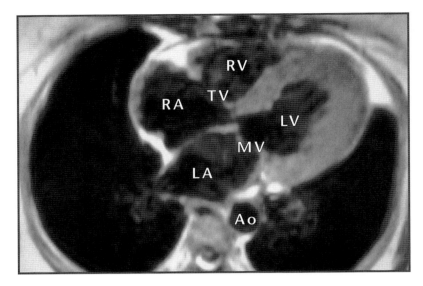

FIGURE 9-1. Oblique spin-echo magnetic resonance imaging in a transverse four-chamber plane. This illustration exemplifies black blood imaging in which the signal from flowing blood is eliminated. This imaging plane is quite useful to assess the size of all four cardiac chambers, function of the left ventricular (LV) septum and lateral walls, and function of the mitral valve (MV) and tricuspid valve (TV). Ao—aorta; LA—left atrium; RA—right atrium; RV—right ventricle.

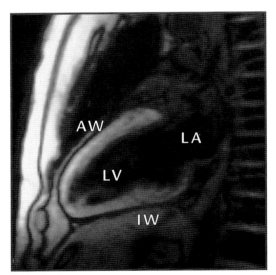

FIGURE 9-2. Oblique spin-echo magnetic resonance imaging in a parasagittal two-chamber plane. This parasagittal imaging plane is helpful in evaluating function in the anterior wall (AW) and inferior wall (IW) of the left ventricle (LV), size of the left atrium (LA), and function of the mitral valve.

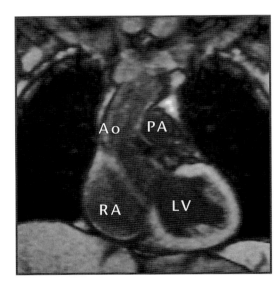

FIGURE 9-3. Spin-echo magnetic resonance imaging in a coronal plane. This plane is helpful in assessment of the left ventricle (LV), aortic valve, and ascending aorta (Ao). PA—pulmonary artery; RA—right atrium.

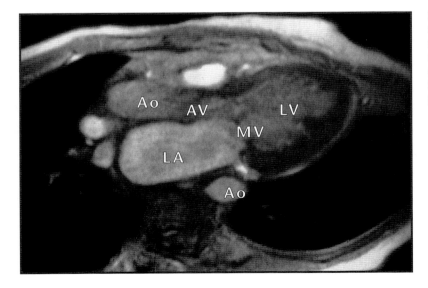

FIGURE 9-4. Oblique gradient-echo magnetic resonance imaging in a transverse three-chamber plane. Gradient-echo imaging produces a white signal from the blood pool, allowing excellent contrast between myocardium and blood. This imaging plane is used to evaluate the structure and function of the anteroseptal and posterior walls of the left ventricle (LV), the LV outflow tract and aortic root, and the function of the mitral valve (MV) and aortic valve (AV). Ao—aorta; LA—left atrium.

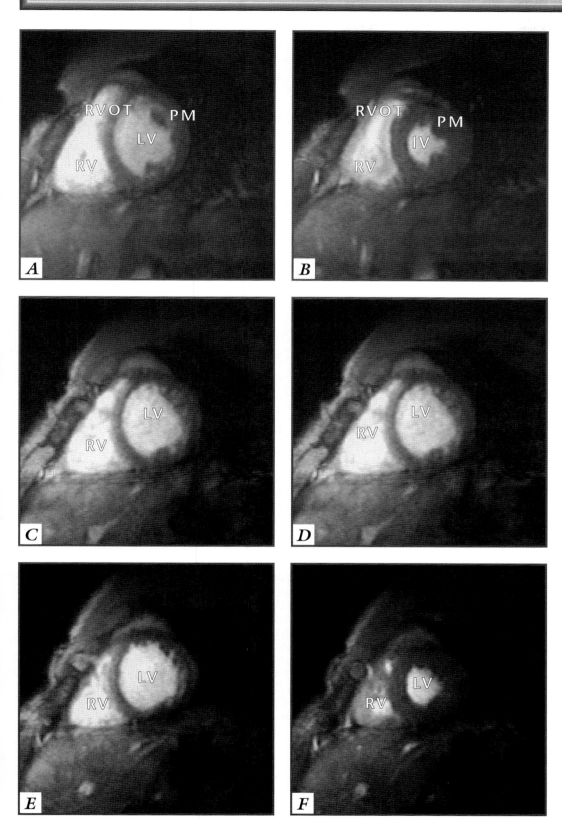

FIGURE 9-5. Gradient-echo cine magnetic resonance imaging in multiple oblique planes in the left ventricular short axis. Cine short-axis imaging is especially helpful in accurate measurements of left ventricular mass [1], volumes [2,3], and ejection fraction [4] from stacked short-axis slices. Regional ventricular function can also be readily assessed using these techniques [5,6]. **A** and **B**, End-diastolic and end-systolic short-axis images at the base of the left ventricle (LV). The right ventricular (RV) outflow tract (RVOT) and the papillary muscles (PMs) are seen on both the end-diastolic and end-systolic images. **C** and **D**, End-diastolic and end-systolic short-axis images at the mid-ventricle. **E** and **F**, End-diastolic and end-systolic short-axis images at the apex of the left ventricle (LV).

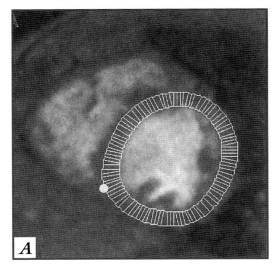

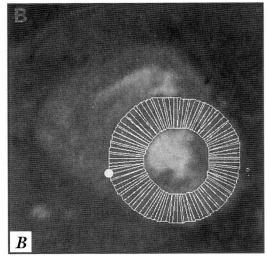

FIGURE 9-6. Gradient-echo short-axis images. These images demonstrate the quantitation of wall thickening from short-axis gradient-echo cine images at the midpapillary level at end-diastole (**A**) and end-systole (**B**) using the centerline method [7]. The endocardial and epicardial contours are shown as well as 100 equidistant chords, each representing the wall thickness at that point, that are placed perpendicular to the endocardial contour. The increase in length of each chord is calculated in order to calculate wall thickening. The starting points (*white dots*) in *A* and *B* are used to correct for rotational motion. (*From* Holman and coworkers [7]; with permission.)

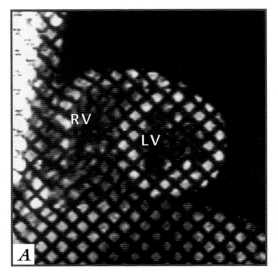

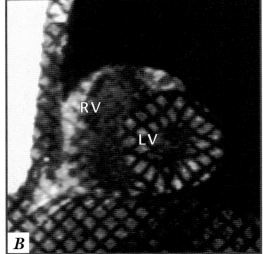

FIGURE 9-7. Gradient-echo tagged short-axis images. Magnetic resonance tagging is a novel approach to understanding left ventricular mechanics [8,9]. Radiofrequency and gradient pulses are applied in a parallel grid pattern using a technique called spatial modulation of magnetization (SPAMM) at end-diastole (**A**), in this case at the base of the left ventricle (LV), and "tag" the myocardium, allowing material points to be tracked throughout the cardiac cycle. The stripes remain embedded in myocardium and deform during systole and, as seen in the end-systolic image (**B**), converge more at the subendocardium than at the subepicardium. Normal values on a topographic basis have been derived for circumferential shortening [10] and two- [11] and three-dimensional deformation [12] from tagged images in normal human volunteers as a reference to compare disease states. RV—right ventricle.

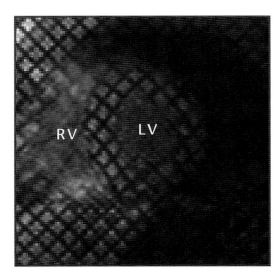

FIGURE 9-8. Gradient-echo tagged mid-diastolic short-axis image. The tagging sequence can be timed to place the tags on the myocardium at end-systole to track myocardial deformation during diastole. Note the stretching of myocardium as the tag stripes expand. Regional myocardial strain or deformation is analyzed using the finite element approach. This technique is based on the assumption that strain within a complex structure may be computed by subdividing it into small "elements" that have homogeneous properties. Using the tag intersections as trackable points, we may calculate intramyocardial strain without including bulk motion of the whole heart. The original position of each tag intersection (in this case end-systole) is compared with the position at a deformed state (in this case end-diastole), and a tensor describing the magnitude and direction (vector) of displacement is defined. By defining a tensor made up of two perpendicular tag segments, the magnitude and direction of maximal deformation may be computed. These values can be transformed to the "heart" coordinate system in which strain in the radial (wall thickening) and circumferential (circumferential shortening) may be determined. In order to determine a strain rate or maximal strain rate, the incremental change in tag position per unit time (the time between image phases) is determined.
LV—left ventricle; RV—right ventricle.

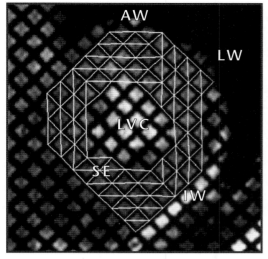

FIGURE 9-9. Spin-echo tagged end-diastolic short-axis image with tag stripe intersections marked and triangulated. To analyze the two-dimensional deformation of the tag stripes, computer software can be applied to mark the stripe intersections, create triangles using the stripe intersections, and track deformation of the triangles during the cardiac cycle. The Lagrangian strain tensors within the triangulated tissue can then be measured [11] as per the discussion in Figure 9-8. AW—anterior wall; IW—inferior wall; LVC—left ventricular cavity; LW—lateral wall; SE—septum.

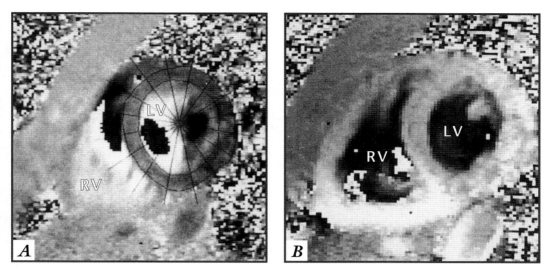

FIGURE 9-10. Velocity maps of left ventricular (LV) long-axis motion [13]. The magnetic resonance (MR) velocity mapping technique encodes the velocity of moving structures quantitatively in the phase of the MR signal, allowing accurate measurements. **A,** Systolic image showing an LV short axis with dark gray pixels demonstrating motion out of plane toward the reader. The endocardial and epicardial contours are drawn and the LV divided into 16 segments for quantitation of regional velocity. **B,** Diastolic image depicting motion away from the reader, and therefore encoded as a lighter gray shade. RV—right ventricle. (*From* Karwatowski and coworkers [13]; with permission.)

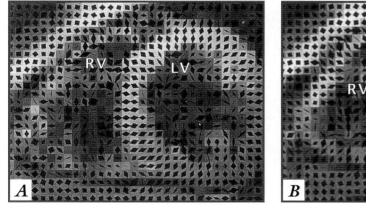

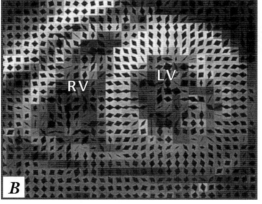

FIGURE 9-11. Motionless movie of myocardial strain rate [14] or the incremental change in deformation per unit time (the time between image phases) is determined from echo planar short-axis images at end-diastole (**A**) and end-systole (**B**). The strain-rate tensor at each pixel is represented by a rhomboid that depicts the effect of the measured strain rate on a square at each locus. In this way the myocardial state of motion at a particular point in time during the cardiac cycle can be displayed without cine images. Strain rates are oriented in a radial direction in the myocardium, consistent with normal thickening and circumferential shortening. LV—left ventricle; RV—right ventricle. (*From* van Wedeen and coworkers [14]; with permission.)

MAGNETIC RESONANCE IMAGING AND CONGENITAL HEART DISEASE

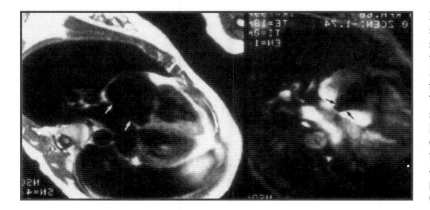

FIGURE 9-12. Spin-echo image (*left*) and cine image (*right*) of a secundum atrial septal defect (ASD) [15] in a four-chamber orientation, similar for both images. The *white arrows* point to the edges detected on the spin echo image, which estimate the size of the ASD as 22 mm. The *black arrows* on the cine image demonstrate the signal void (in *black*) from left-to-right flow of the ASD, which measures only 8 mm wide. These images demonstrate the potential overestimation of ASD size by spin-echo imaging owing to septal thinning adjacent to a secundum defect [15]. Phase-velocity mapping techniques allow more precise estimation of defect size [15,16]. Using phase velocity techniques, the ratio of pulmonary to systemic blood flow (Q_p/Q_s) can be calculated by measuring peak flow and cross-sectional areas of the pulmonary artery and aorta in planes perpendicular to the proximal portions of the respective great vessels. (*From* Holmvang and coworkers [15]; with permission.)

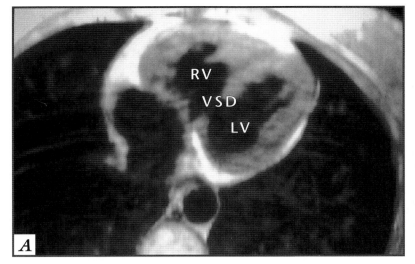

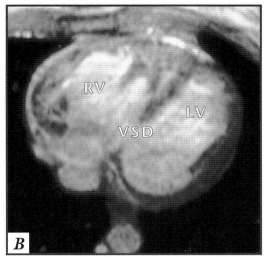

FIGURE 9-13. A, A transverse spin-echo image from a patient with a muscular ventricular septal defect (VSD). The size of the defect can be estimated from the length of the signal loss in the ventricular septum. This image is also useful for sizing the ventricular cavities. The right ventricle (RV) is dilated in this view. **B,** Cine imaging can be used to visualize the defects and in many cases to identify flow across the defects. This example is of a transverse gradient-echo cine image at end-diastole in the same patient as in *A*. The defect size can be estimated as can the size of the chambers. The RV is markedly dilated in this image. In this case, no clear-cut left-to-right flow was identified during systole because the patient had developed Eisenmenger's complex and most of the flow was right to left. In the setting of unidirectional shunts, the pulmonary-to-systemic blood flow ratios can be developed from magnetic resonance phase velocity images to estimate shunt ratios [16]. LV—left ventricle.

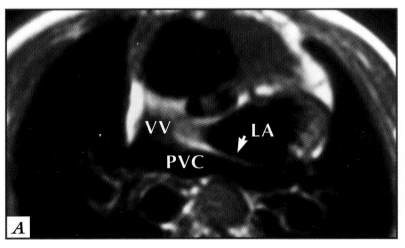

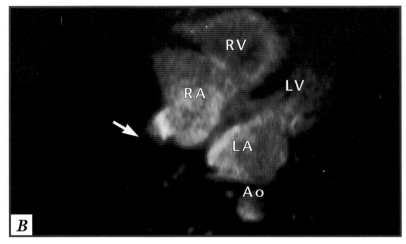

FIGURE 9-14. Axial spin-echo image demonstrating anomalous pulmonary venous return. The pulmonary venous confluence (PVC) is separated from the left atrium (LA) by a membrane (*arrow*) and drains into a right vertical vein (V V), which then drains into the right atrium (RA).

B, Axial gradient-echo image demonstrating the right inferior pulmonary vein (*arrow*) draining into the right atrium (RA), an example of partial anomalous pulmonary venous return. Ao—aorta; LV—left ventricle; RV—right ventricle. (Part A *courtesy of* Luc E. Jutras, Scott D. Flamm, and Charles B. Higgins.)

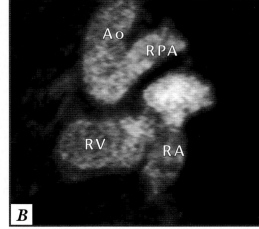

FIGURE 9-15. Axial (**A**) and sagittal (**B**) gradient-echo image in a patient with a conotruncal abnormality. These images demonstrate that the aorta (Ao) is the origin of the right pulmonary artery (RPA), a condition known as hemitruncus. Conotruncal abnormalities are readily evaluated by both spin-echo and gradient-echo magnetic resonance imaging in axial, sagittal, and coronal planes. LPA—left pulmonary artery; LPV—left pulmonary vein; MPA—main pulmonary artery; RA—right atrium; RV—right ventricle.

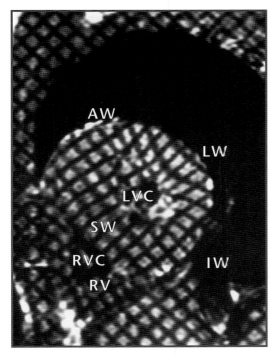

FIGURE 9-16. Spin-echo tagged short-axis image from a patient with hypertrophic cardiomyopathy. The tag lines converge normally in the lateral wall (LW), but demonstrate markedly reduced deformation in the anterior wall (AW), septal wall (SW), and inferior wall (IW), as shown. Using the tag lines to measure intramyocardial circumferential shortening as a marker of intramural function, reduced shortening has been demonstrated in the AW, SW, and IW in patients with hypertrophic cardiomyopathy [17]. LVC—left ventricular cavity; RV—right ventricle; RVC—right ventricular cavity.

MAGNETIC RESONANCE IMAGING AND VALVULAR HEART DISEASE

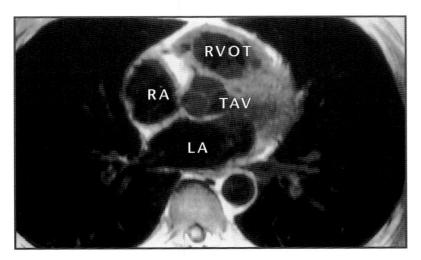

FIGURE 9-17. Normal aortic valve from a spin-echo image in the axial plane. The three leaflets of the aortic valve can be seen clearly. This view is equivalent to the echocardiographic parasternal short-axis view at the aortic level. LA—left atrium; RA—right atrium; RVOT—right ventricular outflow tract; TAV—trileaflet aortic valve.

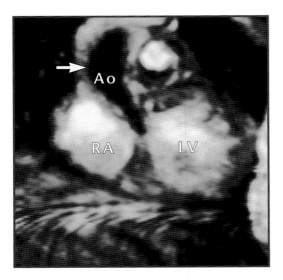

FIGURE 9-18. Valvular aortic stenosis from a gradient-echo image in the coronal plane. There is a marked signal void in the ascending aorta (*arrow*) that has been correlated with the degree of obstruction but does not allow quantitation [18]. Phase-velocity mapping allows more precise quantitation of the valvular gradient [19] because it permits calculation of the velocity of flow across the valve, and then using the modified Bernoulli equation, calculation of the gradient across the valve. Ao—aorta; LV—left ventricle; RA—right atrium.

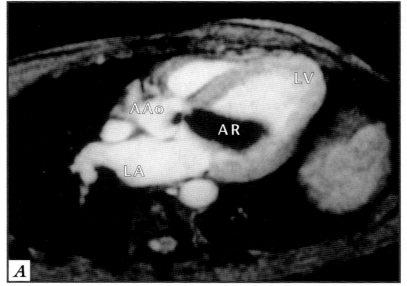 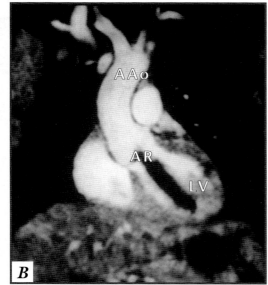

FIGURE 9-19. Severe aortic regurgitation shown in gradient-echo images in a double oblique plane (**A**) and a coronal plane (**B**). The signal void (*black*) represents the regurgitant jet in diastole and correlates with the extent of regurgitation [20], although display and imaging parameters can affect the size of the signal void [21]. Magnetic resonance imaging has been shown to be accurate in assessment of aortic regurgitation (AR) by jet size [22] or velocity mapping methods [23] and of regurgitant orifice area [24], and allows serial examination of chamber dimensions and left ventricular (LV) systolic function. AAo—ascending aorta; LA—left atrium. (*Courtesy of* Gerald G. Blackwell and Gerald M. Pohost.)

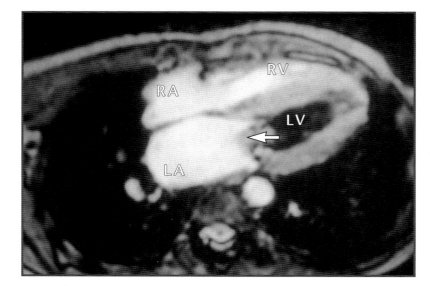

FIGURE 9-20. Mitral stenosis as demonstrated on an axial gradient-echo cine image. In this patient, mitral valve opening (*arrow*) is associated with turbulent left ventricular (LV) inflow, which is seen as a signal void that encompasses the entire LV cavity during diastole. Phase-velocity imaging can be used to quantitate the LV inflow velocity and estimate the severity of mitral stenosis, and it correlates well with Doppler echocardiography [25]. LA—left atrium; RA—right atrium; RV—right ventricle. (*Courtesy of* Gerald G. Blackwell and Gerald M. Pohost.)

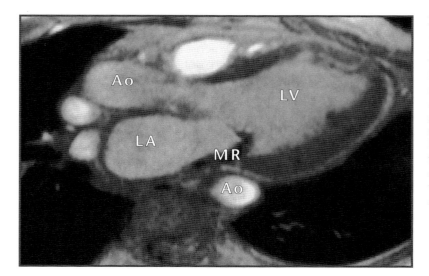

FIGURE 9-21. Oblique gradient-echo systolic image in a three-chamber long-axis plane from a patient with mitral regurgitation (MR). An eccentric turbulent jet represented by a signal void can be seen aimed at the posterior left atrial wall, riding under the posterior mitral leaflet. Magnetic resonance imaging can accurately assess the severity of MR in comparison with Doppler echocardiography [26] or contrast ventriculography using a volumetric analysis of regurgitant fraction [27]. Phase-velocity techniques have been shown to be quite accurate in estimating regurgitant volume and regurgitant fraction [28]. Ao—aorta; LA—left atrium; LV—left ventricular.

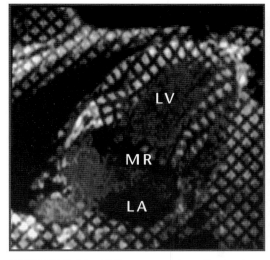

FIGURE 9-22. Oblique tagged gradient-echo image in a two-chamber long-axis plane in late systole from a patient with mitral regurgitation (MR). From this image, both left ventricular intramyocardial function and the severity of MR can be evaluated. The turbulent jet MR is seen coursing under the anterior mitral leaflet (AML) toward the inferior wall and extending to the posterior wall of the left atrium (LA). The cause of the MR in this case is a partially flail AML in the setting of myxomatous valve disease. LV—left ventricle.

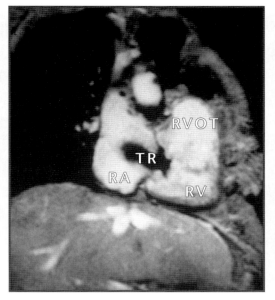

FIGURE 9-23. Right anterior oblique gradient-echo midsystolic cine image. The right ventricle (RV) is seen anteriorly along the chest wall, and the right atrium (RA) is seen posteriorly. The signal void across the tricuspid valve and into the RA in this mid-systolic image represents tricuspid regurgitation (TR). RVOT—right ventricular outflow tract. (*Courtesy of* Gerald G. Blackwell and Gerald M. Pohost.)

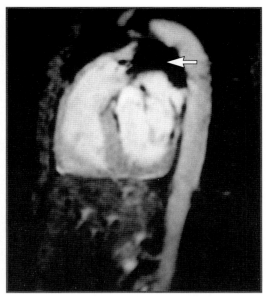

FIGURE 9-24. Parasagittal gradient-echo midsystolic cine image in the plane of the right ventricular outflow tract. This image is taken from a patient with pulmonic stenosis, which usually is a congenital condition. The signal void seen in the proximal main pulmonary artery represents turbulent blood flow across the stenotic pulmonic valve (*arrow*). The gradient across the stenotic orifice can be estimated using phase-velocity techniques. (*Courtesy of* Gerald G. Blackwell and Gerald M. Pohost.)

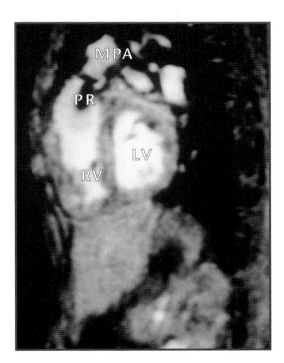

FIGURE 9-25. Parasagittal gradient-echo mid-diastolic cine image in the plane of the right ventricular (RV) outflow tract (RVOT). The signal void seen in the RVOT is that of pulmonary regurgitation (PR), which is often of no clinical significance. However, in patients with postoperative congenital heart disease and severe PR, phase-velocity mapping techniques can be quite helpful in following up with these patients [29]. LV—left ventricle; MPA—main pulmonary artery. (*Courtesy of* Gerald G. Blackwell and Gerald M. Pohost.)

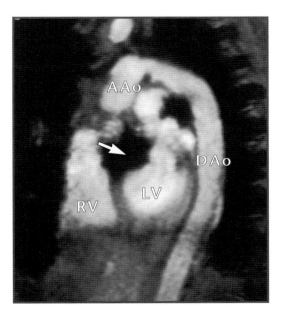

FIGURE 9-26. Parasagittal gradient-echo cine image from a patient after St Jude's aortic valve replacement. On this image, the signal void induced by the prosthesis in the aortic position can be readily identified (*arrow*). With the exception of Starr-Edwards valves, imaging mechanical prosthetic valves by magnetic resonance imaging is safe, even in the early postoperative period. AAo—ascending aorta; DAo—descending aorta; LV—left ventricle; RV—right ventricle.

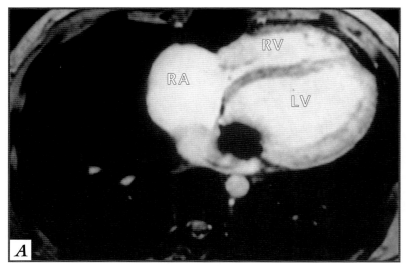

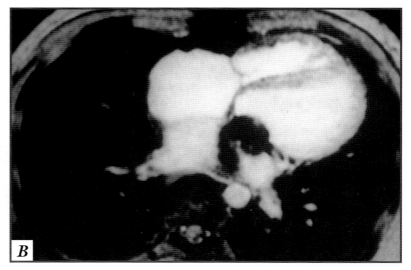

FIGURE 9-27. Axial gradient-echo cine images at end-diastole (**A**) and late systole (**B**). On the end-diastolic image (**A**), the normal signal void induced by a St Jude's mitral valve prosthesis is seen. An eccentric jet of perivalvular magnetic resonance (MR) can be easily identified on the systolic image (**B**). Although transesophageal echocardiography is often used to identify perivalvular regurgitation in the setting of mechanical valvular prostheses, cine MR imaging can be useful in selected patients [30]. LV—left ventricle; RA—right atrium; RV—right ventricle. (*Courtesy of* Gerald G. Blackwell and Gerald M. Pohost.)

MAGNETIC RESONANCE IMAGING AND ACQUIRED HEART DISEASE

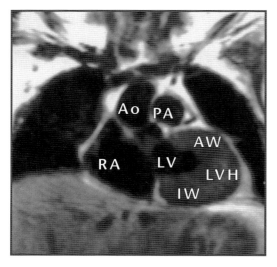

FIGURE 9-28. Coronal spin-echo image from a patient with concentric left ventricular hypertrophy (LVH). Marked hypertrophy of the anterior wall (AW) and inferior wall (IW) can be seen on this coronal image. Cine imaging may demonstrate systolic cavity obliteration in such patients. Ao—aorta; LV—left ventricle; PA—pulmonary artery; RA—right atrium.

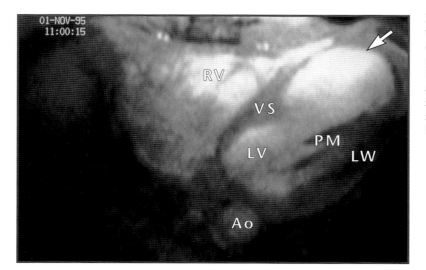

FIGURE 9-29. Oblique end-diastolic gradient-echo cine image in a transverse plane several weeks after anterior wall myocardial infarction. Thinning of the mid and apical septum can be clearly identified (*arrow*), as can preserved wall thickness in the basal septum and lateral wall (LW). Cine imaging can demonstrate systolic bulging of the apex consistent with an anteroapical aneurysm. Quantitative and three-dimensional analyses of systolic wall thickening can be performed on short-axis cine images to assess systolic function [7]. Ao—aorta; LV—left ventricle; PM—papillary muscle; RV—right ventricle; VS—ventricular septum.

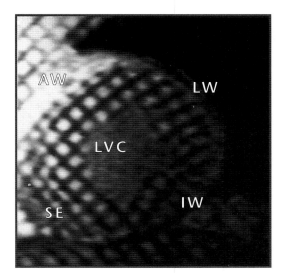

FIGURE 9-30. End-systolic breath-hold gradient-echo tagged short-axis image at the mid–left ventricle (LV) day 4 after anterior wall myocardial infarction (MI). No deformation is seen in the septum (SE) or anterior wall (AW), whereas some motion of the tag stripes toward each other is seen in the lateral wall (LW) and inferior wall (IW). Quantitative analyses of the tagged images from such patients after large anterior MI demonstrate reduced intramyocardial function throughout the LV, including regions remote from the infarcted territory [31]. LVC—left ventricular cavity.

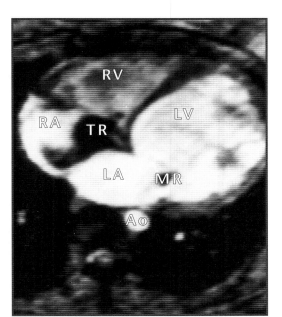

FIGURE 9-31. Mid-systolic gradient-echo cine image in an axial plane in a patient with a dilated cardiomyopathy. All four cardiac chambers are dilated, and the septum, apex, and lateral walls of the left ventricle (LV) are thinned. A small signal void is seen at the mitral valve level into the left atrium (LA) consistent with mitral regurgitation (MR; *see* Fig. 9-21). A larger signal void in the right atrium (RA) is seen and corresponds with significant tricuspid regurgitation (TR; *see* Fig. 9-23). Ao—aorta; RV—right ventricle.

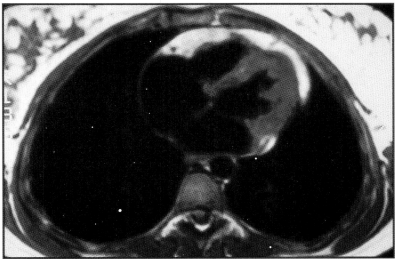

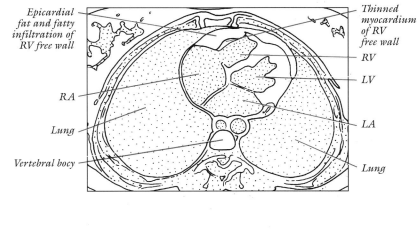

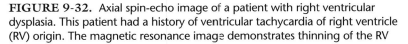

FIGURE 9-32. Axial spin-echo image of a patient with right ventricular dysplasia. This patient had a history of ventricular tachycardia of right ventricle (RV) origin. The magnetic resonance image demonstrates thinning of the RV free wall and replacement of normal myocardium by fatty tissue that can be used to differentiate RV dysplasia from dilated cardiomyopathy [32]. LA—left atrium; LV—left ventricle; RA—right atrium. (*Courtesy of* Adam Fitzpatrick.)

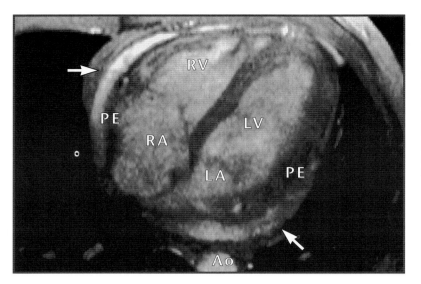

FIGURE 9-33. Axial gradient-echo cine image from a patient with effusive constrictive pericarditis. Magnetic resonance imaging (MRI) can be used to evaluate pericardial thickness and the presence or absence of pericardial effusion (PE) [33]. In this particular image taken several months after cardiac surgery, the pericardium is thickened (*arrows*) anterior to the right ventricle (RV) and right atrium (RA) and posterior to the left atrium (LA). A moderate amount of pericardial fluid is also seen. MRI is more effective in imaging the thickness of the pericardium than is two-dimensional echocardiography. On the basis of clinical symptoms, pressures consistent with constriction on left and right heart catheterization, and the MRI findings, this patient underwent pericardial stripping and was clinically improved postoperatively. Ao—aorta; LV—left ventricle.

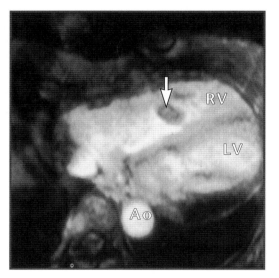

FIGURE 9-34. Axial gradient-echo cine image in a patient with a right ventricular mass. A mass can be seen at the base of the right ventricle (RV) adjacent to the tricuspid valve (*arrow*). Because of underlying risk factors for thrombus formation, the patient was treated presumptively for thrombus with anticoagulation, and repeat imaging studies several weeks later showed no ventricular mass. Ao—aorta; LV—left ventricle.

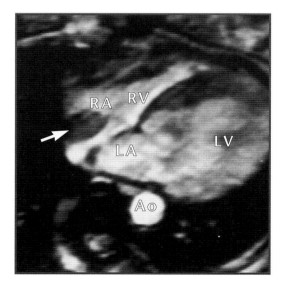

FIGURE 9-35. Axial gradient-echo cine image in a patient demonstrating a right atrial mass (*arrow*). The signal void in the right atrium (RA) in this image is a thrombus attached to the end of a catheter. The catheter and thrombus were removed surgically. Ao—aorta; LA—left atrium; LV—left ventricle; RV—right ventricle.

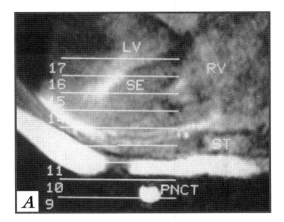

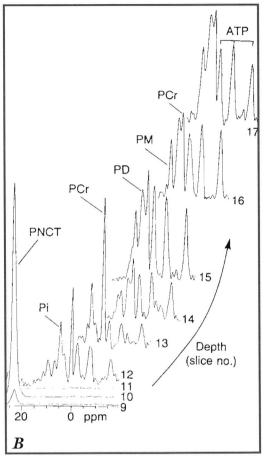

FIGURE 9-36. Magnetic resonance (MR) spectroscopy provides quantitative chemical information about magnetically susceptible materials, *eg*, odd number of protons and neutrons. After stimulation of the material with a radiofrequency pulse, the received signal undergoes Fourier transformation into a spectrum relating signal amplitude to frequency. Whereas MR imaging (MRI) is acquired in the presence of a magetic field gradient and displays the three-dimensional spatial relationship of the signal intensities as an image, MR spectroscopy requires a highly uniform field in order to be sensitive to, and not to alter, local frequencies.

Shown here is an axial surface-coil proton MRI of a patient at rest (**A**) with the corresponding ^{31}P MR spectra (**B**) with the same 10-mm–thick coronal sections indicated in the proton image. MR spectroscopy allows direct quantification of cardiac high-energy phosphates, and spatial localization within the myocardial wall is possible [34]. These spectra were acquired in a 9.1-minute scan. The relative signal gain in slices numbered 12 to 17 is increased 20-fold over that in slices numbered nine to 11. Chemical shift (in parts per million) is relative to the value for phosphocreatine. ATP—adenosine triphosphate; LV—left ventricle; Pcr—phosphocreatine; PD—phosphodiesters; Pi—inorganic phosphate; PM—phosphomonoesters; PNCT—0.5 M phosphonitric chloride trimer in a 0.9-mL vial; RV—right ventricle; SE—septum; ST—sternum. (*From* Weiss and coworkers [34]; with permission.)

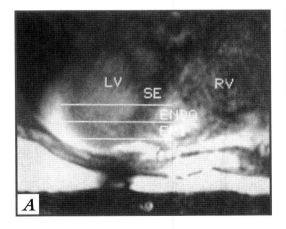

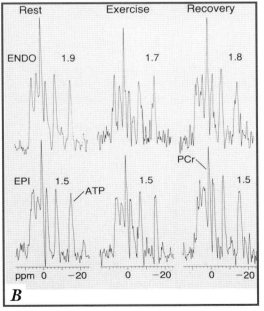

FIGURE 9-37. Axial surface-coil proton magnetic resonance imaging (MRI) of a patient at rest (**A**) and corresponding ^{31}P MR spectra (**B**) from coronal slices in the anterior wall in a patient with anterior ischemia induced by exercise. The ratio of phosphocreatine (PCr) to adenosine triphosphate (ATP) decreases after the onset of severe myocardial ischemia. In the subendocardium (ENDO), the PCr:ATP ratio declines from 1.7 at *rest* to 0.9 with *exercise* and recovers to 1.2 (*recovery*). In the study by Weiss *et al.* [34], five patients, who had anterior ischemia as shown by an exercise-induced decrease in the PCr:ATP ratio in the anterior septum, demonstrated normalization of these ratios after revascularization. Absolute PCr and ATP content can also be measured and correlated with myocardial viability. ATP content has been shown to decrease dramatically in patients with coronary artery disease and nonviable myocardium [35]. EPI—epicardium; Pi—inorganic phosphate; RV—right ventricle; SE—septum. (*From* Weiss and coworkers [34]; with permission.)

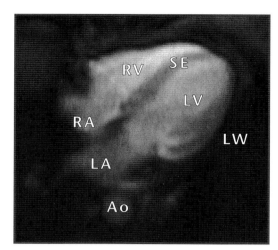

FIGURE 9-38. Oblique T1-weighted inversion-prepared turboflash image in a transverse four-chamber plane obtained using a surface coil after the first pass of an intravenous bolus of gadoteridol contrast medium in a normal human volunteer. T1 weighting is used to maximize signal from the gadoteridol, and Turboflash imaging allows adequate temporal resolution to capture the influx of contrast over a reasonable number of heart beats (in this case, 64). Sufficient images were acquired before the arrival of the prior to contrast medium in the left ventricle (LV) to allow magnetization to reach steady state. The contrast uptake within LV myocardium (septum [SE], apex, and lateral wall [LW]) is uniform. This technique can be used in patients with coronary disease [36] as peak signal intensity after the bolus is lower in regions perfused by a diseased coronary artery and improves after revascularization. This technique can be used before and after infusion of a vasodilator such as dipyridamole or adenosine to assess perfusion reserve [37]. Ao—atrium; LA—left atrium; RA—right atrium; RV—right ventricle.

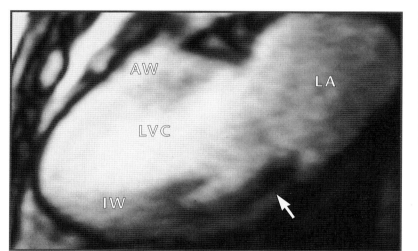

FIGURE 9-39. Oblique T1-weighted inversion-prepared Turboflash image in a two-chamber long-axis orientation obtained using a surface coil after the first pass of an intravenous bolus of gadoteridol contrast medium in a patient 5 days after inferior wall (IW) myocardial infarction. The anterior wall (AW) demonstrates uniform enhancement, whereas a region of hypoenhancement exists in the basal inferior wall (*arrow*). On first pass imaging, these hypoenhanced regions are thought to represent infarcted regions after prolonged obstruction of the infarct-related artery [38] and correlate with regions of no reflow after reperfusion [39]. LA—left atrium; LVC—left ventricular cavity.

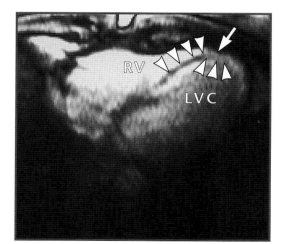

FIGURE 9-40. Oblique T1-weighted inversion-prepared Turboflash image in an transverse four-chamber plane obtained using a surface coil 7 minutes after an intravenous bolus of gadoteridol contrast in a patient 3 days after anterior myocardial infarction. A region of hyperenhancement (*arrow*) is seen in the mid and apical septum and apical lateral walls and surrounds a hypoenhanced region (*arrowheads*) in the septum. Hyperenhancement represents delayed washout of the extravascular contrast medium [40]. Hyperenhancement without hypoenhanced regions may represent infarcts with less regional dysfunction [38] and a greater chance for recovery of function in ensuing weeks [41]. The persistence of hypoenhancement within a hyperenhanced region on delayed imaging, as seen in this patient, corresponds to a lack of functional recovery over time [42] and a greater extent of left ventricular remodeling [41]. LVC—left ventricular cavity; RV—right ventricle.

REFERENCES

1. Shapiro EP, Rogers WJ, Beyar R, *et al.*: MRI determination of left ventricular mass in hearts deformed by acute infarction. *Circulation* 1988, 79:706–711.

2. Sechtem U, Pflugfelder PW, Gould RG, *et al.*: Measurement of right and left ventricular volumes in healthy individuals with cine MR imaging. *Radiology* 1987, 163:697–702.

3. Cranney GB, Lotan CS, Dean L, *et al.*: Left ventricular volume measurement using cardiac axis NMR imaging-validation by calibrated ventricular angiography. *Circulation* 1990, 82:154–163.

4. Buser PT, Aufferman W, Holt WW, *et al.*: Noninvasive evaluation of global left ventricular function with use of cine nuclear magnetic resonance. *J Am Coll Cardiol* 1989, 13:1294–1300.

5. Peshock RM, Rokey R, Malloy CM, *et al.*: Assessment of myocardial systolic wall thickening using nuclear magnetic resonance imaging. *J Am Coll Cardiol* 1989, 14:653–659.

6. Lotan CS, Cranney GB, Bouchard A, *et al.*: The value of cine nuclear magnetic resonance imaging for assessing regional ventricular function. *J Am Coll Cardiol* 1989, 14:1721–1729.

7. Holman ER, Buller VGM, de Roos A, *et al.*: Detection and quantification of dysfunctional myocardium by magnetic resonance imaging. *Circulation* 1997, 95:924–931.

8. Zerhouni E, Parrish D, Rogers WJ, *et al.*: Human heart: tagging with MR imaging—a method for noninvasive measurement of myocardial motion. *Radiology* 1988, 169:59–64.

9. Axel L, Dougherty L: MR imaging of motion with spatial modulation of magnetization. *Radiology* 1989, 171:841–845.

10. Clark N, Reichek N, Bergey P, *et al.*: Normal segmental myocardial function: assessment by magnetic resonance imaging using spatial modulation of magnetization. *Circulation* 1991, 84:67–74.

11. Young AA, Imai H, Chang C-N, Axel L: Two-dimensional left ventricular deformation during systole using magnetic resonance imaging with spatial modulation of magnetization. *Circulation* 1994, 89:740–752.

12. Young AA, Kramer CM, Ferrari VA, *et al.*: Three-dimensional deformation in hypertrophic cardiomyopathy. *Circulation* 1994, 90:854–867.

13. Karwatowski SP, Mohiaddin RH, Yang GZ, *et al.*: Regional myocardial velocity imaged by magnetic resonance in patients with ischaemic heart disease. *Br Heart J* 1994, 72:332–338.

14. van Wedeen VJ, Weisskoff RM, Reese TG, *et al.*: Motionless movies of myocardial strain-rates using stimulated echoes. *Magn Reson Med* 1995, 33:396–408.

15. Holmvang G, Palacios IF, Vlahakes GJ, *et al.*: Imaging and sizing of atrial septal defects by magnetic resonance. *Circulation* 1995, 92:3473–3480.

16. Hundley WG, Li HF, Lange RA, *et al.*: Assessment of left-to-right intracardiac shunting by velocity-encoded, phase-difference magnetic resonance imaging. *Circulation* 1995, 91:2955–2960.

17. Kramer CM, Reichek NR, Ferrari VA, *et al.*: Regional heterogeneity of function in hypertrophic cardiomyopathy. *Circulation* 1994, 90:186–194.

18. Mitchell L, Jenkins JPR, Watson, *et al.*: Diagnosis and assessment of mitral and aortic valve disease by cine-flow magnetic resonance imaging. *Magn Reson Med* 1989, 12:181–197.

19. Sondergaard L, Hildebrandt P, Lindvig K, *et al.*: Valve area and cardiac output in aortic stenosis: quantification by magnetic resonance velocity mapping. *Am Heart J* 1993, 126:1156–1164.

20. Wagner S, Auffermann W, Buser P, *et al.*: Diagnostic accuracy and estimation of the severity of valvular regurgitation from the signal void on cine magnetic resonance imaging. *Am Heart J* 1989, 118:760–767.

21. Suzuki J, Caputo GR, Kondo C, Higgins CB: Cine MR imaging of valvular heart disease: display and imaging parameters affect the size of the signal void caused by valvular regurgitation. *AJR Am J Roentgenol* 1990, 155:723–727.

22. Cranney GB, Benhelloun H, Perry GJ, *et al.*: Rapid assessment of aortic regurgitation and left ventricular function using cine nuclear magnetic resonance imaging and the proximal convergence zone. *Am J Cardiol* 1993, 71:1043–1081.

23. Sondergaard L, Lindvig K, Hildebrandt P, *et al.*: Quantification of aortic regurgitation by magnetic resonance velocity mapping. *Am Heart J* 1993, 125:1081–1090.

24. Reimold SC, Maier SE, Fleischmann KE, *et al.*: Dynamic nature of the aortic regurgitant orifice area during diastole in patients with chronic aortic regurgitation. *Circulation* 1994, 89:2085–2092.

25. Heidenreich PA, Steffens J, Fujita N, *et al.*: Evaluation of mitral stenosis with velocity-encoded cine-magnetic resonance imaging. *Am J Cardiol* 1995, 75:365–369.

26. Aurigemma G, Reichek N, Schiebler M, Axel L: Evaluation of mitral regurgitation by cine magnetic resonance imaging. *Am J Cardiol* 1990, 66:621–625.

27. Hundley WG, Li HF, Willard JE, *et al.*: Magnetic resonance imaging assessment of the severity of mitral regurgitation. *Circulation* 1995, 92:1151–1158.

28. Fujita N, Chazouilleres AF, Hartiala JJ, *et al.*: Quantification of mitral regurgitation by velocity-encoded cine nuclear magnetic resonance imaging. *J Am Coll Cardiol* 1994, 23:951–958.

29. Rebergen SA, Chin JGJ, Oeenkamp J, *et al.*: Pulmonary regurgitation in the late postoperative follow-up of tetralogy of Fallot. *Circulation* 1993, 88:2257–2266.

30. Deutsch HJ, Bachmann R, Sechtem U, *et al.*: Regurgitant flow in cardiac valve prostheses: diagnostic value of gradient echo nuclear magnetic resonance imaging in reference to transesophageal two-dimensional color Doppler echocardiography. *J Am Coll Cardiol* 1992, 19:1500–1507.

31. Kramer CM, Rogers WJ, Theobald TM, *et al.*: Remote noninfarcted region dysfunction soon after first anterior myocardial infarction: a magnetic resonance tagging study. *Circulation* 1996, 94:660–666.

32. Ricci C, Longo R, Pagnan L, *et al.*: Magnetic resonance imaging in right ventricular dysplasia. *Am J Cardiol* 1992, 70:1589–1595.

33. Sechtem U, Tscholakoff D, Higgins CB: MRI of the abnormal pericardium. *AJR Am J Roentgenol* 1986, 147:245–252.

34. Weiss RG, Bottomley PA, Hardy CJ, Gerstenblith G: Regional myocardial metabolism of high-energy phosphates during isometric exercise in patients with coronary heart disease. *N Engl J Med* 1990, 323:1593–1600.

35. Yabe T, Mitsunami K, Inubushi T, Kinoshita M: Quantitative measurements of cardiac phosphorus metabolites in coronary artery disease by ^{31}P magnetic resonance spectroscopy. *Circulation* 1995, 92:15–23.

36. Manning WJ, Atkinson DJ, Grossman W, *et al.*: First pass nuclear magnetic resonance imaging studies using gadolinium-DTPA in patients with coronary artery disease. *J Am Coll Cardiol* 1991, 18:959–965.

37. Walsh EG, Doyle M, Lawson MA, *et al.*: Multislice first-pass myocardial perfusion imaging on a conventional clinical scanner. *Magn Reson Med* 1995, 34:39–47.

38. Lima JAC, Judd RM, Bazille A, *et al.*: Regional heterogeneity of human myocardial infarcts demonstrated by contrast enhanced MRI: potential mechanisms. *Circulation* 1995, 92:1117–1125.

39. Judd RM, Lugo-Olivieri CH, Arai M, *et al.*: Physiological basis of myocardial contrast enhancement in fast magnetic resonance images of 2-day old reperfused canine infarcts. *Circulation* 1995, 92:1902–1910.

40. Kim RJ, Chen E-L, Lima JAC, Judd RM: Myocardial Gd-DTPA kinetics determine MRI contrast enhancement and reflect the extent and severity of myocardial injury after acute reperfused infarction. *Circulation* 1996, 94:3318–3326.

41. Rogers WJ, Kramer CM, Geskin G, *et al.*: Contrast enhanced MRI early after reperfused MI predicts late functional recovery. *Circulation* 1996, 94:I–541.

42. Yakota C, Nonogi H, Miyazaki S, *et al.*: Gadolinium-enhanced magnetic resonance imaging in acute myocardial infarction. *Am J Cardiol* 1995, 75:577–581.

Cardiac Positron Emission Tomography

Richard C. Brunken ~ Ching-yee Oliver Wong
Eric Q. Chen ~ Raymundo T. Go

Positron emission tomography (PET) is a noninvasive, three-dimensional nuclear medicine imaging technique that uses radioactive tracers to depict naturally occurring tissue processes *in vivo* [1–3]. The specific radioactive tracer used for imaging, along with its tissue distribution and disposition, determine the nature of the information provided by the PET imaging study (*see* Figure 10-1).

Positron emission tomography has several advantages relative to single photon emission computed tomography (SPECT) for cardiac imaging, including better temporal and spatial image resolution and correction for attenuation of emitted photons. Current PET tomographs are designed to measure rapidly changing vascular and tissue tracer concentrations and are capable of acquiring multiple cross-sectional images of the heart as frequently as every 10 seconds. Unlike SPECT cameras, the spatial resolution of a PET tomograph depends mainly on the geometry of its detectors and is relatively insensitive to the depth of the scintillation event. PET tomographs have spatial resolutions on the order of 6 to 8 mm full-width, half-maximum (FWHM) in the center of the field of view, as compared with 12 to 15 mm FWHM for SPECT cameras. In addition, PET images are corrected for tissue attenuation by use of individually measured attenuation coefficients [1,2]. The counts observed on PET images therefore reliably reflect true tissue tracer activity concentrations.

Following radioactive tracer administration, PET imaging can be performed at the moment of peak myocardial uptake of the radiopharmaceutical (static image acqui-

sition), or a series of images can rapidly be acquired over time (dynamic image acquisition). The images initially acquired by the PET scanner, the transverse images, are orthogonal to the body. In most imaging centers, the transverse images are "resliced" into standard short-axis and vertical and horizontal long-axis images orthogonal to the long axis of the left ventricle. In addition to visual analysis of the cardiac images, semiquantitative analysis of realigned PET images can be achieved using polar mapping techniques analogous to those used for SPECT perfusion images [4–9]. Gated PET images can also be acquired to provide information about segmental wall motion and thickening and ventricular volumes and ejection fractions [10–14].

Quantitated rates of myocardial perfusion and metabolism can be obtained with PET imaging by examining the change in tissue tracer concentration over time on dynamic images. The dynamic images are usually analyzed by drawing regions of interest on each of the sequential image frames. Because the time of acquisition of each frame is operator-defined, it is possible to generate time–activity curves that depict tissue and vascular tracer activity concentrations as a function of time from the moment of tracer administration. The count data are fitted using a mathematical model that describes the biologic behavior of the radioactive label [3]. The physiologic parameter of interest (*eg*, absolute myocardial blood flow in milliliters per minute per gram of tissue or glucose consumption in micromoles of glucose per minute per gram of tissue) is derived from the equation of the curve used to fit the time–activity data. Application of comparable mathematical operations to each element of a cardiac image using sophisticated computerized image processing techniques permits generation of parametric images and polar maps that display absolute myocardial blood flows and metabolic rates on a pixel-by-pixel basis [15,16].

During the past two decades, PET imaging has contributed substantially to our understanding of myocardial physiology and pathophysiology in a variety of cardiac disorders. As new tracers are synthesized and better PET tomographs are designed, application of this noninvasive imaging technique to a variety of disease processes should provide even more detailed information about the state of the human heart. Our challenge will be to continue to translate this new information into clinical actions that provide better care for and reduce the morbidity and mortality in our patients with heart disease.

BASIC PRINCIPLES OF CARDIAC POSITRON EMISSION TOMOGRAPHY IMAGING

Radioactive Tracers Used for Cardiac Positron Emission Tomography Imaging

	Tracer	Physical Half-life, *min*	Maximum β^+ Energy, *Mev*	Origin	Comments
Perfusion	^{82}Rb	1.26	3.36	Bedside generator	Potassium analogue
	^{13}N ammonia	9.96	1.19	Cyclotron	Metabolically trapped within cardiac myocyte
	^{15}O water	2.07	1.72	Cyclotron	Freely diffusable tracer, with high first-pass extraction
	^{11}C acetate	20.40	0.96	Cyclotron	Initial tissue uptake reflects regional myocardial perfusion
Metabolism	^{11}C acetate	20.40	0.96	Cyclotron	Initial phase of tissue clearance reflects oxidative substrate flux through TCA cycle
	^{11}C palmitate	20.40	0.96	Cyclotron	Initial phase of tissue clearance reflects rate of fatty acid oxidation; second phase of clearance depicts label incorporation into intracellular lipids
	FDG	109.70	0.64	Cyclotron	Glucose analogue that is retained in myocardium in proportion to exogenous glucose utilization
Innervation	^{11}C hydroxyephedrine	20.40	0.96	Cyclotron	Uptake reflects accumulation of norepinephrine in presynaptic sympathetic cardiac neurons

FDG—^{18}F 2-fluoro-2-deoxyglucose; TCA—tricarboxylic acid.

FIGURE 10-1. Radioactive tracers most frequently used for clinical cardiac positron emission tomography (PET) imaging studies. The specific radioactive tracer used for imaging, along with its tissue distribution and disposition, determine the nature of the information provided by the PET imaging study. Carbon, oxygen, and nitrogen each have short-lived radionuclide species that can be incorporated into biologically active molecules and used as tracers for cardiac PET imaging. ^{18}F, similar to the hydroxyl (OH⁻) group in its chemical properties, decays by positron emission and can also be used to label several tracers useful for clinical PET imaging.

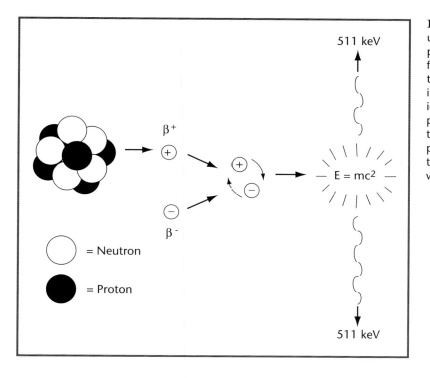

FIGURE 10-2. Annihilation of a positron. Each of the radioactive tracers used for positron emission tomography imaging decays by emitting a positron (or β^+ particle) from a proton-rich nucleus. Positrons are emitted from atomic nuclei with a continuum of energies, up to a maximum energy that is characteristic of the parent atomic species. The emitted positron interacts with atoms in the surrounding medium, producing excitations and ionizations. These slow the positron and decrease its kinetic energy. As the positron slows, it comes into close proximity with one of many electrons in the surrounding medium. After a very brief interaction, the electron and positron mutually annihilate. The energy liberated from the loss of the electron and the positron is released as two 511-keV annihilation photons, which exit from the annihilation site about 180° apart.

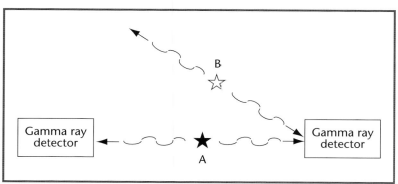

FIGURE 10-3. Annihilation coincidence detection. Positron emission tomographs detect positron-emitting atomic nuclei within the heart by exploiting both the simultaneous creation of the two annihilation photons and the fact that the photons depart from the site of annihilation in opposite directions. Current instruments use gamma-ray detectors connected by sophisticated electronic circuitry to identify paired scintillation events occurring about 180° apart. If two detectors opposite each other simultaneously (within 10 to 20 ns) register photons in coincidence, such as those leaving site *A* in this example, then the annihilation event is effectively localized to the volume between the two detectors. If only one photon is detected, as is the case with the photons originating from site *B* in the illustration, the requirement for coincidence detection is not satisfied, and the scintillation event from this detector pair will not be incorporated into the myocardial image.

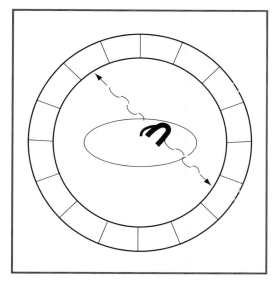

FIGURE 10-4. Positron emission tomography (PET) camera. Current PET instruments use circular rings of gamma-ray detectors to externally detect and localize radioactivity concentrations within the heart, using the principal of annihilation coincidence detection (*see* Fig. 10-3). With the data obtained from millions of positron annihilations, it is possible to use standard back-projection and Fourier reconstruction techniques to reconstruct an image of the tracer distribution within the plane (two dimensions). The three-dimensional spatial distribution of a labeled tracer is obtained by use of multiple rings of detectors adjacent to each other. A detector in one plane can be in the "line of sight" of some of the opposite detectors in the adjacent higher and lower planes. By using *interplane coincidences*, an additional set of interpolated images midway between the direct planes defined by the detector rings is generated.

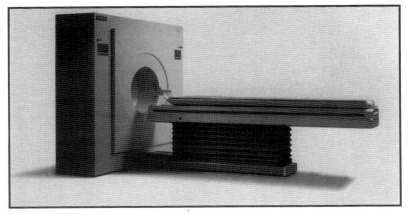

FIGURE 10-5. A current-generation positron emission tomograph. Multiple rings of gamma-ray detectors are located around the circular opening in the instrument. The patient bed slides into the circular opening so the heart is positioned in the center of the field of view. The instrument depicted is capable of simultaneously obtaining 47 cross-sectional images in a 16.2-cm axial field of view. For clinical imaging, individualized attenuation correction factors are determined for each patient on a pixel-by-pixel basis. A scan is first performed using a ring source of a positron-emitting agent placed about the edge of the field of view of the tomograph ("blank scan"). The scan is then repeated with the patient in the field of view (the "transmission scan"). The attenuation correction factors are generated by dividing the blank scan by the transmission scan. Following either inhalation or intravenous administration of the radioactive tracer(s), static or dynamic emission myocardial images are obtained. The calculated attenuation correction factors are then used to correct the patient's emission scan count data for photon attenuation by the structures of the thorax. (*Courtesy of* CTI, Inc, Knoxville, TN.)

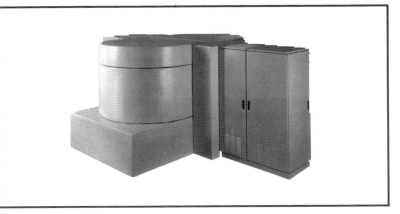

FIGURE 10-6. Mini-cyclotron. The physical half-lives of the radioactive tracers used for clinical cardiac positron emission tomography (PET) imaging are short, necessitating the on-site production of most of these radioactive substances. Although early investigators used large cyclotrons to produce these isotopes, smaller self-shielded "mini-cyclotrons" are now commercially available for use in medical imaging centers. The radioisotope delivery system depicted in this illustration bombards specific targets with 11 million electron Volt protons to produce ^{15}O, ^{13}N, ^{11}C, and ^{18}F. A radioisotope generated in this cyclotron can then be incorporated into the appropriate radiopharmaceutical for imaging (*eg*, ^{13}N into ^{13}N ammonia) by use of automated synthesis modules. (*Courtesy of* CTI, Inc, Knoxville, TN.)

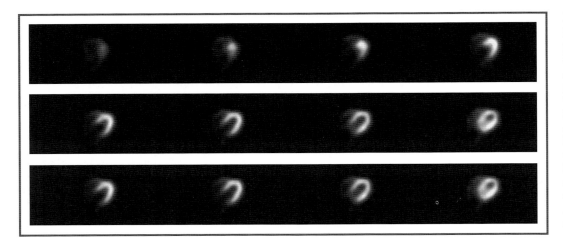

FIGURE 10-7. Normal ^{82}Rb perfusion study. The myocardial emission images initially acquired by positron emission tomography are orthogonal to the body. Whereas *image 1* is the most superior (cranial), *image 11* is the most inferior (caudal) of the imaging planes. In this display, the heart is oriented so that the left ventricle (LV) points to the right and upward in the images. The LV has a crescent-shaped appearance in the more superior images and assumes a horseshoe appearance on the images at midventricular level. Thinning of myocardial activity is normal in the apical area, representing the slightly (1 to 2 mm) smaller thickness of the tissue in this region. On the more inferior images, the ventricle assumes an ellipsoid appearance and then becomes a single collection of activity in the lowest image planes.

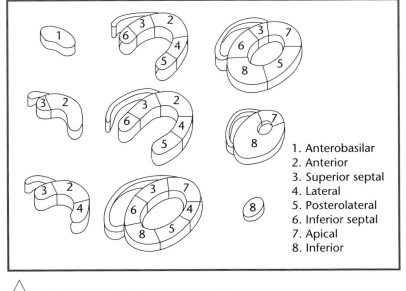

1. Anterobasilar
2. Anterior
3. Superior septal
4. Lateral
5. Posterolateral
6. Inferior septal
7. Apical
8. Inferior

FIGURE 10-8. An eight-segmental myocardial model using transverse positron emission tomography (PET) images. The most superior (cranial) plane, traversing the anterobasilar segment, is represented by the *upper left image*. In the first column, the *second* and *third images* are the next most inferior (caudal) images, and the *second* and *third columns* of images depict progressively lower images, with the lowest plane traversing the inferior segment. The right ventricle can usually be identified on the PET images and assists in defining the interventricular septum.

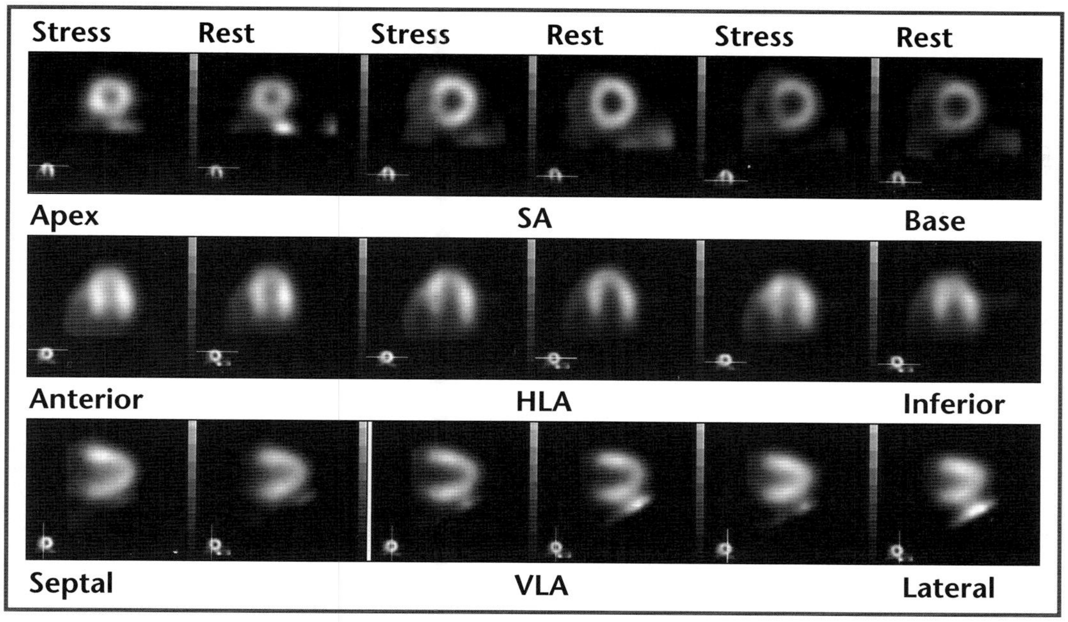

FIGURE 10-9. ^{82}Rb perfusion images from a normal study that have been reoriented into short-axis (SA), horizontal long-axis (HLA), and vertical long-axis (VLA) image sets. "Reslicing" of the initially acquired transverse myocardial images into SA, HLA and VLA sets, which are orthogonal to the major axis of the left ventricle, enhances the localization of segmental abnormalities by minimizing interpatient differences in cardiac position within the thorax and reduces partial volume–related regional variability in observed tissue activity. Visualization of the anterobasilar and inferior segments is also improved. The reoriented images can also be used to generate polar maps of relative myocardial perfusion, at rest and with stress, analogous to the maps used for analysis of single photon emission tomographic ^{201}Tl perfusion images.

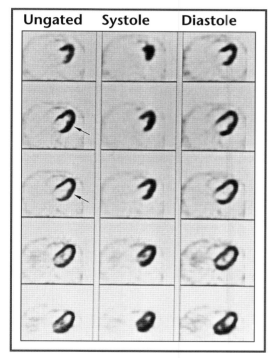

FIGURE 10-10. Representative gated transverse ^{18}F 2-fluoro-2-deoxyglucose metabolic images from a normal volunteer. The more superior image planes are at the *top* and the more inferior imaging planes are displayed at the *bottom*. The *arrows* point to the papillary muscle. During systole, both left ventricular and right ventricular volumes decrease, and there is an increase in the apparent wall thickness of the myocardium of both the right and left ventricles. The increase in count density reflects the increase in wall thickness during ventricular contraction. From the gated images, it is possible to assess regional function, wall thickening, and ventricular volumes and ejection fractions. (*Courtesy of Heinrich R. Shelbert.*)

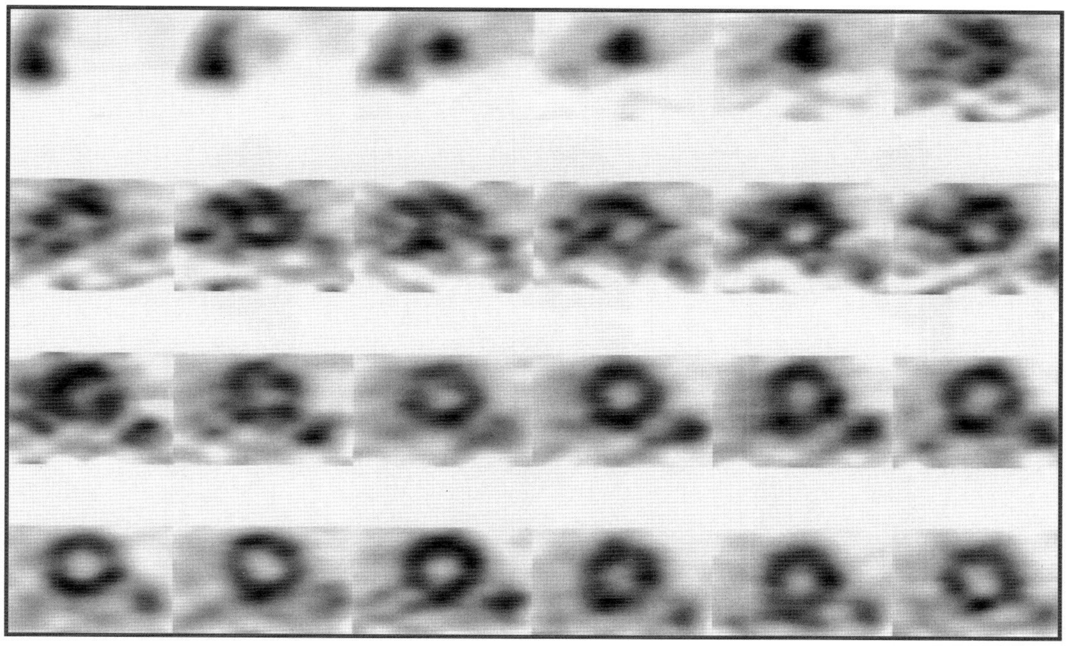

FIGURE 10-11. Dynamic ^{82}Rb short-axis perfusion images from a patient with a history of coronary artery disease and prior percutaneous transluminal coronary angioplasty. The *upper left panels* depict early activity in a crescent-shaped right ventricle. Activity then appears in lung and subsequently in the left ventricular cavity. As time progresses there is progressive accumulation of activity within the myocardium.

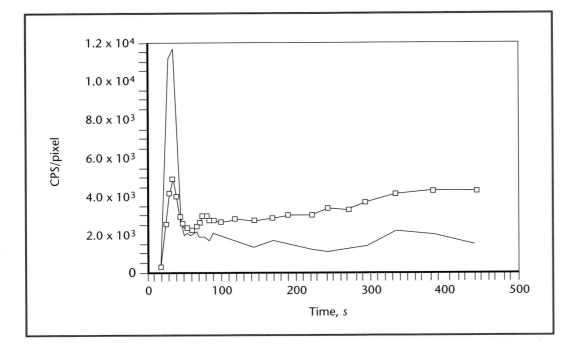

FIGURE 10-12. Blood pool (*solid line*) and myocardial (*line with boxes*) time–activity curves obtained from the dynamic [82]Rb images illustrated in Figure 10-11. Blood pool activity was obtained from a left atrial region of interest. The blood pool curve shows an abrupt increase early following tracer injection and a rapid decline as the tracer is extracted from the vascular space. The initial upstroke of the myocardial curve reflects in part spillover of blood pool activity into the myocardial region of interest. With time, there is a progressive accumulation of [82]Rb activity within the myocardium. Analysis of the time–activity curves permits calculation of the absolute rate of myocardial blood flow, in milliliters per minute per gram of tissue [17]. CPS—counts per second.

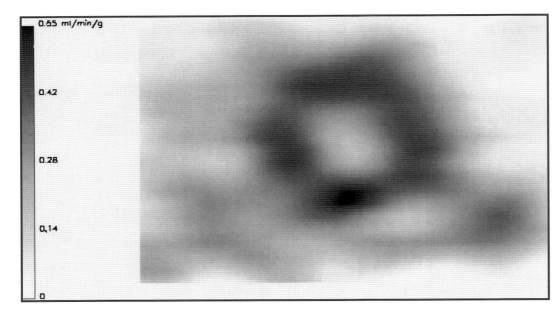

FIGURE 10-13. A parametric image of myocardial blood flow obtained from applying the appropriate tracer kinetic model to the dynamic [82]Rb cardiac images in Figure 10-11. A parametric image displays a calculated or derived physiologic parameter of interest on a pixel-by-pixel basis. In this case, absolute rates of myocardial blood flow in milliliters per minute per gram of tissue are displayed. For a given pixel value, the corresponding myocardial blood flow measurement can be obtained from the gray scale at the *left* of the figure. CPS—counts per second.

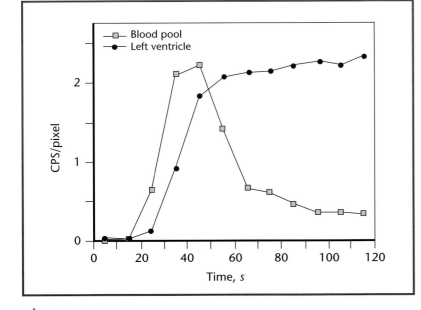

FIGURE 10-14. Time–activity curves derived from a dynamic ^{13}N ammonia positron emission tomography imaging study. The blood pool curve was generated by applying a region of interest drawn over the center of the left ventricular (LV) cavity on a basal short-axis image to each of the corresponding short-axis images in the dynamic image set. This curve depicts the amount of the tracer within the circulating blood as a function of time, and demonstrates that the clearance of ^{13}N activity from blood is relatively prompt. The LV time–activity curve was obtained by applying a region of interest drawn over the LV free wall to each of the sequential images within the dynamic image set. Following the intravenous administration of ^{13}N ammonia, the tracer concentration within the myocardium increases over time, reflecting the "trapping" of ^{13}N activity within the tissue via the glutamic acid–glutamine reaction [18]. CPS—counts per second.

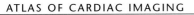

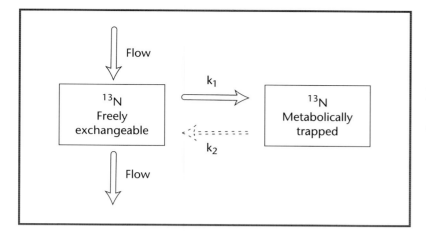

FIGURE 10-15. Two-compartment ^{13}N ammonia ($^{13}NH_3$) tracer–kinetic model used in conjunction with dynamic positron emission tomographic (PET) imaging to quantitate myocardial perfusion. In this model, ^{13}N activity is considered to be in either a freely exchangeable compartment or in a compartment in which the tracer is metabolically trapped as glutamine. k_1 and k_2 are the effective rate constants for the transfer of label between the two compartments. Once trapped, only a very small portion of the label returns to the freely exchangeable compartment, and k_2 is virtually negligible during the period of PET imaging.

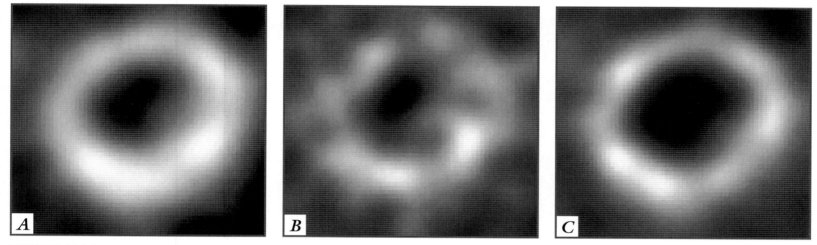

FIGURE 10-16. Parametric myocardial perfusion images. These images can also be generated using a dynamic ^{13}N ammonia ($^{13}NH_3$) imaging study. Several approaches to performing the calculations have been described. **A,** A static $^{13}NH_3$ short-axis perfusion image. **B,** A parametric image of myocardial blood flow calculated using a Patlak graphical analysis. **C,** A short-axis parametric image in which absolute blood flows have been calculated using factor analysis of dynamic structures. This technique is based on principle component analysis and assumes that the pixel activity as a function of time in a dynamic positron emission tomographic imaging study is a linear combination of a limited number of physiologic fundamental time–activity curves [19]. As illustrated in this example, the parametric image generated by use of the factor analysis of dynamic structures is less noisy than that obtained using the Patlak graphic approach. (*Courtesy of* Carl Hoh.)

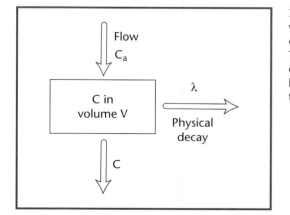

FIGURE 10-17. Single-compartment model for quantitation of myocardial blood flow with ^{15}O water. In this tracer-kinetic model, it is assumed that ^{15}O water freely and rapidly exchanges across the capillary membrane and that the partition coefficient between plasma and myocardium is constant. The relative distribution of the tracer between blood and myocardium is then a function of the hematocrit and the water content of the myocardial tissue. In most models, the water content is assumed to be equal to 0.7 g water per gram of muscle. λ—constant value that reflects physical decay of ^{15}O; C—tracer concentration; C_a—arterial tracer concentration; V—volume of distribution in tissue.

Study	PET tracer	Myocardial Perfusion, mL/min/g			Findings
		Rest	Exercise	Hyperemia	
Cardiac Transplant					
Krivokapich et al. [44]	$^{13}NH_3$	1.05 ± 0.39	1.56 ± 0.71	—	Myocardial blood flow in transplants increases commensurate with exercise.
Rechavia et al. [45]	$H_2^{15}O$	1.16 ± 0.26	—	2.73 ± 1.03	Perfusion is homogeneous at rest and during dipyridamole-induced hyperemia in transplants with no evidence of rejection.
Senneff et al. [46]	$H_2^{15}O$	1.63 ± 0.51	—	3.49 ± 1.70	In allografts with normal coronary arteries on angiography, blood flows during dipyridamole stress are similar to those of normal volunteers.
Chan et al. [47]	$^{13}NH_3$	1.7 ± 0.2 (AR) 1.2 ± 0.3 (Rx)	—	2.5 ± 0.9 (AR) 3.9 ± 1.1 (Rx)	In allografts with acute rejection, resting perfusion is increased and dipyridamole stress flows are decreased, reducing perfusion reserve. Both resting and hyperemic flows improve with treatment.
Kofoed et al. [48]	$^{13}NH_3$	0.94 ± 0.26	—	1.69 ± 0.78	In patients with cardiac allograft vasculopathy, dipyridamole-induced hyperemic blood flows are inversely related to the severity of intimal thickness on intravascular ultrasound.
Hyperlipidemia					
Dayanikli et al. [49]	$^{13}NH_3$	0.76 ± 0.18	—	2.17 ± 0.56	In asymptomatic men with cardiac risk factors, adenosine-induced hyperemic flows are significantly smaller than those of age-matched controls. Myocardial perfusion reserve is negatively correlated with total cholesterol levels, with LDL levels, and with total-to-HDL cholesterol ratios.
Yokoyama et al. [50]	$^{13}NH_3$	0.81 ± 0.31	—	1.29 ± 0.19	In response to IV dipyridamole, patients with familial hypercholesterolemia have significantly lower myocardial perfusion reserves than do normal subjects.
Pitkanen et al. [51]	$H_2^{15}O$	0.92 ± 0.24	—	3.19 ± 1.59	During pharmacologic vasodilation with dipyridamole, young (31 ± 8 y) men with familial hypercholesterolemia have coronary flow reserves that are 35% lower than those of control subjects.
Czernin et al. [52]	$^{13}NH_3$	0.78 ± 0.18 (Pre Rx) 0.69 ± 0.14 (Post Rx)	—	2.06 ± 0.35 (Pre Rx) 2.25 ± 0.40 (Post Rx)	Cardiovascular conditioning and a diet deriving less than 10% of its caloric content from fat significantly lowers resting blood flows and increases dipyridamole-induced hyperemic flows in patients with increased risk for or known coronary artery disease.
Aging					
Senneff et al. [53]	$H_2^{15}O$	1.17 ± 0.35	—	3.12 ± 1.09	Adults aged 55 ± 9 y have significantly lower hyperemic flows with dipyridamole stress than do younger adults with a mean age of 25 ± 4 y (4.25 ± 1.54 mL/min/g).
Czernin et al. [54]	$^{13}NH_3$	0.92 ± 0.25	—	2.64 ± 0.58	Adults at a mean age of 64 ± 9 y have coronary flow reserves in response to dipyridamole stress that are significantly smaller than those of younger adults aged 31 ± 9 y: 3.0 ± 0.7 vs 4.1 ± 0.9.
Chest Pain, Normal Coronary Artery					
Geltman et al. [55]	$H_2^{15}O$	1.61 ± 0.38	—	2.26 ± 0.92	Approximately half of patients with angina and angiographically normal coronary arteries have elevated resting blood flows and a blunted hyperemic response to dipyridamole.
Camici et al. [56]	$^{13}NH_3$	0.88 ± 0.13	—	1.48 ± 0.29	Approximately one third of patients with chest pain, angiographically normal coronary arteries, and ST segment depression on stress ECG have a blunted hyperemic response to dipyridamole and an impaired myocardial perfusion reserve.

ECG—electrocardiogram; HDL—high-density lipoprotein; IV—intravenous; LDL—low-density lipoprotein; Rx—treatment.

FIGURE 10-18. Several examples of the clinical utility of quantitative perfusion measurements made with dynamic positron emission tomography (PET) imaging. Conventional planar or single-photon emission tomography (SPECT) perfusion or metabolic images, as well as static PET perfusion or metabolic images, depict proportionate tissue tracer concentrations and therefore only relative myocardial perfusion or metabolism. In patients with "balanced" coronary artery disease or homogeneous myocardial pathophysiology (nonischemic cardiomyopathies, heart transplant rejection, chest pain with normal coronary arteries), conventional imaging techniques may offer little additional useful information because frequently there are no regional disparities in the disease process.

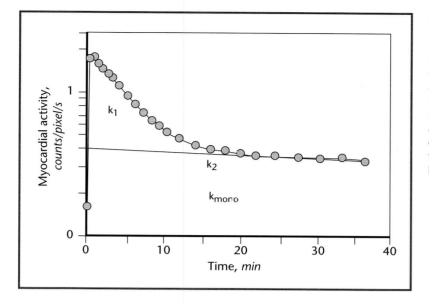

FIGURE 10-19. Myocardial time–activity curve obtained from a dynamic $^{11}C11$ acetate positron emission tomography (PET) imaging study. The myocardial time–activity curve demonstrates prompt tissue uptake of the activity and a biexponential pattern of clearance from the myocardium. The curve can be fit using a biexponential curve-fitting technique, to derive both k_1 and k_2. k_1, the constant for the first component of the exponential curve-fit, is linearly related to myocardial oxygen consumption. The second smaller exponential component, k_2, probably reflects incorporation of a label into an amino acid pool. In situations of low myocardial oxygen demand, a monoexponential curve fit can be performed. As illustrated, k_{mono}, the rate constant derived from the monoexponential curve-fitting process, slightly underestimates k_1 but is less affected by the statistical noise associated with low count rates.

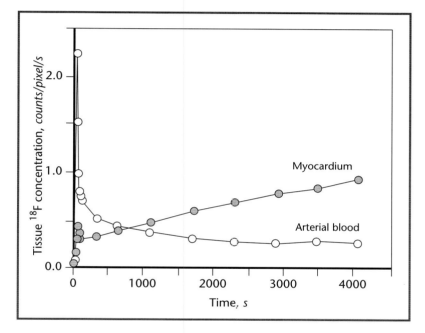

FIGURE 10-20. Myocardial and arterial ^{18}F activity following the intravenous administration of ^{18}F 2-fluoro-2-deoxyglucose (FDG). The initial vascular concentration increases abruptly and then declines over time as the tracer is cleared from the vascular space. FDG concentration within the myocardium progressively increases over time as the radiopharmaceutical is metabolically trapped within the cardiac myocytes. The ratio of the myocardial-to-arterial curves provides an index of tissue-to-background activity. As can be observed from these curves, the target-to-background activity continually improves during the course of the imaging study.

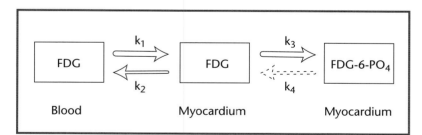

FIGURE 10-21. The tracer kinetic model used for quantitation of rates of myocardial glucose consumption with ^{18}F-2-fluoro-2-deoxyglucose (FDG). Following its transport into the myocardium, hexokinase phosphorylates FDG at the 6-carbon position. In contrast to other tissues, such as liver, the dephosphorylation of FDG-6-phosphate (PO_4) in myocardium is an extremely slow process relative to its rate of phosphorylation. Once phosphorylated, FDG is essentially irreversibly bound within the cardiac myocyte because the phosphorylated moiety is virtually impermeable to the cell membrane. Quantitative analysis of the myocardial FDG time–activity curves, using this tracer-kinetic model, yields a quantitative measurement of the rate of consumption of exogenous glucose by tissue in micromoles per minute per gram. k_1 and k_2 are the forward and backward rate constants for transport of FDG into myocardium. k_3 and k_4 represent the rate constants for the phosphorylation and dephosphorylation of FDG, respectively. In myocardium, k_4 is virtually negligible relative to the other rate constants.

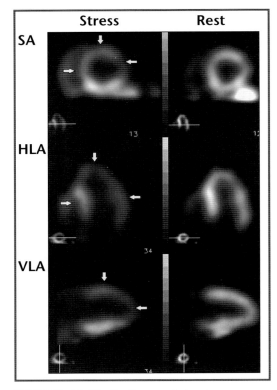
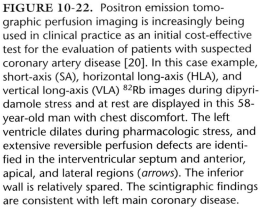

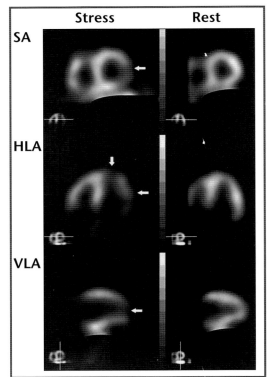
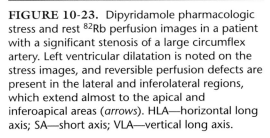

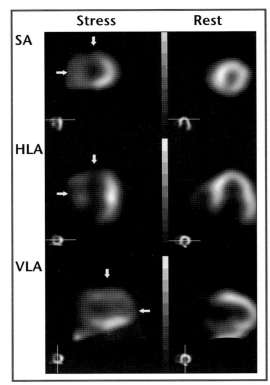

FIGURE 10-22. Positron emission tomographic perfusion imaging is increasingly being used in clinical practice as an initial cost-effective test for the evaluation of patients with suspected coronary artery disease [20]. In this case example, short-axis (SA), horizontal long-axis (HLA), and vertical long-axis (VLA) [82]Rb images during dipyridamole stress and at rest are displayed in this 58-year-old man with chest discomfort. The left ventricle dilates during pharmacologic stress, and extensive reversible perfusion defects are identified in the interventricular septum and anterior, apical, and lateral regions (*arrows*). The inferior wall is relatively spared. The scintigraphic findings are consistent with left main coronary disease.

FIGURE 10-23. Dipyridamole pharmacologic stress and rest [82]Rb perfusion images in a patient with a significant stenosis of a large circumflex artery. Left ventricular dilatation is noted on the stress images, and reversible perfusion defects are present in the lateral and inferolateral regions, which extend almost to the apical and inferoapical areas (*arrows*). HLA—horizontal long axis; SA—short axis; VLA—vertical long axis.

FIGURE 10-24. Dipyridamole stress and rest [82]Rb images demonstrating reversible perfusion defects in the interventricular septal and anterior and apical regions (*arrows*) in this patient with disease of the left anterior descending coronary artery. Moderate left ventricular dilatation is noted on the stress images. HLA—horizontal long axis; SA—short axis; VLA—vertical long axis.

EDV	ESV

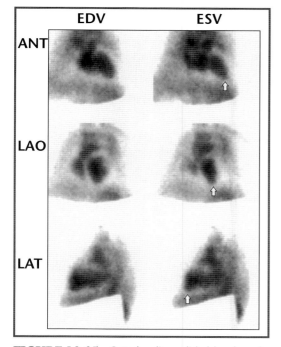

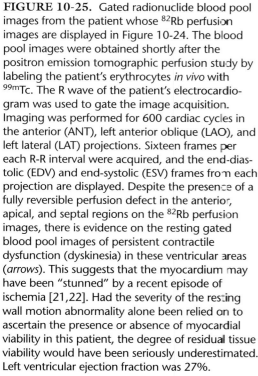

FIGURE 10-25. Gated radionuclide blood pool images from the patient whose [82]Rb perfusion images are displayed in Figure 10-24. The blood pool images were obtained shortly after the positron emission tomographic perfusion study by labeling the patient's erythrocytes *in vivo* with [99m]Tc. The R wave of the patient's electrocardiogram was used to gate the image acquisition. Imaging was performed for 600 cardiac cycles in the anterior (ANT), left anterior oblique (LAO), and left lateral (LAT) projections. Sixteen frames per each R-R interval were acquired, and the end-diastolic (EDV) and end-systolic (ESV) frames from each projection are displayed. Despite the presence of a fully reversible perfusion defect in the anterior, apical, and septal regions on the [82]Rb perfusion images, there is evidence on the resting gated blood pool images of persistent contractile dysfunction (dyskinesia) in these ventricular areas (*arrows*). This suggests that the myocardium may have been "stunned" by a recent episode of ischemia [21,22]. Had the severity of the resting wall motion abnormality alone been relied on to ascertain the presence or absence of myocardial viability in this patient, the degree of residual tissue viability would have been seriously underestimated. Left ventricular ejection fraction was 27%.

Stress	Redistribution

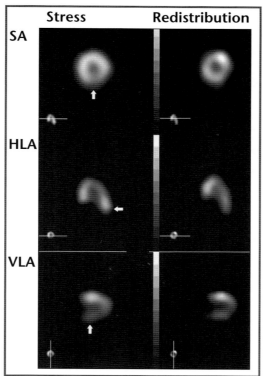

FIGURE 10-26. Stress and redistribution ^{201}Tl tomographic images in the short axis (SA), horizontal long-axis (HLA), and vertical long-axis (VLA) projections. Positron emission tomography has several advantages that improve the diagnostic accuracy relative to single photon emission tomography thallium scintigraphy for coronary artery disease detection. The study demonstrates a persistent reduction in tracer activity involving the inferior and the adjacent inferolateral (*arrows*) area of left ventricle in a pattern, which may reflect soft-tissue attenuation. No reversible defects to suggest stress-induced ischemia were noted.

Stress	Rest

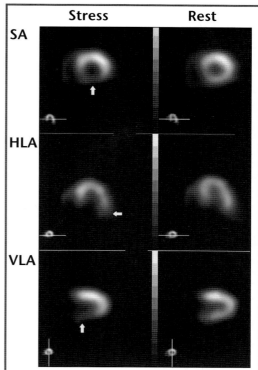

FIGURE 10-27. Dipyridamole stress and rest [82]Rb cardiac positron emission tomography (PET) images in the patient whose single photon emission computed tomography (SPECT) thallium images were shown in Figure 10-26. A reversible perfusion defect is noted in the inferior and adjacent inferolateral myocardial areas (*arrows*), which is consistent with disease of the right coronary artery. The enhanced contrast resolution with PET, along with the ability to accurately correct for soft tissue attenuation by means of individualized transmission imaging, provides an incremental benefit for the detection of coronary artery disease relative to SPECT perfusion imaging. Figure 10-28 is an analysis of the sensitivity, specificity, and diagnostic accuracy of both SPECT and PET images in the same patient populations with angiographic correlation. HLA—horizontal long axis; SA—short axis; VLA—vertical long axis.

PET versus ^{201}Tl SPECT for Detection of Coronary Artery Disease in Same Patients

Imaging Center	Patients, n	PET, n/n(%)	SPECT, n/n(%)	Probability
A. Sensitivity (Patients with Angiographic CAD)				
Kyoto University, Japan [57]	48	47/48(98)	46/48(96)	NS
University of Michigan [58]	60	52/60(87)	52/60(87)	NS
Cleveland Clinic [59]	98	93/98(95)	77/98(79)	< 0.002
Total	206	192/206(93)	175/206(85)	< 0.005
B. Specificity (Patients with No CAD on Angiography)				
Kyoto University, Japan [57]	3	3/3(100)	3/3(100)	NS
University of Michigan [58]	21	17/21(82)	11/21(52)	< 0.025
Cleveland Clinic [59]	34	28/34(82)	26/34(76)	NS
Total	55	45/55(82)	37/55(67)	< 0.05
C. Overall Accuracy				
Kyoto University, Japan [57]	51	50/51(98)	49/51(96)	NS
University of Michigan [58]	81	69/81(85)	63/81(78)	NS
Cleveland Clinic [59]	132	121/132(92)	103/132(78)	< 0.002
Total	264	240/264(91)	215/264(81)	< 0.001

NS—not significant.

FIGURE 10-28. Clinical studies comparing positron emission tomography (PET) with single photon emission tomography (SPECT) for detection of coronary artery disease (CAD) in the same patients. Although PET perfusion imaging is slightly more costly than SPECT ^{201}Tl scintigraphy, the total costs borne by the health care system reflect not only those of the imaging procedures themselves, but also the indirect costs associated with establishing (or missing) the diagnosis of CAD. For example, a false-positive imaging study may result in an inappropriate referral for coronary angiography, generating additional costs for the patient's health care provider. Alternatively, a false-negative result could delay or prevent appropriate medical treatment in an individual with actual CAD, which may lead to earlier morbidity or mortality from the disease process.

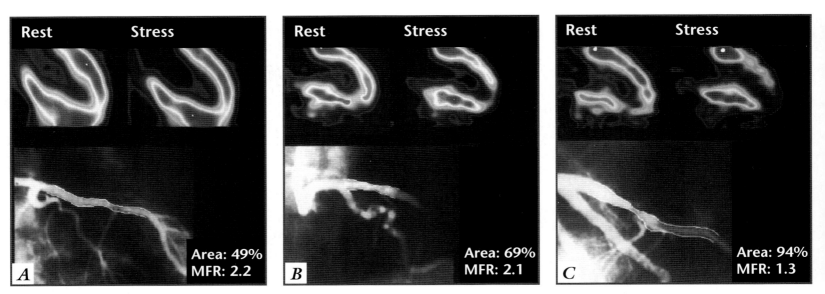

FIGURE 10-29. In individuals with coronary arterial stenoses, rest and stress positron emission tomographic perfusion imaging can provide additional information about the physiologic significance of the lesions. **A,** This patient has a 49% percent area left anterior descending coronary artery (LAD) stenosis on quantitative coronary arteriography. Although a reversible perfusion defect is not clearly present on the rest and dipyridamole stress ^{13}N ammonia perfusion images, quantitative measurements of regional blood flow reveal a slightly decreased myocardial flow reserve (MFR) of 2.2 in the affected region (normal is typically greater than 2.6). **B,** This patient's quantitative angiogram revealed a 69% area stenosis of the LAD. A small reversible perfusion defect is present in the anteroapical area of the ventricle on the stress and rest images, and the calculated myocardial perfusion reserve was decreased at 2.1. **C,** This patient's quantitative coronary angiography revealed a LAD arterial area stenosis of 94%, which was associated with an extensive reversible perfusion defect on the stress and rest ^{13}N ammonia perfusion images and a markedly reduced perfusion reserve of 1.3. (*Courtesy of* Marcelo Di Carli.)

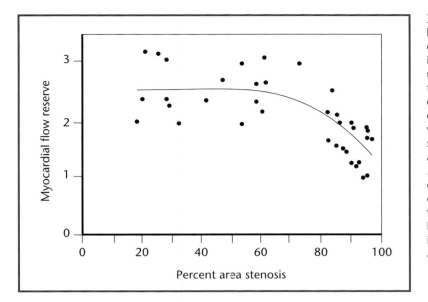

FIGURE 10-30. Relationship between coronary artery disease (CAD) lesion severity and myocardial flow reserve (MFR). Di Carli et al. [23] examined the relationship between coronary stenosis severity and MFR in patients with CAD. Noninvasive measurements of MFR were obtained using rest and dipyridamole ^{13}N ammonia dynamic positron emission tomographic (PET) perfusion imaging studies in regions supplied by diseased vessels. Measurements of percent luminal area stenosis were derived from quantitative coronary angiography, using biplane orthogonal views of each lesion. As the luminal percent area stenosis increases and the severity of a coronary lesion becomes more pronounced, there is an inverse and nonlinear decrease in MFR in the affected vascular territory ($r = 0.78$; $P < 0.00001$). These authors suggested that flow reserve measurements derived from noninvasive ^{13}N ammonia PET perfusion imaging could distinguish lesions of 50% to 70% area stenosis from those of 70% to 90% area stenosis. PET perfusion imaging thus affords the greatest clinical benefit when used to assess the physiologic impact of lesions appearing intermediate in severity on coronary angiography. (*Adapted from* Di Carli and coworkers [23]; with permission.)

EVALUATION OF LEFT VENTRICULAR DYSFUNCTION BY POSITRON EMISSION TOMOGRAPHY IMAGING

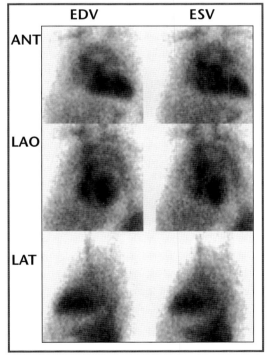

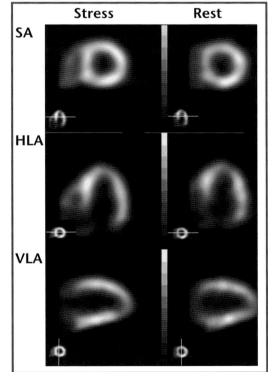

FIGURE 10-31. Gated radionuclide blood pool images from a patient who was referred for evaluation of symptoms of congestive heart failure. The blood pool images were obtained by labeling the patient's erythrocytes *in vivo* with [99m]Tc. Imaging was performed for 600 cardiac cycles in the anterior (ANT), left anterior oblique (LAO), and left lateral (LAT) projections, using the R wave of the patient's electrocardiogram to gate the image acquisition. Sixteen frames per R-R interval were acquired, and the end-diastolic (EDV) and end-systolic (ESV) frames from each projection are displayed. Both ventricles appear dilated, and there is diffuse left and right ventricular systolic dysfunction. Left ventricular ejection fraction (LVEF) was 25%.

FIGURE 10-32. Dipyridamole stress and rest [82]Rb positron emission tomography (PET) perfusion images from the patient whose gated blood pool images are displayed in Figure 10-31. Dilatation of the right and left ventricles is noted on both the stress and rest images. No reversible defects are identified to suggest pharmacologic stress-induced ischemia. Although there is heterogeneity in [82]Rb activity on both the stress and rest images with thinning of counts in the inferoapical region, no large fixed perfusion defects are noted to suggest prior infarction. The findings in this patient are consistent with idiopathic dilated cardiomyopathy, and on angiography the coronary arteries appeared normal. The findings on the [82]Rb PET perfusion images are consistent with prior clinical imaging studies using single photon imaging with [201]Tl [24–26], in which a normal perfusion pattern or only small-to-moderate perfusion defects favored the diagnosis of idiopathic dilated cardiomyopathy whereas extensive perfusion defects were frequently associated with ischemic cardiomyopathy. HLA—horizontal long axis; SA—short axis; VLA—vertical long axis.

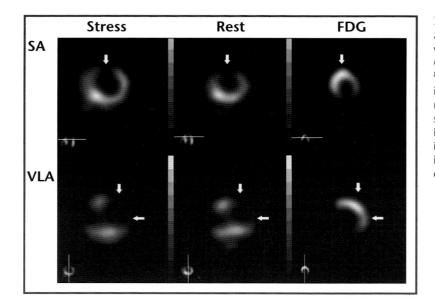

	Stress	Rest	FDG
SA			
VLA			

FIGURE 10-33. Dipyridamole stress and rest [82]Rb perfusion images, along with [18]F 2-fluoro-2-deoxyglucose (FDG) metabolic images in a patient with coronary artery disease and a history of prior myocardial infarction. On the short axis (SA) and vertical long axis (VLA) images, extensive fixed [82]Rb perfusion defects are identified in the septal, anterior, apical, and inferoapical regions (*arrows*). On the FDG metabolic images, matching metabolic defects are noted in the ventricular regions with the fixed perfusion defects. This pattern of matching perfusion and FDG metabolic defects is termed *PET infarction* by some authors because ventricular function rarely improves if revascularization is performed (*see* Figure 10-34). The images indicate a completed infarction in the distribution of the left anterior descending coronary artery.

Relationship of PET FDG Metabolic Activity to Improvement in Function after Coronary Revascularization

Patients, *n*	Segments, *n*	Procedure	Segments with Improved WM, *n/n*(%)		LVEF, %		Study
			With FDG Uptake	No FDG Uptake	Pre	Post	
17	67	CABG	35/41(85)	2/26(8)	32 ± 14	41 ± 15	Tillisch *et al.* [60]
22	46	CABG	18/23(78)*	5/23(22)	NR	NR	Tamaki *et al.* [61]
11	56	CABG	40/50(80)*	0/6(0)	NR	NR	Tamaki *et al.* [62]
16	85	PTCA, CABG	25/37(68)	10/48(21)	NR	NR	Marwick *et al.* [63]
14	54	CABG	37/39(95)*	3/15(20)	38 ± 5	48 ± 4	Lucignani *et al.* [64]
21	23	CABG	16/19(84)	1/4(25)	34 ± 14	52 ± 11	Carrel *et al.* [65]
34	116	CABG, PTCA	38/73(52)	8/43(19)	NR	NR	Gropler *et al.* [66,67]
48	90	PTCA, CABG	23/27(85)	10/63(16)	53 ± 11	NR	Knuuti *et al.* [68]
37	110	PTCA, CABG	24/59(41)†	7/51(14)†	34 ± 10	36 ± 10	vom Dahl *et al.* [69]
43	130	CABG, PTCA	45/59(76)*	6/71(9)	41	NR	Tamaki *et al.* [70]
12‡	12	PTCA, CABG	12/12(100)	—	55 ± 7	65 ± 8	Vanoverschelde *et al.* [71]
20‡	20	CABG	8/12(67)	2/8(25)	49 ± 9	56 ± 9	Maes *et al.* [72]
25	25	CABG, PTCA	16/19(84)§	1/6(17)	49 ± 11	57 ± 15	Grandin *et al.* [73]
24‡	24	CABG	7/9(78)	9/15(60)	39 ± 15	42 ± 19	Depre *et al.* [74]
39	39	CABG, PTCA	18/23(78)	6/16(38)	33 ± 10	40 ± 10	Gerber *et al.* [75]
42	371	CABG, PTCA	167/180(93)	65/191(34)	40 ± 13	NR	Baer *et al.* [76]
52	55	CABG, PTCA	19/28(68)	2/27(7)	47 ± 10	52 ± 11	vom Dahl *et al.* [77]
Total							
477	1323		548/710(77)	137/613(22)	39	46	

* Metabolic imaging performed in the fasting state.
†Segments with moderate hypokinesis or worse function.
‡Histopathologic correlation performed.
§FDG metabolic imaging results were incorporated into a discriminant model that also included absolute measurements of myocardial blood flow.
CABG—coronary artery bypass graft; LVEF—left ventricular ejection fraction; NR—not reported; PET—positron emission tomography;
PTCA—percutaneous transluminal coronary angioplasty; WM—wall motion.

FIGURE 10-34. Relationship of positron emission tomography (PET) [18]F 2-fluoro-2-deoxyglucose (FDG) metabolic activity to improvement in function after coronary revascularization. Accumulating clinical studies indicate that the presence of tissue glucose metabolism in hypoperfused ventricular segments on FDG PET metabolic images can be used to predict improvement in regional contractile function following interventional restoration of blood flow.

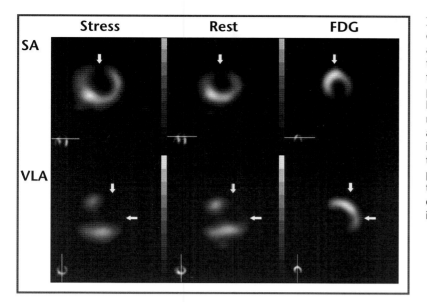

FIGURE 10-35. Dipyridamole stress and rest ^{82}Rb images in this patient demonstrate a fixed perfusion defect involving the septal, anterior, apical, and inferoapical regions. The perfusion images suggest prior infarction in the distribution of the left anterior descending coronary artery. In contrast to the case example in Figure 10-33, however, glucose metabolism is well preserved in the myocardial areas with the fixed perfusion defects, as shown by the prominent uptake of ^{18}F 2-fluoro-2-deoxyglucose (FDG) on the myocardial metabolic images. The "mismatch" between resting perfusion and glucose metabolism on the positron emission tomography (PET) images is termed *PET ischemia* by some authors. In this individual, considerable tissue viability remains in the hypoperfused ventricular regions, and the probability is high that coronary revascularization will benefit regional function (*see* Figure 10-34). In this case example, PET FDG metabolic imaging distinguished viable but jeopardized tissue from the scar of completed infarction.

POSITRON EMISSION TOMOGRAPHIC TISSUE CHARACTERIZATION: HISTOPATHOLOGIC CORRELATION

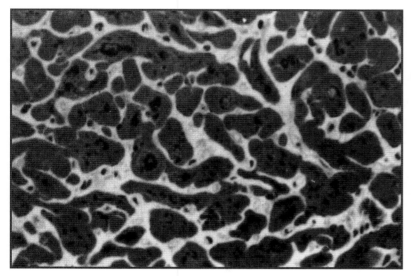

FIGURE 10-36. Light microscopic findings in a myocardial biopsy taken from the distal anterior left ventricular wall at the time of coronary artery bypass surgery in a 66-year-old woman with chronic stable angina. The patient had a 90% stenosis of the left anterior descending coronary artery and normal regional wall motion on contrast ventriculography prior to revascularization. Preoperative positron emission tomographic imaging demonstrated normal perfusion and glucose metabolism. On quantitative analysis of dynamic ^{13}N ammonia perfusion and ^{18}F 2-fluoro-2-deoxyglucose metabolic images, myocardial blood flow averaged 0.88 mL/min/g and glucose utilization 0.50 µmol/min/g in the area. The biopsy specimen was stained with periodic acid–Schiff (PAS), which identifies glycogen as a darkly colored amorphous collection of the stain. The biopsy specimen demonstrates a paucity of PAS-positive cells and relatively normal-appearing cardiac myocytes (*From* Maes and coworkers [27]; with permission.)

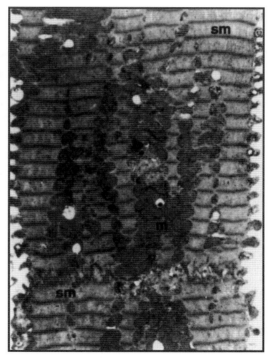

FIGURE 10-37. Electron microscopic findings in the patient whose light microscopic findings are presented in Figure 10-36. Sarcomeres (sm) are abundant and uniformly positioned throughout the myocytes. The number and appearance of mitochondria (m) are normal. On quantitative analysis of the biopsy specimens in this patient, the endocardium had 17% fibrosis, whereas the epicardium had 12% fibrosis. When examined for the number of myocytes in which glycogen stores had replaced more than 10% of the cell's sarcomeres, 9% of the endocardial cells and 4.5% of the epicardial cells exhibited this finding. Following revascularization, the regional ejection fraction on gated radionuclide ventriculography was 88%, essentially unchanged from the normal preoperative regional ejection fraction of 85%. This patient thus demonstrated only minor histologic changes in a myocardial region that was considered normal on positron emission tomographic ^{13}N ammonia perfusion and ^{18}F 2-fluoro-2-deoxyglucose metabolic images. (*From* Maes and coworkers [27]; with permission.)

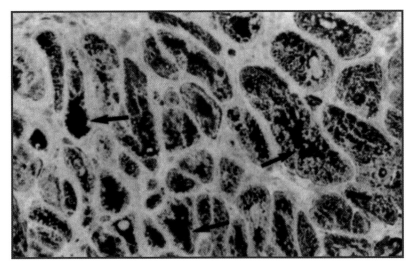

FIGURE 10-38. Light microscopic findings in a myocardial biopsy obtained from the distal anterior wall at the time of coronary revascularization in a 48-year-old man with stable angina and a 70% stenosis of the left anterior descending coronary artery. The anterior wall was hypokinetic on contrast ventriculography and preoperative positron emission tomographic (PET) imaging with ^{13}N ammonia and [18]F 2-fluoro-2-deoxyglucose demonstrated a perfusion-metabolism mismatch. Quantitative analysis of the dynamic PET images yielded an average blood flow of 0.63 mL/min/g in the anterior region, about 64% of the 0.98 mL/min/g noted in normal myocardium. Glucose consumption in the affected region was 0.46 μmol/min/g, slightly higher than the 0.41 μmol/min/g noted in remote myocardium. On the periodic acid–Schiff–stained biopsy specimen, several prominent accumulations of glycogen are noted (*arrows*). Although cell volume appears preserved, some myocytes appear to exhibit a loss of contractile protein from the cytoplasm. (*From* Maes and coworkers [27]; with permission.)

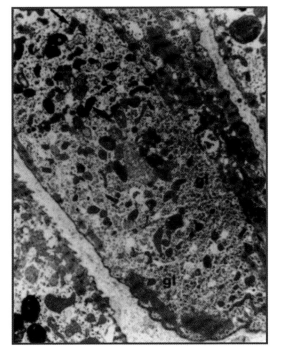

FIGURE 10-39. Electron microscopic results in the patient with the perfusion-metabolism mismatch on preoperative positron emission tomographic (PET) images whose light microscopic findings are illustrated in Figure 10-38. Electron microscopy confirms that there is a loss of contractile proteins, with sarcomeres (sm) identifiable only at the periphery of the cell. Accumulation of glycogen (gl) is noted in the cytosol, and the mitochondria are small and primitive in appearance (*arrows*). On quantitative analysis, the endocardium had 15% fibrosis, whereas the epicardium had 3% fibrosis. When examined for the number of myocytes in which glycogen had replaced more than 10% of the cell's sarcomeres, 15% of the endocardial and epicardial cells exhibited this finding. Following successful revascularization, the regional ejection fraction increased from 46% to 55%, and the global left ventricular ejection fraction increased from 54% to 62%. Thus, significant improvement in regional and global left ventricular function was noted after revascularization, despite the histologic abnormalities present in the region with the perfusion-metabolism mismatch on preoperative PET imaging. (*From* Maes and coworkers [27]; with permission.)

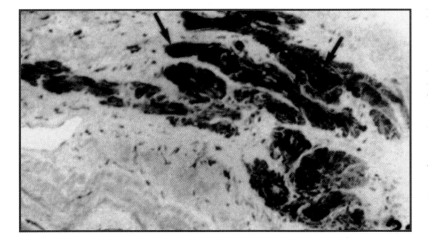

FIGURE 10-40. Light microscopic findings in an anterior wall myocardial biopsy obtained at the time of coronary bypass surgery in a 70-year-old man with stable angina and matching perfusion and metabolic defects on preoperative positron emission tomographic (PET) images. Coronary angiography demonstrated an occlusion of the left anterior descending coronary artery and a 90% stenosis of the circumflex artery. Contrast ventriculography revealed anterior wall hypokinesis prior to surgical revascularization. Extensive connective tissue (scar) is apparent on this periodic acid–Schiff–stained specimen, and glycogen deposition is noted in a number of the myocytes (*arrows*) associated with a loss of contractile protein. Myocardial blood flows averaged 0.63 mL/min/g in the anterior wall on the preoperative PET perfusion images, or about 72% of the 0.88 mL/min/g observed in normal myocardium. Absolute rates of glucose consumption in the affected area averaged 0.43 μmol/min/g, considerably less than the 0.69 μmol/min/g noted in reference myocardium. (*From* Maes and coworkers [27]; with permission.)

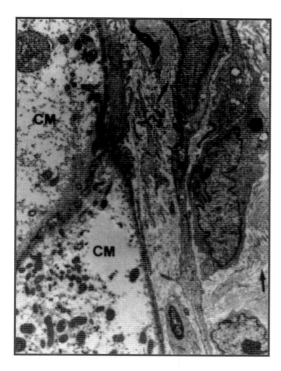

FIGURE 10-41. Electron microscopic findings in the biopsy of the patient with anterior wall hypokinesis and matching perfusion and metabolic defects on positron emission tomographic (PET) imaging. The myocytes (CM) exhibit a profound depletion of sarcomeres, and there is extensive connective tissue (scar; *arrows*). The relative amount of fibrosis averaged 55% in the endocardium and 40% in the epicardium in this patient. None of the cells in the epicardium had more than 10% of their sarcomeres replaced by glycogen, whereas 32% of the myocytes in the endocardium were reported to have this finding. Following successful revascularization, the regional ejection fraction dropped to 17% from a preoperative value of 23%, and there was a modest increase in global ejection fraction from 50% to 55%. Measures of relative and absolute perfusion therefore could not have distinguished this patient without recovery of regional function from the individual whose biopsy findings were shown in Figures 10-38 and 10-39, in whom regional wall motion substantially improved after revascularization. In contrast, positron emission tomographic metabolic imaging with ^{18}F 2-fluoro-2-deoxyglucose readily distinguished between the patients with and without recovery of regional function. (*From* Maes and coworkers [27]; with permission.)

POSITRON EMISSION TOMOGRAPHIC ^{18}F 2-FLUORO-2-DEOXYGLUCOSE METABOLIC IMAGING VERSUS OTHER CLINICAL TESTS FOR MYOCARDIAL VIABILITY

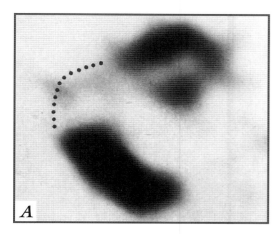

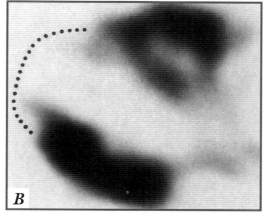

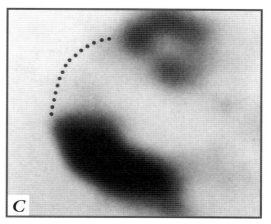

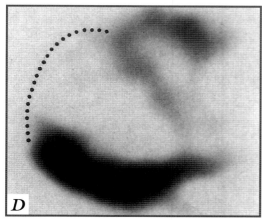

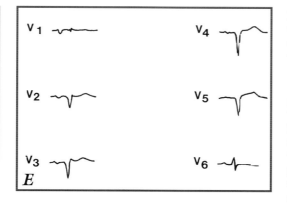

FIGURE 10-42. Representative ^{13}N ammonia transverse images (**A** and **B**), ^{18}F 2-fluoro-2-deoxyglucose metabolic images (**C** and **D**), and the precordial electrocardiogram in a 68-year-old man with a history of myocardial infarction 5 months prior to study. A matching reduction in perfusion and glucose metabolism is noted on the positron emission tomography (PET) images involving the anterior (*dotted lines*) and septal regions of the ventricle. The PET images were, therefore, consistent with the electrocardiographic (**E**) diagnosis of chronic anterior and septal myocardial infarction. (*From* Brunken and coworkers [28]; with permission.)

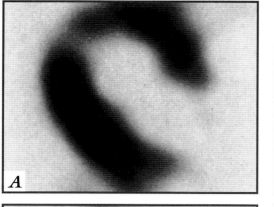

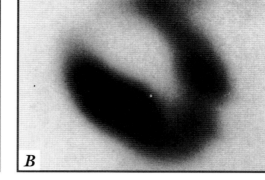

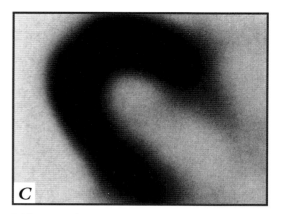

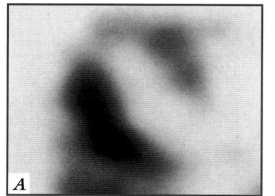

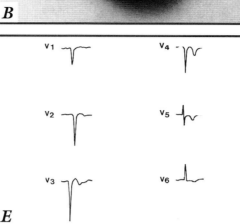

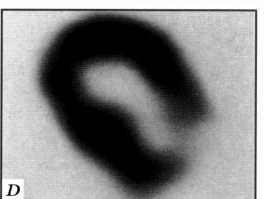

FIGURE 10-43. Positron emission tomographic ^{13}N ammonia perfusion images (A and B), metabolic images (C and D), and the precordial electrocardiogram (E) in a 59-year-old man who sustained a myocardial infarction 1 year before the study. Although pathologic Q waves are noted on the electrocardiogram in leads V_1 through V_4, the scintigraphic study demonstrates a perfusion-metabolism mismatch indicative of residual tissue viability. (*From* Brunken *and coworkers* [28]; with permission.)

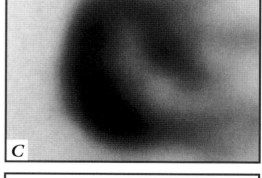

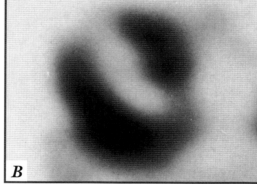

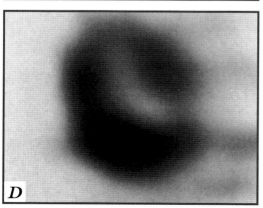

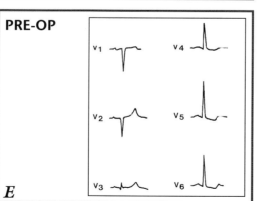

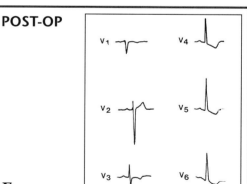

PRE-OP

POST-OP

FIGURE 10-44. Pre- and postoperative precordial electrocardiograms from a 73-year-old woman with a history of two previous myocardial infarctions and recurrent angina. The positron emission tomographic (PET) perfusion images (A and B) demonstrate a perfusion defect involving the anterior region of the ventricle. Preserved glucose utilization is noted in the same ventricular region on the PET metabolic images (C and D). The preoperative (PRE-OP) electrocardiographic (E) tracings demonstrate Q waves in leads V_1 and V_2 and a small Q wave in lead V_3. Following successful coronary artery bypass surgery, the Q waves were replaced by R waves on the postoperative (POST-OP) electrocardiographic tracing (F). Associated with the change in the patient's electrocardiogram was an improvement in regional wall motion in the anteroapical area of the ventricle from akinesis to severe hypokinesis and an improvement in global left ventricular ejection fraction from 25% to 45% after coronary bypass surgery. Thus, electrographic Q waves do not necessarily imply the absence of myocardial viability. PET imaging with ^{18}F 2-fluoro-2-deoxyglucose has identified tissue metabolic viability in up to 54% of chronic electrocardiographic Q wave infarct regions [28]. (*From* Brunken and coworkers [28]; with permission.)

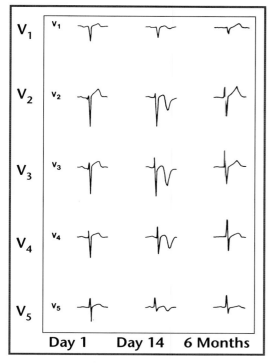

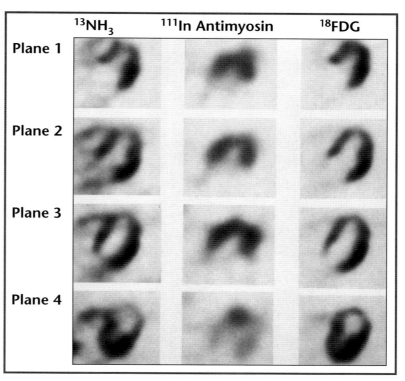

FIGURE 10-45. Serial precordial electrocardiographic tracings in a 64-year-old man who presented with substernal chest discomfort of 60 minutes duration and on serial laboratory tests was noted to have an increase in peak creatine kinase and creatine kinase myocardial band levels. The initial tracings demonstrate a loss of anterior R-wave voltage, ST elevation in leads V_1 to V_5, and small Q waves in leads V_2 and V_3. The patient was treated with thrombolytic therapy, and on day 14 the tracing demonstrated persistent ST segment elevation and T-wave inversion in leads V_2 to V_6. By 6 months, however, there is further improvement in R-wave progression and residual minor ST changes. (*From* Brunken and Schelbert [29]; with permission.)

FIGURE 10-46. Representative ^{13}N ammonia perfusion images, ^{111}In antimyosin single photon emission tomography (SPECT) images and ^{18}F 2-fluoro-2-deoxyglucose (FDG) metabolic positron emission tomographic (PET) images in the patient whose electrocardiographic tracings were shown in Figure 10-45. Whereas the SPECT images were acquired 48 hours after presentation, the PET images were acquired on the fifth hospital day. The ^{13}N ammonia perfusion images demonstrate a perfusion defect involving the superior septal, anterior, and apical ventricular segments. ^{111}In antimyosin activity, a marker of acute myocardial necrosis, is identified in the hypoperfused ventricular regions. Metabolic imaging, however, demonstrates preserved FDG activity in most of the hypoperfused ventricular regions. Echocardiography in the coronary care unit early after clinical presentation revealed severe anterior and apical hypokinesis with an estimated left ventricular ejection fraction (LVEF) of 40%. At 6 months, echocardiography revealed akinesis to dyskinesis of a small portion of the apical area with normal function in the remaining ventricular segments. Resting LVEF had improved to 58%. Thus, despite the presence of an acute myocardial infarction, which was identified both by conventional laboratory criteria and by an accumulation of a labeled antibody specific for acute necrosis, the presence of preserved metabolic activity in the hypoperfused infarct region identified significant tissue viability. Most of the initial ventricular dysfunction, therefore, must have represented myocardial stunning, and PET metabolic imaging identified correctly tissue that subsequently demonstrated functional improvement. (*From* Brunken and Shelbert [29]; with permission.)

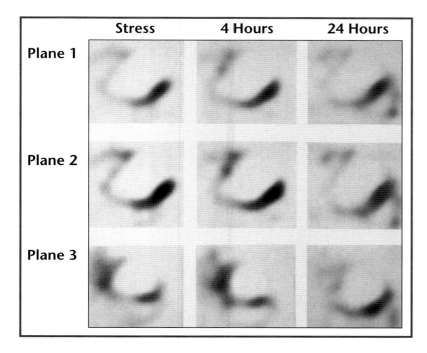

FIGURE 10-47. Stress, 4-hour, and 24-hour redistribution transverse single photon emission computed tomographic ^{201}Tl myocardial perfusion images in a 66-year-old man with congestive heart failure (left ventricular ejection fraction, 18%), prior myocardial infarction, and angina. Extensive fixed perfusion defects are noted in the anterior, apical, inferior, and posterolateral segments, and a partially reversible defect is noted in the superior septum. The left ventricle is markedly dilated. (*From* Brunken and coworkers [30]; with permission.)

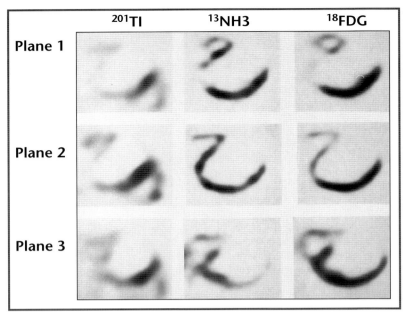

FIGURE 10-48. Twenty-four-hour redistribution single photon emission tomographic ^{201}Tl images from the patient in Figure 10-47 as well as the resting ^{13}N ammonia perfusion and ^{18}F 2-fluoro-2-deoxyglucose (FDG) metabolic cardiac positron emission tomographic (PET) images. Matching perfusion and metabolic defects consistent with irreversible injury are noted in the anterior and apical segments as well as in the superior septal segment, with a partially reversible thallium defect. In contrast, the hypoperfused inferior and posterolateral regions exhibit preserved glucose metabolism denoting PET ischemia. (*From* Brunken and coworkers [30]; with permission.)

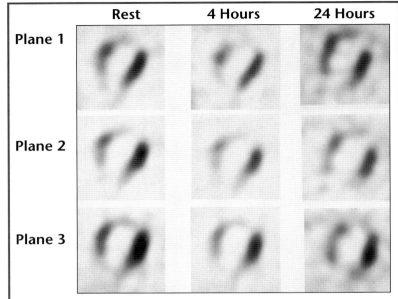

FIGURE 10-49. Rest, 4-hour, and 24-hour redistribution single photon emission tomography ^{201}Tl images from a 75-year-old man with two prior myocardial infarctions and congestive heart failure (left ventricular ejection fraction, 23%). Extensive fixed thallium defects are identified in the anterior, septal, and inferior segments in a dilated left ventricle. (*From* Brunken and coworkers [30]; with permission.)

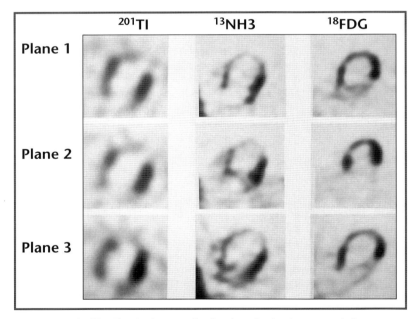

FIGURE 10-50. The 24-hour redistribution single photon emission tomographic (SPECT) ^{201}Tl images along with the corresponding ^{13}N ammonia perfusion and ^{18}F 2-fluoro-2-deoxyglucose (FDG) metabolic images from the patient whose SPECT study is shown in Figure 10-49. On the ^{13}N ammonia perfusion images, perfusion defects similar to those identified on the SPECT ^{201}Tl images are noted. Preserved glucose metabolism is identified in the anterior and septal segments, in a perfusion-metabolism mismatch indicating viable tissue. A matching concordant reduction of FDG uptake is noted in the hypoperfused inferior segment, which is consistent with PET infarction. (*From* Brunken and coworkers [30]; with permission.)

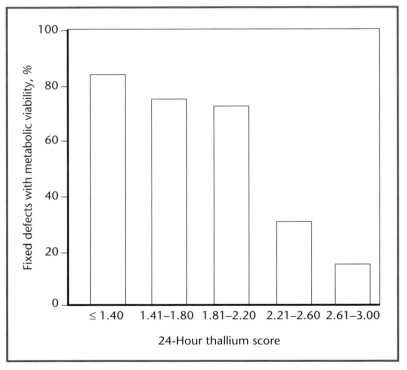

FIGURE 10-51. The relative proportion of fixed ^{201}Tl defects on 24-hour redistribution single photon emission computed tomography (SPECT) images, which exhibit preserved tissue metabolic viability on positron emission tomography (PET) imaging with ^{18}F 2-fluoro-2-deoxyglucose relative to the severity of the ^{201}Tl perfusion defect. A thallium score of 1 was considered indicative of a mild but definite defect; 2, a severe defect; and 3, a complete defect (one in which only background activity was identified). As the severity of the ^{201}Tl defect increases, the relative proportion of fixed SPECT defects with metabolic tissue viability declines. However, even for the most profound defects, there was a one in seven likelihood that metabolic viability would be identified on PET imaging. (*Adapted from* Brunken and coworkers [30].)

Effect of Revascularization on Perfusion, Metabolism, and Function

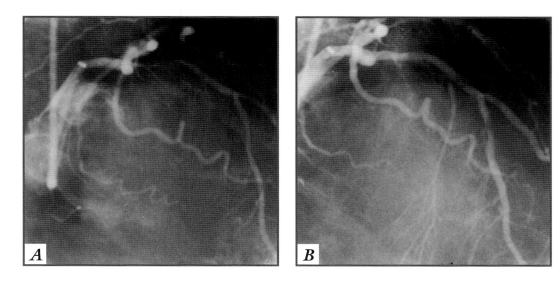

FIGURE 10-52. A, Coronary angiogram obtained in the right arterial oblique projection with cranial angulation demonstrating a severe lesion of the left anterior descending artery (stenosis area, 0.28 mm²). **B,** Coronary angiogram obtained following successful angioplasty of the culprit lesion. The angiogram demonstrates a marked improvement in blood flow in the coronary artery, and on quantitative angiography, the stenotic area had increased to 3.46 mm² following revascularization. (*From* Nienaber and coworkers [31]; with permission.)

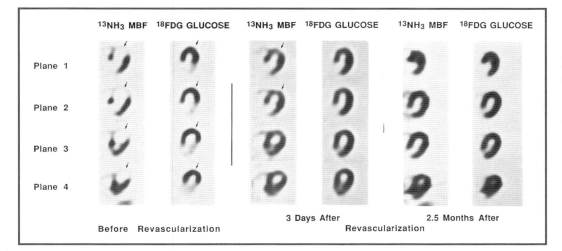

FIGURE 10-53. Serial ^{13}N ammonia perfusion and ^{18}F 2-fluoro-2-deoxyglucose (FDG) glucose metabolic positron emission tomographic (PET) images obtained in the patient whose angiographic results were shown in Figure 10-52. The initial PET study was obtained on the day of angioplasty, with follow-up PET scans obtained at 3 days and at 2.5 months. The pre-angioplasty ^{13}N ammonia perfusion images demonstrate an extensive perfusion defect involving the anterior, anteroseptal, and apical segments (*arrows*). Preserved glucose metabolism was noted in the hypoperfused vascular territory, indicating an extensive perfusion-metabolism mismatch. On the study performed 3 days after the procedure, perfusion had improved substantially in the risk territory, although a small deficit still remained (*arrows*). At this time, glucose metabolism was still enhanced relative to perfusion. On the late follow-up scan, both perfusion and metabolism have normalized. Thus,

recovery of regional myocardial perfusion preceded recovery of tissue glucose metabolism. Echocardiography before angioplasty demonstrated virtual akinesis of most of the risk territory and a depressed left ventricular ejection fraction (LVEF) of 32%. Little improvement in regional function was noted at 3 days, and the LVEF remained depressed at 36%. By the late follow-up study, however, substantial improvement in regional function was noted in the anterior wall with residual mild-to-moderate hypokinesia in the apical and periapical area. LVEF had improved to 62%.

In this investigation of 11 patients undergoing percutaneous transluminal coronary angioplasty (PTCA) who had perfusion-metabolism mismatches on PET images, early recovery in echocardiographic indices of regional contractile function after revascularization were unrelated to pre-PTCA perfusion or mismatch defect extent or severity. Late functional recovery, however, was linearly related to the extent and severity of the perfusion-metabolism mismatch on the pre-PTCA PET images, meaning that patients who had the most pronounced mismatches had the greatest improvement in wall motion following successful revascularization. (*From* Nienaber and coworkers [31]; with permission.)

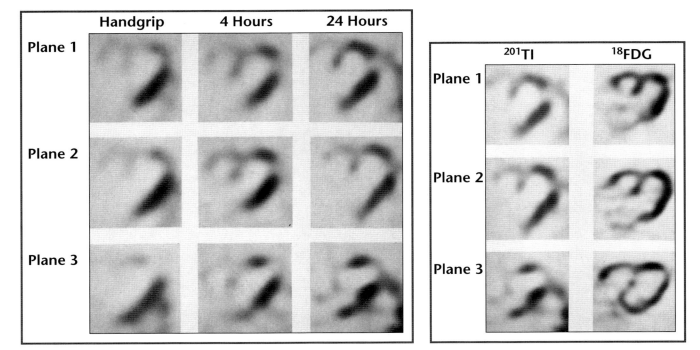

FIGURE 10-54. The temporal delay between coronary revascularization and recovery of function that can be observed in "hibernating myocardium." **A,** Handgrip, 4-hour, and 24-hour redistribution single photon emission computed tomography ²⁰¹Tl perfusion images in a 45-year-old man with angina and congestive heart failure. Extensive fixed perfusion defects are identified in the anterolateral, anteroseptal, septal, inferior, and inferolateral regions. **B,** ¹⁸F 2-fluoro-2-deoxyglucose (FDG) positron emission tomography (PET) metabolic images in the same patient. Preserved FDG activity is noted in the hypoperfused regions, indicating substantial residual tissue viability. Further, enhanced FDG activity relative to perfusion is identified in the right ventricle, suggesting a perfusion-metabolism mismatch in this region as well. (*From* Luu and coworkers [32]; with permission.)

Recovery of Left Ventricular Function after Revascularization

	LVEF (RNV), %		
Time	Rest	Exercise	LV EDD (Echo), *mm*
Preoperative	16	15	66
1 month	26	24	68
6 months	33	34	52
12 months	40	47	52

EDD—end-diastolic dimension; LVEF—left ventricular ejection fraction; RNV—radionuclide ventriculography.

FIGURE 10-55. Recovery of left ventricular (LV) function after revascularization. In the patient whose images are provided in Figure 10-54, coronary revascularization was successfully performed. As this sequence of noninvasive studies obtained in this individual demonstrates, there was a progressive improvement in LV function over time. As indicated by this case example, profound LV dysfunction may require a substantial period of time for the ultimate recovery of contractile function following restoration of coronary blood flow. (*Adapted from* Luu and coworkers [32].)

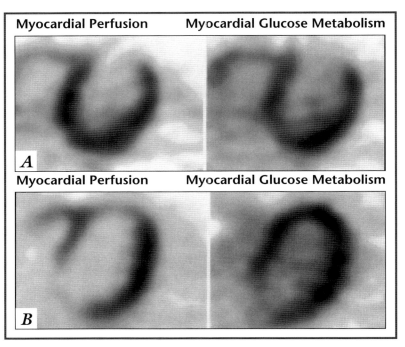

FIGURE 10-56. ¹³N ammonia perfusion and ¹⁸F 2-fluoro-2-deoxyglucose glucose metabolic positron emission tomography (PET) images from two patients with congestive heart failure (CHF). The patients' estimated exercise capacities (in metabolic equivalents) were quantitated before and after coronary artery bypass surgery using the Goldman Specific Activity Scale [33]. **A,** A small perfusion-metabolism mismatch (6%). Following successful coronary revascularization, only a modest improvement (24%) in Goldman activity scale estimated exercise capacity is noted. **B,** Contrasting case of a patient with a perfusion-metabolism mismatch involving 72% of the left ventricle. Successful revascularization resulted in a substantial improvement (200%) in the patient's estimated exercise capacity. (Case examples *courtesy of* Marcelo Di Carli.)

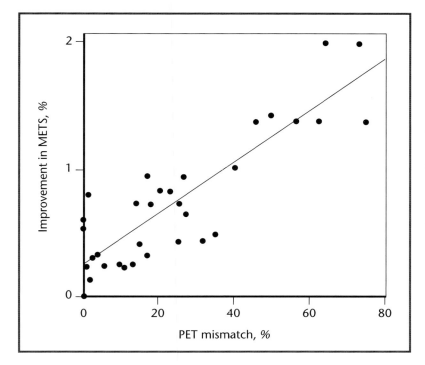

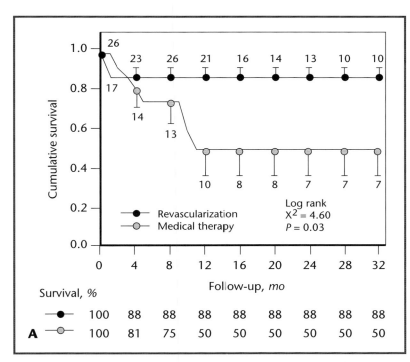

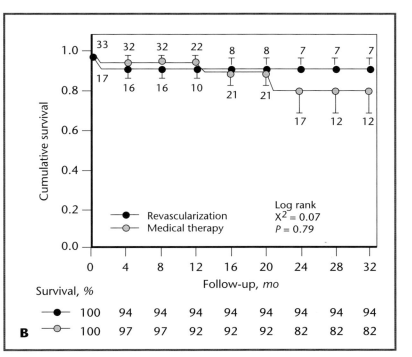

FIGURE 10-57. Improvement in exercise capacity (in metabolic equivalents [METS]) versus pre–coronary artery bypass graft (CABG) positron emission tomography (PET) mismatch. In a study of 36 patients with ischemic cardiomyopathy, Di Carli et al. [34] performed PET imaging with ^{13}N ammonia and ^{18}F 2-fluoro-2-deoxyglucose prior to coronary artery bypass surgery. The percent of the left ventricular myocardium exhibiting a perfusion-metabolism mismatch on the PET images was correlated with the change in reported exercise capacity obtained using the Goldman Specific Activity Scale [33]. A linear and highly significant correlation was observed between the extent of the preoperative perfusion-metabolism mismatch and the reported improvement in exercise capacity ($r = 0.87$; $P < 0.0001$). The presence or absence of angina was not related to the amount of myocardium exhibiting the perfusion-metabolism mismatch. A perfusion-metabolism mismatch involving 18% or more of the left ventricle predicted an improvement in functional class postoperatively of at least one grade, with a sensitivity of 76% and a specificity of 78%. This study thus demonstrates that the larger the perfusion-metabolism mismatch on PET imaging, the greater the functional benefit derived from successful revascularization. (*Adapted from* Di Carli and coworkers [34].)

FIGURE 10-58. Patients with coronary artery disease (CAD) and left ventricular (LV) dysfunction who exhibit perfusion-metabolism mismatches on positron emission tomographic (PET) imaging appear to be at higher risk for subsequent cardiac events. In 93 patients with CAD and LV dysfunction (mean LV ejection fraction [EF], 25 ± 6%), Di Carli et al. [35] reported that patients with perfusion-metabolism mismatches had a significantly better cumulative survival if treated surgically than those treated medically. **A,** Survival curves for patients with perfusion-metabolism mismatches according to type of treatment. *Solid circles* indicate patients who underwent coronary revascularization; *open circles* indicate those treated medically. The survival of the individuals with mismatches who were treated medically was only 50% at 1 year, which is significantly lower than the 88% noted in the individuals treated surgically.

B, Survival curves for the patients who had matching perfusion and metabolic defects on the positron emission tomography (PET) images. In these individuals, no significant difference was noted in survival up to 32 months. The survival curves for these individuals were comparable to those of the patients with mismatches who were treated surgically. In this study, the relative risk of

death increased by 3.5% for each percent increase in the amount of the LV affected by the perfusion-metabolism mismatch. Thus, individuals with the largest mismatches had the highest risk for cardiac death. Conversely, the risk of cardiac death was reduced by 28% in those who were treated surgically. In five clinical reports [35–39] involving 423 patients (mean LVEF, 37%), the risk of all adverse cardiac events over an average follow-up period of 18 months in those with mismatches treated medically was approximately threefold higher (41%) than in individuals with mismatches treated surgically (13%) or those with only matching defects treated either medically (12%) or surgically (11%). The risk of cardiac death in patients with perfusion-metabolism mismatches was approximately twofold higher (16.5%) than those with mismatches treated surgically (8.3%) or those with matching defects only treated either medically (9%) or surgically (7%). A perfusion-metabolism mismatch on PET imaging in patients with coronary artery disease and LV dysfunction thus identifies an individual who will benefit symptomatically, functionally, and prognostically from revascularization. The larger and more pronounced the perfusion-metabolism mismatch, the greater the anticipated benefit from coronary revascularization.

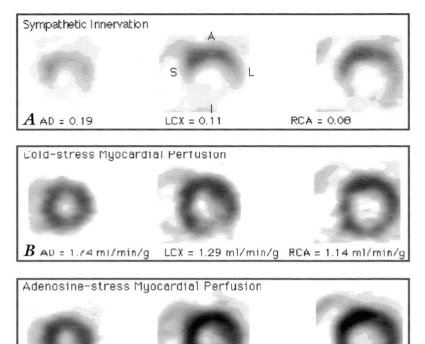

Sympathetic Innervation

A AD = 0.19   LCX = 0.11   RCA = 0.08

Cold-stress Myocardial Perfusion

B AD = 1.74 ml/min/g   LCX = 1.29 ml/min/g   RCA = 1.14 ml/min/g

Adenosine-stress Myocardial Perfusion

C AD = 3.3 ml/min/g   LCX = 3.2 ml/min/g   RCA = 3.1 ml/min/g

FIGURE 10-59. Representative apical, midventricular, and basal short-axis PET images (*left to right*) in a patient with previous cardiac transplantation. Future clinical investigations using cardiac positron emission tomographic (PET) imaging offer the promise of additional important insights into myocardial and coronary physiology. **A,** Image obtained using ^{11}C hydroxyephedrine, an analogue of norepinephrine. [11]C hydroxyephedrine is taken up and stored in cardiac sympathetic nerves in a manner identical to that of norepinephrine [40]. Images obtained with this tracer therefore reflect the density of sympathetic neurons in each myocardial region. Following cardiac transplantation, reinnervation of the myocardium is a regional process, typically favoring the territory of the left anterior descending coronary artery (LAD) [41,42]. Because of the regional differences in myocardial reinnervation, transplanted hearts provide a unique model for studying adrenergic control of the coronary circulation. In this case example, the proportion of the injected tracer that was taken up in the myocardium perfused by the LAD (19%) was about twice that of the tissue supplied by either the left circumflex artery (LCX; 11%) or right coronary artery (RCA; 8%), indicating a regional disparity in sympathetic innervation. **B,** On dynamic ^{13}N ammonia imaging, measurements of blood flow obtained during the cold pressor test demonstrate a 35% higher increase in regional perfusion in the LAD territory, suggesting a regional sympathetic neuronal effect. **C,** In contrast, myocardial blood flows during pharmacologic vasodilation with adenosine, a direct coronary vasodilator, show no regional differences. In a study of 14 cardiac transplant recipients, Di Carli *et al.* [43] concluded that increases in coronary blood flow in response to sympathetic stimulation are related in part to regional norepinephrine content in sympathetic nerve terminals, and that regional adrenergic innervation may play an important role in regulating local myocardial perfusion. (*Courtesy of* Marcelo Di Carli.)

REFERENCES

1. Hoffman EJ, Phelps ME: Positron emission tomography: principles and quantitation. In *Positron Emission Tomography and Autoradiography: Principles and Applications for the Brain and Heart*. Edited by Phelps ME, Mazziotta JC, Schelbert HR. New York: Raven Press; 1986:237–286.

2. Bacharach SL: The physics of positron emission tomography. In *Positron Emission Tomography of the Heart*. Edited by Bergmann SR, Sobel BE. Mount Kisco, NY: Futura Publishing Company; 1992:13–44.

3. Schelbert HR: Principles of positron emission tomography. In *Marcus Cardiac Imaging: A Companion to Braunwald's Heart Disease*, edn 2. Edited by Skorton DJ, Schelbert HR, Wolf GL, Brundage BH. Philadelphia: WB Saunders Company; 1996:1063–1112.

4. Hicks K, Ganti G, Mullani N, Gould KL: Automated quantitation of three-dimensional cardiac positron emission tomography for routine clinical use. *J Nucl Med* 1989, 30:1787–1797.

5. Miller TR, Wallis JW, Geltman EM, Bergmann SR: Three-dimensional functional images of myocardial oxygen consumption from positron tomography. *J Nucl Med* 1990, 31:2064–2068.

6. Kuhle WG, Porenta G, Huang SC, *et al.*: Issues in the quantitation of reoriented PET images. *J Nucl Med* 1992, 33:1235–1242.

7. Ratib O, Bidaut L, Nienaber C, *et al.*: Semiautomatic software for quantitative analysis of cardiac positron tomography studies. *SPIE* 1988, 914:412–419.

8. Porenta G, Kuhle WG, Czernin J, *et al.*: Semiquantitative assessment of myocardial blood flow and viability using polar map displays of cardiac PET images. *J Nucl Med* 1992, 33:1628–1636.

9. Sun KT, De Groof M, Yi J, *et al.*: Quantification of the extent and severity of perfusion defects in canine myocardium by PET polar mapping. *J Nucl Med* 1994, 35:2031–2040.

10. Hoffman EJ, Phelps ME, Wisenberg G, *et al.*: Electrocardiographic gating in positron emission tomography. *J Comput Assist Tomogr* 1979, 3:733–739.

11. Yamashita K, Tamaki N, Yonekura Y, *et al.*: Quantitative analysis of regional wall motion by gated myocardial positron emission tomography: validation and comparison with left ventriculography. *J Nucl Med* 1989, 30:1775–1786.

12. Yamashita K, Tamaki N, Yonekura Y, *et al.*: Regional wall thickening of left ventricle evaluated by gated positron emission tomography in relation to myocardial perfusion and glucose metabolism. *J Nucl Med* 1991, 32:679–685.

13. Miller TR, Wallis JW, Landy BR, *et al.*: Measurement of global and regional left ventricular function by cardiac PET. *J Nucl Med* 1994, 35:999–1005.

14. Porenta G, Kuhle W, Sinha S, *et al.*: Parameter estimation of cardiac geometry by ECG-gated PET imaging: validation using magnetic resonance imaging and echocardiography. *J Nucl Med* 1995, 36:1123–1129.

15. Choi Y, Hawkins RA, Huang SC, *et al.*: Parametric images of myocardial metabolic rate of glucose generated from dynamic cardiac PET and 2-[^{18}F]fluoro-2-deoxy-d-glucose studies. *J Nucl Med* 1991, 32:733–738.

16. Blanksma PK, Willemsen ATM, Meeder JG, *et al.*: Quantitative myocardial mapping of perfusion and metabolism using parametric polar map displays in cardiac PET. *J Nucl Med* 1995, 36:153–158.

17. Chen EQ, MacIntyre WJ, Go RT, *et al.*: Quantitative resting myocardial blood flow measurement by Rb-82: Sapirstein's method compared to a two-compartmental model. *J Nucl Med* 1995, 36:37.

18. Schelbert HR, Phelps ME, Huang SC, *et al.*: N-13 ammonia as an indicator of myocardial blood flow. *Circulation* 1981, 63:1259–1272.

19. Wu HM, Hoh CK, Buxton DB, *et al.*: Quantification of myocardial blood flow using dynamic nitrogen-13-ammonia PET studies and factor analysis of dynamic structures. *J Nucl Med* 1995, 36:2087–2093.

20. Patterson RE, Eisner RL, Horowitz SF: Comparison of cost-effectiveness and utility of exercise ECG, single photon emission computed tomography, positron emission tomography, and coronary angiography for diagnosis of coronary artery disease. *Circulation* 1995, 91:54–65.

21. Braunwald E, Kloner RA: The stunned myocardium: prolonged, postischemic

ventricular dysfunction. *Circulation* 1982, 66:1146–1149.

22. Kloner RA, Przyklenk K: Hibernation and stunning of the myocardium. *N Engl J Med* 1991, 325:1877–1879.

23. Di Carli M, Czernin J, Hoh CK, *et al.*: Relation among stenosis severity, myocardial blood flow, and flow reserve in patients with coronary artery disease. *Circulation* 1995, 91:1944–1951.

24. Bulkley BH, Hutchins GM, Bailey I, *et al.*: Thallium-201 imaging and gated cardiac blood pool scans in patients with ischemic and idiopathic congestive cardiomyopathy: a clinical and pathologic study. *Circulation* 1977, 55:753–760.

25. Iskandrian AS, Hakki AH, Kane S: Resting thallium-201 myocardial perfusion patterns in patients with severe left ventricular dysfunction: differences between patients with primary cardiomyopathy, chronic coronary artery disease, or acute myocardial infarction. *Am Heart J* 1986, 111:760–767.

26. Eichhorn EJ, Kosinski EJ, Lewis SM, *et al.*: Usefulness of dipyridamole-thallium-201 perfusion scanning for distinguishing ischemic from nonischemic cardiomyopathy. *Am J Cardiol* 1988, 62:945–951.

27. Maes A, Flameng W, Nuyts W, *et al.*: Histologic alterations in chronically hypoperfused myocardium: correlation with PET findings. *Circulation* 1994, 90:735–745.

28. Brunken R, Tillisch J, Schwaiger M, *et al.*: Regional perfusion, glucose metabolism and wall motion in patients with chronic electrocardiographic Q-wave infarctions: evidence for persistence of viable tissue in some infarct regions by positron emission tomography. *Circulation* 1986, 73:951–963.

29. Brunken RC, Schelbert HR: Acute myocardial infarction: a case for metabolic imaging. *The Leading Edge: Cardiology* 1989, 3:1–11.

30. Brunken RC, Mody FV, Hawkins RA, *et al.*: Positron emission tomography detects metabolic viability in myocardium with persistent 24-hour single photon emission computed tomography ^{201}Tl defects. *Circulation* 1992, 86:1357–1369, 1992.

31. Nienaber CA, Brunken RC, Sherman CT, *et al.*: Metabolic and functional recovery of ischemic human myocardium after coronary angioplasty. *J Am Coll Cardiol* 1991, 18:966–978.

32. Luu M, Stevenson LW, Brunken RC, *et al.*: Delayed recovery of revascularized myocardium after referral for cardiac transplantation. *Am Heart J* 1990, 119 (part I):668–670.

33. Goldman L, Hashimoto B, Cook EF, *et al.*: Comparative reproducibility and validity of systems for assessing cardiovascular functional class: advantages of a new specific activity scale. *Circulation* 1981, 64:1227–1234.

34. Di Carli MF, Asgarzadie F, Schelbert HR, *et al.*: Quantitative relation between myocardial viability and improvement in heart failure symptoms after revascularization in patients with ischemic cardiomyopathy. *Circulation* 1995, 92:3436–3444.

35. Di Carli MF, Davidson M, Little R, *et al.*: Value of metabolic imaging with positron emission tomography for evaluating prognosis in patients with coronary artery disease and left ventricular dysfunction. *Am J Cardiol* 1994, 73:527–533.

36. Eitzman D, Al-Aouar Z, Kanter HL, *et al.*: Clinical outcome of patients with advanced coronary artery disease after viability studies with positron emission tomography. *J Am Coll Cardiol* 1992, 20:559–565.

37. Yoshida K, Gould KL: Quantitative relation of myocardial infarct size and myocardial viability by positron emission tomography to left ventricular ejection fraction and 3-year mortality with and without revascularization. *J Am Coll Cardiol* 1993, 22:984–997.

38. Tamaki N, Kawamoto M, Takahashi N, *et al.*: Prognostic value of an increase in fluorine-18 deoxyglucose uptake in patients with myocardial infarction: comparison with stress thallium imaging. *J Am Coll Cardiol* 1993, 22:1621–1627.

39. Lee KS, Marwick TH, Cook SA, *et al.*: Prognosis of patients with left ventricular dysfunction, with and without viable myocardium after myocardial infarction: relative efficacy of medical therapy and revascularization. *Circulation* 1994, 90:2687–2694.

40. Schwaiger M, Kalff V, Rosenspire K, *et al.*: Noninvasive evaluation of sympathetic nervous system in human heart by positron emission tomography. *Circulation* 1990, 82:457–464.

41. Schwaiger M, Hutchins GD, Kalff V, *et al.*: Evidence for regional catecholamine uptake and storage sites in the transplanted human heart by positron emission tomography. *J Clin Invest* 1991, 87:1681–1690.

42. Wilson RF, Laxson DD, Christensen BV, *et al.*: Regional differences in sympathetic reinnervation after human orthotopic cardiac transplantation. *Circulation* 1993, 88:165–171.

43. Di Carli MF, Tobes MC, Mangner T, *et al.*: Effects of cardiac sympathetic innervation on coronary blood flow. *N Engl J Med* 1997, 336:1208–1215.

44. Krivokapich J, Stevenson LW, Kobashigawa J, *et al.*: Quantification of absolute perfusion at rest and during exercise with positron emission tomography after human cardiac transplantation. *J Am Coll Cardiol* 1991, 18:512–517.

45. Rechavia E, Araujo LI, De Silva R, *et al.*: Dipyridamole vasodilator response after human orthotopic heart transplantation: quantification by oxygen-15-labeled water and positron emission tomography. *J Am Coll Cardiol* 1992, 19:100–106.

46. Senneff MJ, Hartman J, Sobel B, *et al.*: Persistence of coronary vasodilator responsivity after cardiac transplantation. *Am J Cardiol* 1993, 71:333–338.

47. Chan SY, Kobashigawa J, Stevenson LW, *et al.*: Myocardial blood flow at rest and during pharmacological vasodilatation in cardiac transplants during and after successful treatment of rejection. *Circulation* 1994, 90:204–212.

48. Kofoed KF, Czernin J, Johnson J, *et al.*: Effects of cardiac allograft vasculopathy on myocardial blood flow, vasodilatory capacity, and coronary vasomotion. *Circulation* 1997, 95:600–606.

49. Dayanikli F, Grambow D, Muzik O, *et al.*: Early detection of abnormal coronary flow reserve in asymptomatic men at high risk for coronary artery disease using positron emission tomography. *Circulation* 1994, 90:808–817.

50. Yokoyama I, Ohtake T, Momomura S, *et al.*: Reduced coronary flow reserve in hypercholesterolemic patients without overt coronary stenosis. *Circulation* 1996, 94:3232–3238.

51. Pitkanen O, Raitakari OT, Miinikoski H, *et al.*: Coronary flow reserve is impaired in young men with familial hypercholesterolemia. *J Am Coll Cardiol* 1996, 28:1705–1711.

52. Czernin J, Barnard RJ, Sun KT, *et al.*: Effect of short-term cardiovascular conditioning and low-fat diet on myocardial blood flow and flow reserve. *Circulation* 1995, 92:197–204.

53. Senneff MJ, Geltman EM, Bergmann SR, Hartman J: Noninvasive delineation of the effects of moderate aging on myocardial perfusion. *J Nucl Med* 1991, 32:2037–2042.

54. Czernin J, Muller P, Chan S, *et al.*: Influence of age and hemodynamics on myocardial blood flow and flow reserve. *Circulation* 1993, 88:62–69.

55. Geltman EM, Henes CG, Senneff MJ, *et al.*: Increased myocardial perfusion at rest and diminished perfusion reserve in patients with angina and angiographically normal coronary arteries. *J Am Coll Cardiol* 1990, 16:586–595.

56. Camici P, Gistri R, Lorenzoni R, *et al.*: Coronary reserve and exercise ECG in patients with chest pain and normal coronary angiograms. *Circulation* 1992, 86:179–186.

57. Tamaki N, Yonekura Y, Senda M, *et al.*: Value and limitation of stress thallium-201 single photon emission computed tomography: comparison with nitrogen-13 ammonia positron tomography. *J Nucl Med* 1988, 29:1181–1188.

58. Stewart RE, Schwaiger M, Molina E, *et al.*: Comparison of rubidium-82 positron emission tomography and thallium-201 SPECT imaging for detection of coronary artery disease. *Am J Cardiol* 1991, 67:1303–1310.

59. Go RT, Marwick TH, MacIntyre WJ, *et al.*: A prospective comparison of rubidium-82 PET and thallium-201 SPECT myocardial perfusion imaging utilizing a single dipyridamole stress in the diagnosis of coronary artery disease. *J Nucl Med* 1990, 31:1899–1905.

60. Tillisch J, Brunken R, Marshall R, *et al.*: Reversibility of cardiac wall motion abnormalities predicted by positron tomography. *N Engl J Med* 1986, 314:884–888.

61. Tamaki N, Yonekura Y, Yamashita K, *et al.*: Positron emission tomography using fluorine-18 deoxyglucose in evaluation of coronary artery bypass grafting. *Am J Cardiol* 1989, 64:860–865.

62. Tamaki N, Ohtani H, Yamashita K, *et al.*: Metabolic activity in the areas of new fill-in after thallium-201 reinjection: comparison with positron emission tomography using fluorine-18 deoxyglucose. *J Nucl Med* 1991, 32:673–678.

63. Marwick TH, MacIntyre WJ, Lafont A, *et al.*: Metabolic responses of hibernating and infarcted myocardium to revascularization: a follow-up study of regional perfusion, function and metabolism. *Circulation* 1992, 85:1347–1353.

64. Lucignani G, Paolini G, Landoni C, *et al.*: Presurgical identification of hibernating myocardium by combined use of technetium-99m hexakis 2-methoxy-isobutylisonitrile single photon emission tomography and fluorine-18 fluoro-2-deoxy-D-glucose positron emission tomography in patients with coronary artery disease. *Eur J Nucl Med* 1992, 19:874–881.

65. Carrel T, Jenni R, Haubold-Reuter S, *et al.*: Improvement of severely reduced left ventricular function after surgical revascularization in patients with preoperative myocardial infarction. *Eur J Cardio-Thorac Surg* 1992, 6:479–484.

66. Gropler RJ, Geltman EM, Sampathkumaran K, *et al.*: Functional recovery after

coronary revascularization for chronic coronary artery disease is dependent on maintenance of oxidative metabolism. *J Am Coll Cardiol* 1992, 20:569–577.

67. Gropler RJ, Geltman EM, Sampathkumaran K, *et al.*: Comparison of carbon-11-acetate with fluorine-18-fluorodeoxyglucose for delineating viable myocardium by positron emission tomography. *J Am Coll Cardiol* 1993, 22:1587–1597.

68. Knuuti MJ, Saraste M, Nuutila P, *et al.*: Myocardial viability: fluorine-18-deoxyglucose positron emission tomography in prediction of wall motion recovery after revascularization. *Am Heart J* 1994, 127:785–796.

69. vom Dahl J, Eitzman DT, Al-Aouar ZR, *et al.*: Relation of regional function, perfusion, and metabolism in patients with advanced coronary artery disease undergoing surgical revascularization. *Circulation* 1994, 90:2356–2366.

70. Tamaki N, Kawamoto M, Tadamura E, *et al.*: Prediction of reversible ischemia after revascularization: perfusion and metabolic studies with positron emission tomography. *Circulation* 1995, 91:1697–1705.

71. Vanoverschelde JLJ, Wijns W, Depre C, *et al.*: Mechanisms of chronic regional postischemic dysfunction in humans: new insights from the study of noninfarcted collateral-dependent myocardium. *Circulation* 1993, 87:1513–1523.

72. Maes A, Flameng W, Nuyts J, *et al.*: Histologic alterations in chronically hypoperfused myocardium: correlation with PET findings. *Circulation* 1994, 90:735–745.

73. Grandin C, Wijns W, Melin JA, *et al.*: Delineation of myocardial viability with

PET. *J Nucl Med* 1995, 36:1543–1552.

74. Depre C, Vanoverschelde JLJ, Melin J, *et al.*: Structural and metabolic correlates of the reversibility of chronic left ventricular ischemic dysfunction in humans. *Am J Physiol* 1995, 268:H1265–1275.

75. Gerber BL, Vanoverschelde JLJ, Bol A, *et al.*: Myocardial blood flow, glucose uptake, and recruitment of inotropic reserve in chronic left ventricular dysfunction: implications for the pathophysiology of chronic myocardial hibernation. *Circulation* 1996, 94:651–659.

76. Baer FM, Voth E, Deutsch HJ, *et al.*: Predictive value of low dose dobutamine transesophageal echocardiography and fluorine-18 flurorodeoxyglucose positron emission tomography for recovery of regional left ventricular function after successful revascularization. *J Am Coll Cardiol* 1996, 28:60–69.

77. vom Dahl J, Altehoefer C, Sheehan FH, *et al.*: Recovery of regional left ventricular dysfunction after coronary revascularization: impact of myocardial viability assessed by nuclear imaging and vessel patency at follow-up angiography. *J Am Coll Cardiol* 1996, 28:948–958.

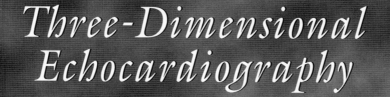

Three-Dimensional Echocardiography

Tsui-Lieh Hsu ~ Jiefen Yao
Stefano De Castro ~ Natesa G. Pandian

Cardiac anatomy and pathology, every part and structure in the heart, and every facet of cardiac flow and function are three-dimensional. Most imaging techniques used in cardiology today yield two-dimensional information only in a given view or projection. By examining a number of two-dimensional views, the physician attempts to mentally reconstruct the three-dimensional nature of the disease. Rapid advances during the past decade in image acquisition and computerized image processing have led to the development of three-dimensional cardiac imaging. Efforts are being made in almost every area of cardiac imaging to obtain, visualize, and quantify the cardiovascular problem in three dimensions. Image information from most techniques such as electron beam tomography, magnetic resonance imaging, and nuclear imaging are currently obtained in a digital mode; when acquired otherwise, as in echocardiography, the video data can be quickly transformed into digital data. This capability then allows for further digital manipulation and processing to develop three-dimensional images.

Faster progress in three-dimensional imaging has occurred in echocardiography. It is now possible to perform three-dimensional echocardiography at the patient's bedside and obtain qualitative three-dimensional data. Initial experience with three-dimensional echocardiography explored means of accurately measuring ventricular volumes and myocardial mass without the need for geometric assumptions [1–5]. Recent developments in ultrasound instrumentation and image reconstruction

have led to the practicality of volume-rendered three-dimensional echocardiography that yields tissue-depiction images in a more realistic manner [6–13].

The major steps involved in three-dimensional imaging include optimal acquisition of image data with temporal and spatial registration, image processing and reconstruction, development of three-dimensional image projections or sections, and derivation of quantitative data. The development of three-dimensional imaging that could be performed in real time with on-line three-dimensional display in one heartbeat would be advantageous. Efforts toward this goal are in progress, specifically the development of a prototype ultrasound instrument that can acquire data in a three-dimensional pyramidal volume; however, this approach does not deliver three-dimensional images at the moment. Therefore, all approaches require off-line reconstruction. Such off-line reconstruction, however, is becoming faster and easier, hence the feasibility of bedside three-dimensional echocardiography. A considerable body of work in progress using dynamic, volume-rendered three-dimensional echocardiography strongly suggests that this modality can aid in a better delineation of cardiac pathology, yield accurate quantitative data, and provide new quantitative information that has not been available so far in almost all forms of cardiovascular disorders. In addition, three-dimensional echocardiographic data sets can be used for solid modeling and holography [14,15]. This chapter illustrates the methods and application of three-dimensional echocardiography.

METHODOLOGY

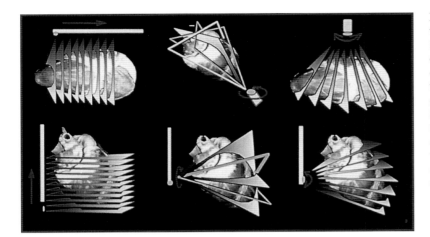

FIGURE 11-1. Commonly used modes of two-dimensional image acquisition [6,7,16]. Volume-rendered three-dimensional echocardiography (3DE) is performed from sets of two-dimensional images, acquired with electrocardiographic and respiration gating. For transthoracic 3DE, motorized carriage devices are mounted to a conventional two-dimensional echocardiographic transducer; for transesophageal 3DE, special transesophageal echocardiographic probes are needed. **Top,** Image acquisition for transthoracic 3DE. Sequential two-dimensional images are collected in a parallel slicing mode (equidistant images at 1- to 5-mm intervals), a rotational mode (equiangled at 1° to 5° intervals). **Bottom,** Modes of image collection are similar for transesophageal 3DE. However, rotational mode is easier and more commonly used because of the easy availability of multiplane transesophageal echocardiography transducers.

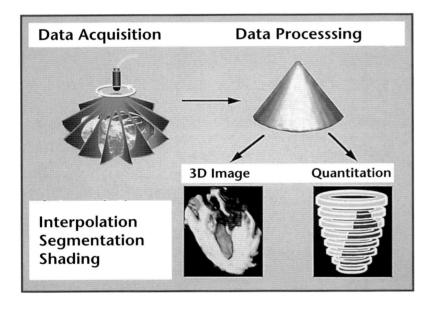

Data Acquisition   **Data Processsing**

Interpolation
Segmentation
Shading

3D Image   **Quantitation**

FIGURE 11-2. Image-processing method for three-dimensional echocardiography (3DE). The two-dimensional echocardiography (2DE) data set acquired (a conical data set from rotational imaging is shown here) is digitally reformatted. Interpolation fills in the gaps between images. Segmentation allows further processing of desired regions or objects in the data set. Various shading techniques are used to imply a three-dimensional nature of the image and codify distances [18]. Then, using a reference image, multiple 3DE projections are derived. For quantification of the area and volume, the selected object (left ventricular myocardium and a region of dysfunction in this illustration) is contoured and labeled in multiplane paraplane 2DE images. Measurement of the area multiplied by slice thickness yields the volume of the given slice. Addition of such volumes provides the total volume of the selected region or object. This approach allows for calculation of chamber volumes and thus function, area of defects, and size of lesions such as intracardiac masses.

VALVULAR HEART DISEASE

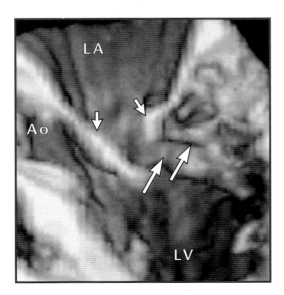

FIGURE 11-3. Longitudinal three-dimensional echocardiography (3DE) projection of the left heart from a patient with mitral stenosis. Left atrial (LA) cavity, left ventricle (LV) and LV outflow region are seen as well as the mitral valve (MV). The thickened mitral leaflets (*small arrows*) and fused chordae (*large arrows*) are well visualized. 3DE exhibits, in a dynamic mode, alterations in morphology and motion and function in a much more realistic manner than does two-dimensional echocardiography. Ao—aorta.

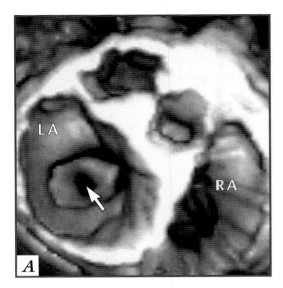

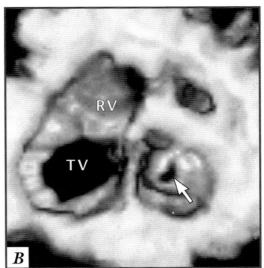

FIGURE 11-4. Three-dimensional echocardiographic (3DE) images of mitral valve (MV) from a patient with mitral stenosis. **A,** The MV as seen from above the left atrium (LA). The right atrium (RA) is seen to the right of LA and aorta anteriorly adjoining both atria. This type of 3DE sections displays MV and the narrowed MV orifice (*arrow*) in a view that stimulates intraoperative visualization [14]. **B,** The MV is visualized from below. The domed, stenotic MV (*arrow*) and normally open tricuspid valve (TV) are brought into view. In this view, right ventricle (RV) outflow region also is seen.

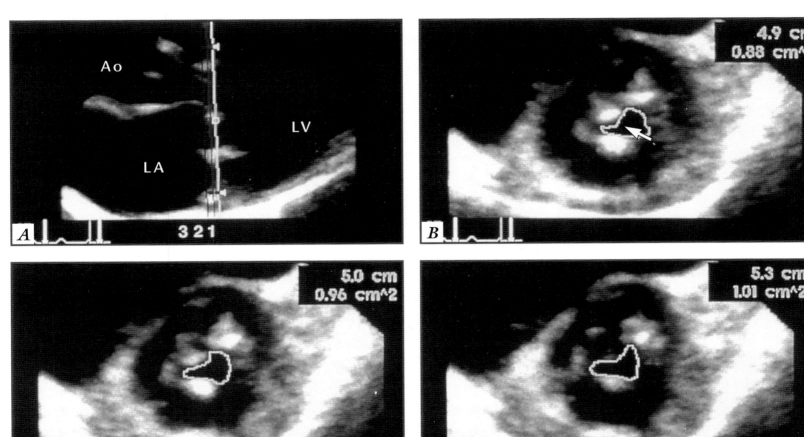

FIGURE 11-5. Method of measuring mitral valve (MV) area. **A** to **D,** Using a reference frame from the three-dimensional echocardiographic (3DE) data set, multiple paraplane two-dimensional echocardiography images are extracted and MV orifice (*arrow*) area is measured. Studies correlating 3DE assessment of MV area with surgical measurements have demonstrated that 3DE yields accurate data. Ao—aorta; LA—left atrium; LV—left ventricle.

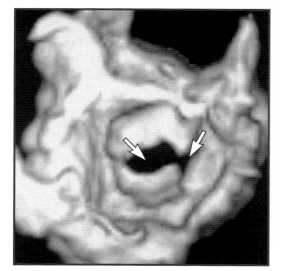

FIGURE 11-6. Three-dimensional echocardiographic (3DE) image of mitral valve orifice (*left arrow*) following balloon mitral valvuloplasty. 3DE aids in the assessment of the effects and complications of interventions and surgery. In this patient, only one commissure has been split (*right arrow*).

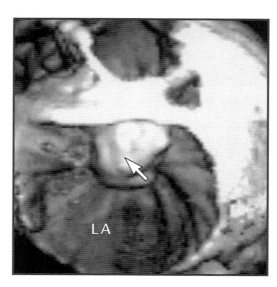

FIGURE 11-7. Left atrium (LA) as viewed from above. In this patient with mitral valvular disease, a large mass (thrombus) (*arrow*) is attached to the anterior wall of the LA. Three-dimensional echocardiography reveals the size and shape, precise location, and site of attachment of intracardiac masses such as clots, tumors, and vegetations. In addition, the size (volume) of the masses can be determined [17].

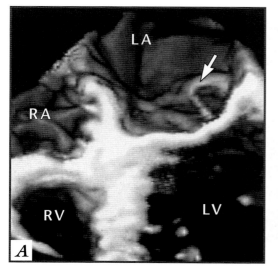

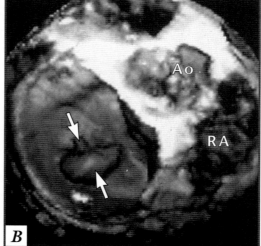

FIGURE 11-8. Flail mitral valve. **A,** In this patient, the four-chamber projection displays the chambers and the prolapsing leaflet (*arrow*) of the mitral valve (MV). **B,** The view from the left atrium (LA) provides even more specific information regarding the particular portion of MV leaflet that is flail (*lower arrow*), in this case the middle scallop of posterior leaflet. The loose end of a ruptured chord (*upper arrow*) is also seen. Systematic studies comparing three-dimensional echocardiography (3DE) with two-dimensional echocardiography (2DE) have shown that 3DE is more accurate than is multiplane transesophageal echocardiography in the precise identification of prolapsing portions of MV. This information is of value in planning MV repair. LV—left ventricle; RA—right atrium; RV—right ventricle.

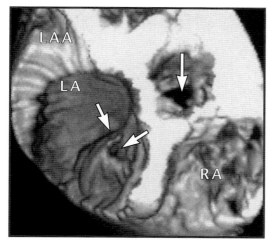

FIGURE 11-9. Another case of flail mitral valve (*small arrows*). In this patient, the medial portion of the posterior leaflet is flail. Abnormalities such as this are better appreciated in real-time dynamic three-dimensional echocardiography studies. *Large arrow* indicates the aortic valve opening. LA—left atrium; LAA—left atrial appendage; RA—right atrium.

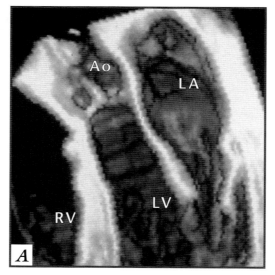

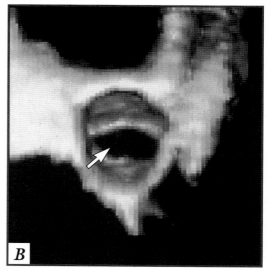

FIGURE 11-10. Three-dimensional echocardiographic images of aortic valve. Longitudinal and tomographic images are useful in assessing aortic valve anatomy and pathology. **A,** The aortic valve, subaortic region, and aortic root are displayed in a study from a normal subject. **B,** This cut section from a patient demonstrates that the aortic valve (*arrow*) is bicuspid. Ao—aorta; LA—left atrium; LV—left ventricle; RV—right ventricle.

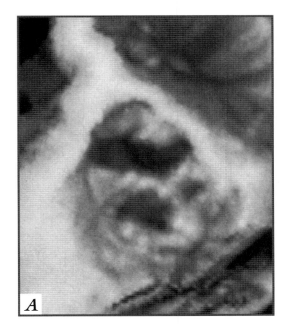

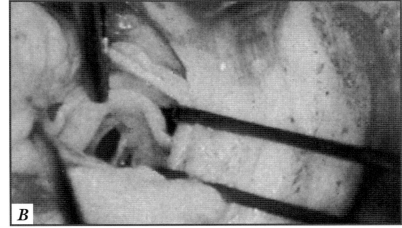

FIGURE 11-11. Aortic valve endocarditis. Intraoperative photograph and a three-dimensional echocardiographic (3DE) cut section from a patient with bicuspid aortic valve with perforations caused by endocarditis. Preoperative 3DE (A) displays the opening of the aortic valve and two perforations (a large and small one) that appear identical to those seen at surgery. (B).

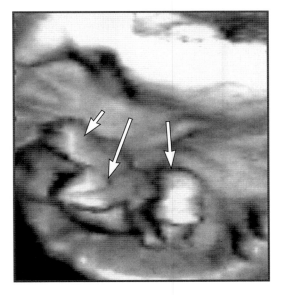

FIGURE 11-12. Three-dimensional echocardiographic (3DE) image from a patient with mitral valve endocarditis. In this view of the mitral valve from above, multiple large vegetations (*arrows*) are noted attached to the valve. Preliminary clinical studies indicate that 3DE might be more accurate than two-dimensional echocardiography in defining the number and size of vegetations and perforations in endocarditis.

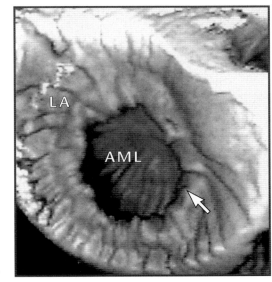

FIGURE 11-13. Rapid data acquisition and fast processing now permit performance of three-dimensional echocardiographic (3DE) studies in the operating room. This 3DE image from the left atrium (LA) from a patient following mitral valve (MV) repair and ring placement shows a well-placed MV ring (*arrow*) and a closing anterior mitral valve leaflet (AML).

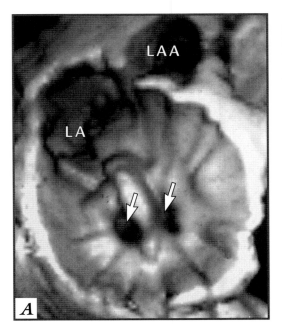

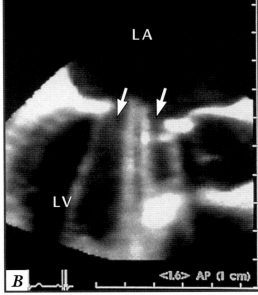

FIGURE 11-14. Three-dimensional echocardiographic projection (A) and two-dimensional echocardiographic (B) image following placement of a bileaflet mechanical (St. Jude) mitral valve prosthesis. The two openings of the St. Jude valve are well seen (*arrows*). LA—left atrium; LAA—left atrial appendage; LV—left ventricle.

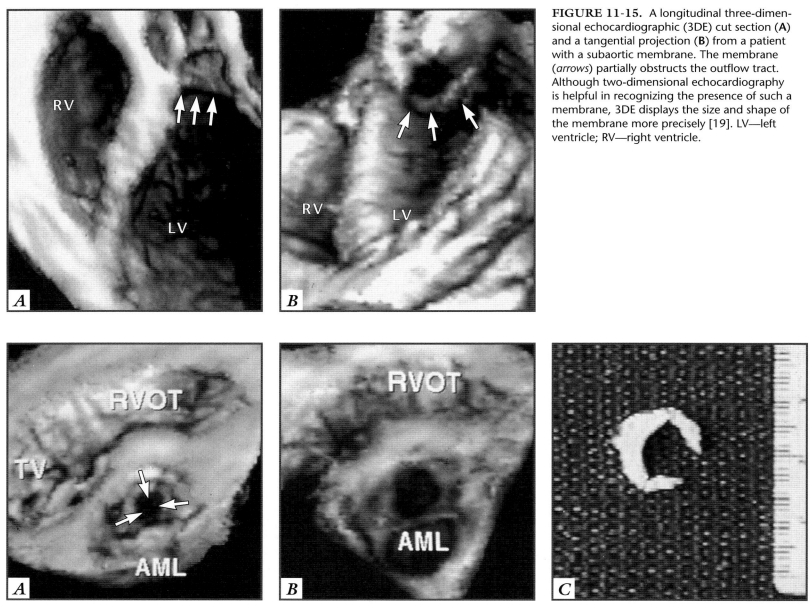

FIGURE 11-15. A longitudinal three-dimensional echocardiographic (3DE) cut section (**A**) and a tangential projection (**B**) from a patient with a subaortic membrane. The membrane (*arrows*) partially obstructs the outflow tract. Although two-dimensional echocardiography is helpful in recognizing the presence of such a membrane, 3DE displays the size and shape of the membrane more precisely [19]. LV—left ventricle; RV—right ventricle.

FIGURE 11-16. Intraoperative three-dimensional echocardiographic (3DE) images before (**A**) and after (**B**) surgical resection of subaortic membrane (*arrows*). The preoperative image is a projection in which the left ventricular outflow region is viewed from below from the left ventricle.

C, The crescent-shaped subaortic membrane (identical to resected specimen) is narrowing the outflow tract. The postoperative image demonstrates the enlarged outflow tract. AML—anterior mitral valve leaflet; RVOT—right ventricular outflow tract; TV—tricuspid valve.

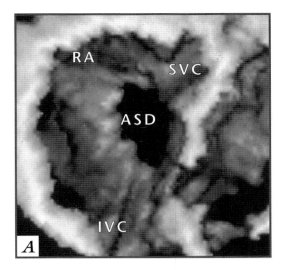

A

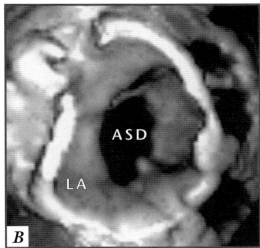

B

FIGURE 11-17. Three-dimensional echocardiographic (3DE) images of the interatrial septum as viewed from the right atrium (**A**) and the left atrium (**B**) showing a large atrial septal defect. 3DE helps in delineating the site, shape, and size of atrial septal defects (ASD) as well as in measuring the span of the septal tissue surrounding the defect [20]. Such information is of value in planning catheter-based closure of septal defects. IVC—inferior vena cava; LA—left atrium; RA—right atrium; SVC—superior vena cava.

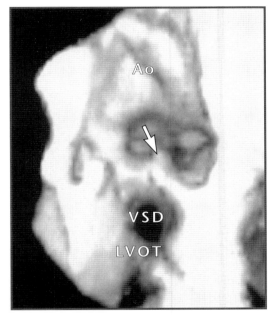

FIGURE 11-18. Muscular and membranous ventricular septal defects (VSDs) are well defined by three-dimensional echocardiography (3DE). The longitudinal image in this figure shows a subaortic VSD as viewed from the left ventricle. The dimensions and area of VSDs can be measured as well from the 3DE data set. *Arrow* indicates aortic valve cusps. LVOT—left ventricular outflow tract.

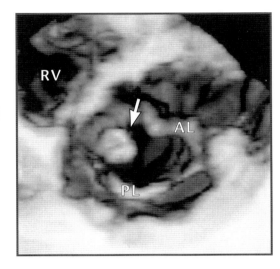

FIGURE 11-19. Three-dimensional echocardiographic (3DE) image of cleft mitral valve as viewed from below (*arrow*). Whereas two-dimensional echocardiography can help in diagnosing the presence of a cleft valve, 3DE delineates not only the presence but also the longitudinal span of the cleft. AL—anterior leaflet; PL—posterior leaflet; RV—right ventricle.

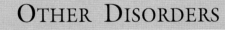

OTHER DISORDERS

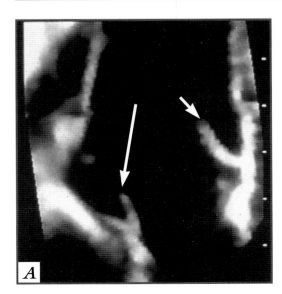

A

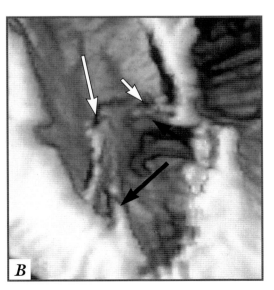

B

FIGURE 11-20. Aortic dissection. Longitudinal two-dimensional echocardiographic image (**A**), longitudinal upright three-dimensional echocardiographic (3DE) image (**B**),

(Continued on next page)

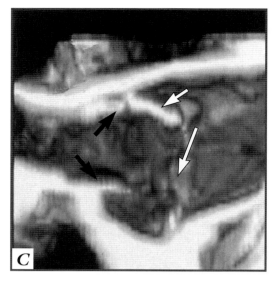 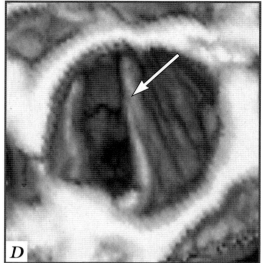

FIGURE 11-20. (*Continued*) another longitudinal cut-section (**C**), and a 3DE view from above (**D**). The 3DE images delineate the origin of the intimal flap (*white arrows*) and the size of the true and false lumens [21]. *Black arrows* indicate the aortic valve cusps.

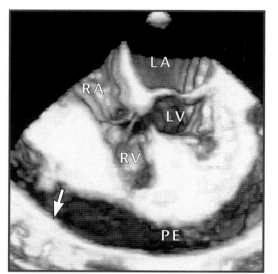

FIGURE 11-21. Three-dimensional echocardiographic (3DE) image from a patient with pericardial effusion (PE). This four-chamber view shows a circumferential PE. Two-dimensional echocardiography has proven to be extremely valuable in the assessment of PE. 3DE better demonstrates metastatic deposits, particularly in electronically simulated pericardiectomy. *Arrow* indicates parietal pericardium. LA—left atrium; LV—left ventricle; RA—right atrium; RV—right ventricle.

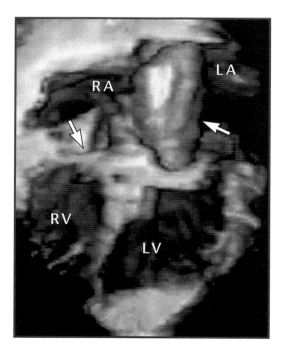

FIGURE 11-22. Three-dimensional reconstruction of flow jets. Color Doppler flow data can be acquired along with B-mode echocardiographic images and processed to yield three-dimensional images of flow jets [22]. In this four-chamber view, a mitral regurgitation jet (*right arrow*) and a tricuspid regurgitation jet (*left arrow*) are seen. Three-dimensional echocardiography (3DE) displays the origin, size, and shape of the flow jets and aids in understanding the morphologic and functional mechanism of abnormal flow jets. Preliminary work suggests that 3DE may be of value in quantifying regurgitant flow. LA—left atrium; LV—left ventricle; RA—right atrium; RV—right ventricle.

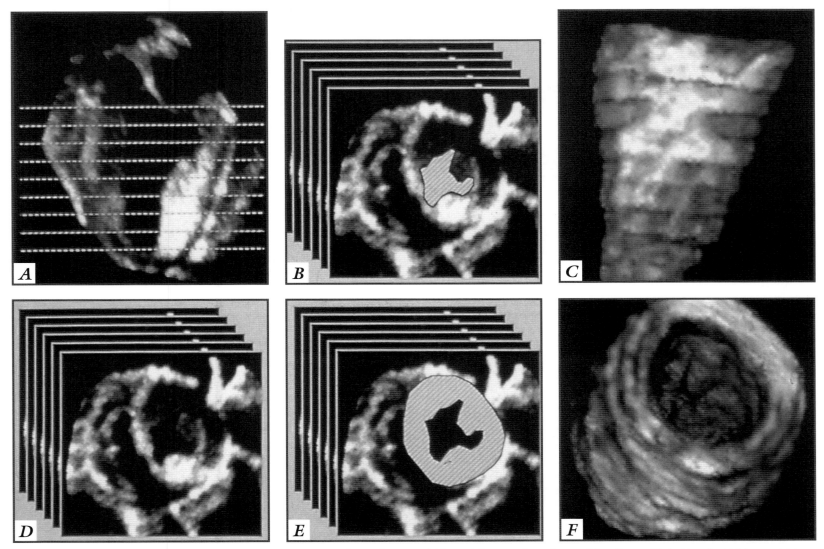

FIGURE 11-23. Determination of left ventricular (LV) volume and mass by three-dimensional echocardiography (3DE). From the three-dimensional data set, a reference longitudinal image is chosen (**A**). Using that image, multiple paraplane (parallel) tomographic two-dimensional images are derived at desired intervals (**B**). The cavity borders are semiautomatically extracted and the cavity area labeled. From this labeling process, the cast of the cavity is obtained, providing a visual appreciation of the size and shape of the cavity (**C**). In addition, the cavity area measurement in each slice is available. Because the slice thickness is known, the volume of the slice multiplied by slice thickness yields the cavity volume in each slice. Addition of these volumes provides the total cavity volume. Using this approach, end-diastolic and end-systolic LV volumes as well as LV ejection fraction are obtained. The LV myocardium can be labeled as well (**D** to **F**) and the volume of myocardium derived. Myocardial volume multiplied by assumed myocardial density yields myocardial mass. *In vitro* and human *in vivo* studies have validated the accuracy of 3DE in the determination of LV volumes, ejection fraction, and LV mass [23].

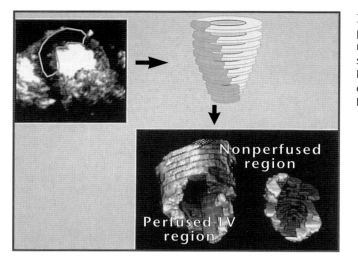

FIGURE 11-24. Estimation of perfused and nonperfused myocardial territories can be performed coupling contrast echocardiography with three-dimensional echocardiography [24]. In the setting of coronary occlusion, perfused areas exhibit enhanced, bright signals whereas nonperfused areas appear dark (*left*). Using the method described in Figure 11-23, perfused (contrast-enhanced) and nonperfused (nonenhanced) regions can be labeled, extracted in three dimensions (*bottom*), and also quantified in grams. LV—left ventricle.

VASCULAR STRUCTURES

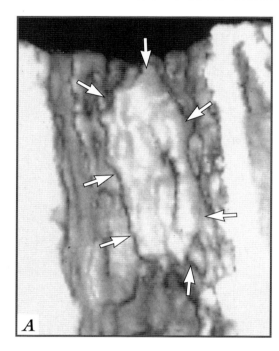

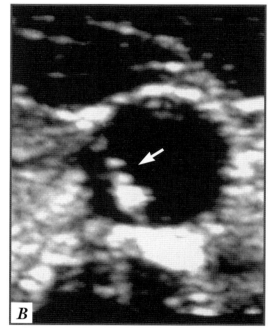

FIGURE 11-25. Three-dimensional imaging of vascular structures such as carotid arteries can be performed with a higher frequency ultrasound transducer using various two-dimensional image acquisition approaches. In patients with carotid atherosclerosis, the atherosclerotic plaque (*arrows*) can be delineated in three dimensions (**A**) better than by two-dimensional imaging (**B**); in addition, the plaque volume can be quantified.

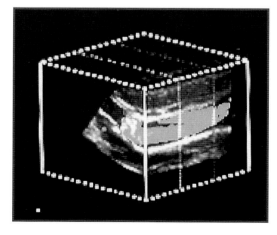

FIGURE 11-26. Visualization of carotid artery and flow within the artery. Advances in three-dimensional imaging technology now allow acquisition and visualization color (not shown) Doppler data in its true form instead of converting it to gray-scale images. Currently such imaging can be performed to study vascular flow. Work is in progress to apply a similar approach to cardiac flow.

REFERENCES

1. Ghosh A, Nanda NC, Maurer G: Three-dimensional reconstruction of echocardiographic images using the rotation method. *Ultrasound Med Biol* 1982, 6:655–661.

2. Nikravesh PE, Skorton DJ, Chandran KB, *et al.*: Computerized three-dimensional finite element reconstruction of the left ventricle from cross-sectional echocardiograms. *Ultrason Imaging* 1984, 6:48–59.

3. Ariet M, Geiser EA, Lupkiewicz SM, *et al.*: Evaluation of a three-dimensional reconstruction to compute left ventricular volume and mass. *Am J Cardiol* 1984, 54:415–420.

4. Handschumacher MD, Lethor JP, Siu SC, *et al.*: A new integrated system for three-dimensional echocardiographic reconstruction: development and validation for ventricular volume with application in human subjects. *J Am Coll Cardiol* 1993, 21:743–753.

5. Sapin PM, Schroedr KD, Smith MD, *et al.*: Three-dimensional echocardiographic measurement of left ventricular volume in vitro: comparison with two-dimensional echocardiography and cineventriculography. *J Am Coll Cardiol* 1993, 22:1530–1537.

6. Pandian NG, Nanda NC, Schwartz SL, *et al.*: Three-dimensional and four-dimensional transesophageal echocardiographic imaging of the heart and aorta in humans using a computed tomographic imaging probe. *Echocardiography* 1992, 9:677–687.

7. Pandian NG, Roelandt J, Nanda NC, *et al.*: Dynamic three-dimensional echocardiography: methods and clinical potential. *Echocardiography* 1994, 11:237–259.

8. Fulton DR, Marx G, Pandian NG, *et al.*: Dynamic three-dimensional echocardiographic imaging of congenital heart defects in infants and children by computer-controlled tomographic parallel slicing using a single integrated ultrasound instrument. *Echocardiography* 1994, 11:155–164.

9. Marx G, Fulton DR, Pandian NG, *et al.*: Delineation of site, relative size and dynamic geometry of atrial septal defects by real-time three-dimensional echocardiography. *J Am Coll Cardiol* 1995, 25:482–490.

10. Belohlavek M, Foley DA, Gerber TC, *et al.*: Three-dimensional ultrasound imaging of the atrial septum: normal and pathologic anatomy. *J Am Coll Cardiol* 1993, 22:1673–1678.

11. Vogel M, Lösch S: Dynamic three-dimensional echocardiography with a computed tomography imaging probe: initial clinical experience with transthoracic application in infants and children with congenital heart defects. *Br Heart J* 1994, 71:462–467.

12. Roelandt JRTC, Cate FJ, Vletter WB, Taams MA: Ultrasonic dynamic three-dimensional visualization of the heart with a multiplane transesophageal imaging transducer. *J Am Soc Echocardiogr* 1994, 7:217–229.

13. Ludomirsky A, Vermilion R, Nesser J, *et al.*: Transthoracic real-time three-dimensional echocardiography using the rotational scanning approach for data acquisition. *Echocardiography* 1994, 11:599–606.

14. Schwartz SL, Cao QL, Azevedo J, Pandian NG: Simulation of intraoperative visualization of cardiac structures and study of dynamic surgical anatomy with real-time three-dimensional echocardiography. *Am J Cardiol* 1994, 73:501–507.

15. Vannan MA, Cao QL, Pandian NG, *et al.*: Volumetric multiplexed transmission holography of the heart with echocardiographic data. *J Am Soc Echocardiogr* 1995, 8:567–575.

16. Delabays A, Pandian NG, Cao QL, *et al.*: Transthoracic real-time three-dimensional echocardiography using a fan-like scanning approach for data acquisition: methods, strength, problems, and initial clinical experience. *Echocardiography* 1995, 12:49–59.

17. Kupferwasser I, Mohr-Kahaly S, Erbel R, *et al.*: Three-dimensional imaging of cardiac mass lesions by transesophageal echocardiographic computed tomography. *J Am Soc Echocardiogr* 1994, 7:561–570.

18. Cao QL, Pandian NG, Azevedo J, *et al.*: Enhanced comprehension of dynamic cardiovascular anatomy by three-dimensional echocardiography with the use of mixed shading techniques. *Echocardiography* 1994, 11:627–633.

19. Fyfe DA, Ludomirsky A, Sandhu S, *et al.*: Left ventricular outflow tract obstruction defined by active three-dimensional echocardiography using rotational transthoracic acquisition. *Echocardiography* 1994, 11:607–615.

20. Magni G, Cao QL, Sugeng L, *et al.*: Volume-rendered three-dimensional echocardiographic determination of the size, shape and position of atrial septal defects: validation in an in vitro model. *Am Heart J* 1996, 132:376–381.

21. Sugeng L, Cao QL, Delabays A, *et al.*: Three-dimensional echocardiographic evaluation of aortic disorders with rotational multiplanar imaging. *J Am Soc Echocardiogr* 1997, 10:120–132.

22. Delabays A, Sugeng L, Pandian NG, *et al.*: Dynamic three-dimensional echocardiographic assessment of intracardiac blood flow jets. *Am J Cardiol* 1995, 76:1053–1058.

23. Yao J, Cao QL, Masani N, *et al.*: Three-dimensional echocardiographic estimation of infarct mass based on quantification of dysfunctional left ventricular mass. *Circulation* 1997, 96:1660–1666.

24. Delabays AK, Cao QL, Yao J, *et al.*: Contrast three-dimensional echocardiography in acute myocardial infarction: 3-D reconstruction of perfusion defects yields accurate estimate of infarct mass and extent [abstract 718-4]. *J Am Coll Cardiol* 1996, 27(suppl A):63.

12

Angiography

Adhip Mukerjee ~ Krishna Kandarpa

The potential of demonstrating the vascular tree was quickly recognized after Roentgen's discovery of x-rays in 1896. Angiography—the use of radiographic methods to image the luminal aspects of veins and arteries in living subjects with the aim of diagnosing disease states—began in earnest in the 1920s after many earlier cadaveric and animal studies [1]. Lower extremity arteriography (Brooks, 1924), pulmonary arteriography (Forsmann, 1931), direct carotid arteriography (Moniz, 1928) angiocardiography (Ameuille, 1936), and direct abdominal aortography (Dos Santos, 1928) were early important milestones in the development of the discipline.

This development was fueled on the one hand by the discovery of contrast agents that could be applied *in vivo*, and on the other by the elaboration of catheter techniques and improved radiographic techniques. Early agents such as sodium iodide were found to be too toxic. Organic iodides began to be used after Swick's description of the use of Selectan in 1929. The extensive pharmaceutical research that then began has continued to this day, providing newer generations of contrast agents that approximate the necessary features: solubility in aqueous solution, appropriate viscosity, adequate radiopacity, chemical stability, biologic inertness with rapid and complete elimination, ready availability, and low cost. Current contrast media are all derivatives of a triiodinated benzoic acid skeleton in which the aromatic entity is fully substituted to decrease reactivity, and in which side chains have been constructed to maximize hydrophilicity while decreasing protein binding [2]. Presently, ionic monomers (diatrizoate, iothalamate) and a dimer (ioxaglate), nonionic monomers (iopamidol, iohexol, ioversol, ioxilan) and a dimer (iodixanol) are all in use.

In 1928, Forsmann first described the technique of cardiac catheterization from an antecubital vein, making possible catheter approaches to angiography. Catheter thoracic aortography (Radner, 1948), and retrograde femoral aortography (Farina, 1941) were further developed into the percutaneous transfemoral approach by Seldinger in 1953, the basis of the majority of vascular and nonvascular procedures performed today.

These developments and technical advances (especially image amplification, rapid filming, and real-time digital subtraction) have allowed widespread application of angiography to medical diagnosis. Over the past decade, other technologies (ultrasound with Doppler and color mapping, magnetic resonance imaging, computed tomography) have made noninvasive vascular imaging a reality and have (with fine-needle biopsy) obviated many arteriographic diagnostic studies. However, the same developments that allowed vascular diagnosis also gave rise to the pioneering of vascular intervention by Dotter, Gruentzig, and others. Now, balloon angioplasty, transcatheter atherectomy and biopsy, thrombolytic or other therapeutic infusion, intravascular stenting, and vascular occlusion, retrieval, and access, as well as nonvascular intervention, are essential parts of peripheral angiographic training and practice.

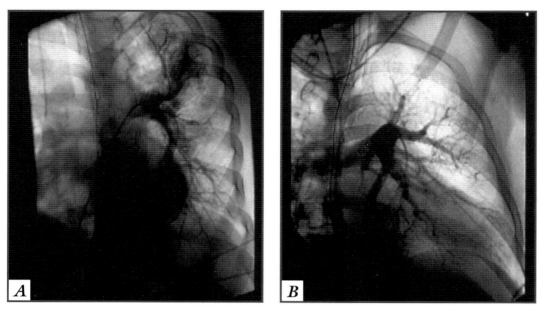

FIGURE 12-1. Pulmonary arteriography for pulmonary embolism (PE). Left pulmonary arteriogram in a patient who presented with sudden onset of shortness of breath, confusion, seizure, and hypotension, soon requiring intubation and pressor support. A, Initial diagnostic study demonstrating large filling defect of the descending left pulmonary artery (PA) extending into lateral and anteromedial segmental arteries, and into the upper lobe artery, with occlusion of the anterior segmental and lingular arteries.

Flow is significantly decreased; echocardiogram demonstrated right ventricular dysfunction and tricuspid regurgitation measures consistent with severely elevated PA pressures, confirmed at arteriography. B, Repeat right anterior oblique arteriogram performed a few hours after the intravenous administration of 100 mg recombinant tissue plasminogen activator over 2 hours showing significant lysis of clot and much improved flow. Mental and clinical status improved rapidly and the patient was extubated the following day. Pulmonary arteriography for PE is generally now reserved for those who fall into the category of nondiagnostic V/Q scan with negative compression duplex ultrasound examination of the lower extremity veins and continued suspicion of PE [3], for those at high risk for anticoagulation and less than two risk factors for PE [4], and for recurrent PE and chronic PE, even though pulmonary arteriography has an overall low rate of complications [5]. Although prophylaxis and treatment with intravenous heparin and 6 months of coumadin therapy remain the mainstay, lytic therapy and transcatheter thromboembolectomy [6,7] have a role in the management of acute hemodynamic instability or severely reduced cardiac or pulmonary reserve.

Pulmonary Angiographic Findings in Thromboembolism

Primary Signs

Filling defect
   Persistent intraluminal radiolucency, central or marginal, without complete obstruction of blood flow
   Proximal edge of an intraluminal radiolucency when there is complete obstruction of distal blood flow (convex meniscus)

Secondary Signs

Abrupt occlusion ("cut-off") of a pulmonary artery without visualization of an intraluminal filling defect
Perfusion defect (asymmetric filling)
   Areas of oligemia or avascularity
   Focal areas in which the arterial phase is prolonged (especially lower lobes); usually accompanied by slow filling and emptying of the pulmonary veins

FIGURE 12-2. Pulmonary angiography. Pulmonary angiography is the definitive test for acute pulmonary thromboembolism. The examination must be of high quality for accurate diagnosis. If areas are suspicious after two views have been obtained, balloon occlusion or superselective angiograms may clarify the area in question. (Legend *adapted from* Skibo and Goldhaber [8]; figure *adapted from* Sagel and Greenspan [9].)

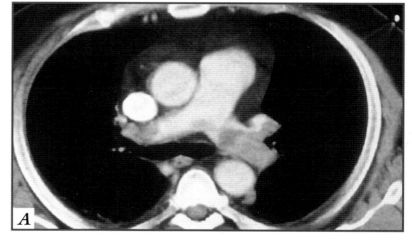

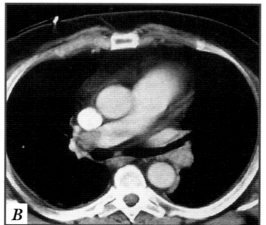

FIGURE 12-3. Dynamic contrast computed tomography (CT) displayed at mediastinal windows showing low attenuation thromboembolus in contrast-enhanced left (A) and right (B) pulmonary arteries (PAs).
(*Continued on next page*)

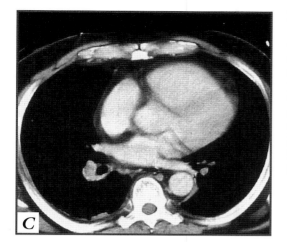

FIGURE 12-3. (*Continued*) Thrombus is also evident in the right interlobar pulmonary artery (**C**). Dynamic contrast-enhanced CT is an excellent modality to assess the central pulmonary vasculature. Cardiac motion does not degrade images substantially because of fast imaging times. Helical CT uses a new technique in which continuous scanning is performed while the patient is moved through the scanning plane. It allows for imaging of sections of the body during a single breath-hold (provided the patient can suspend respiration for 24 to 40 seconds), eliminating respiratory misregistration. The volume of contrast material can usually be reduced relative to conventional CT. With high injection rates (5 to 7 mL/s), the central PAs can be displayed optimally. Electron-beam CT is another new CT modality that can perform axial scans in 100 ms, thereby eliminating the need for breath-holding. Potential exists to visualize the proximal segmental arteries using helical dynamic CT and electron-beam CT. Accuracy for pulmonary embolism using these methods appears to be high [10–13]. (Legend *adapted from* Skibo and Goldhaber [8]; figure *courtesy of* James Fraser.)

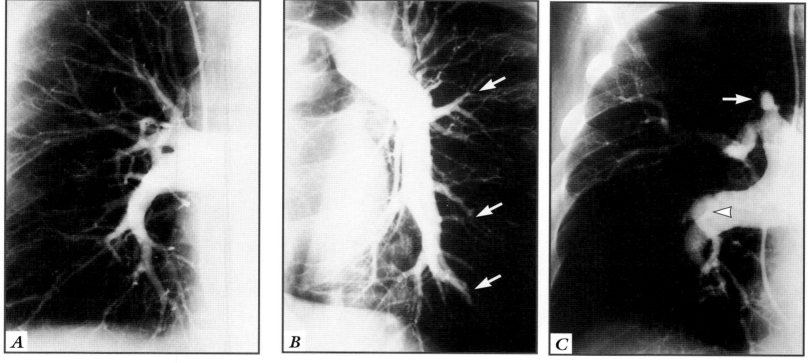

FIGURE 12-4. Pulmonary angiography. **A,** Normal angiogram demonstrating a diffuse branching pattern with smoothly tapering vessels and branches leading to the periphery of the lung. **B,** In primary pulmonary hypertension, pulmonary angiography demonstrates marked "pruning" of small vessels (*arrows*) with absent peripheral flow. No segmental or larger vascular abnormalities are noted. **C,** In contrast, the angiogram in a patient with chronic thromboembolic pulmonary hypertension characteristically demonstrates proximal pulmonary artery (PA) irregularity (*arrowhead*), abnormal narrowing of the proximal vessel (*arrow*), and large areas with absent flow. (*Courtesy of* Richard N. Channick.)

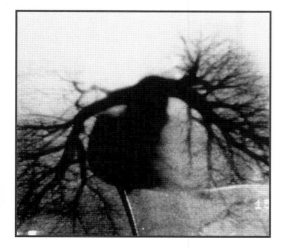

FIGURE 12-5. Intravenous digital subtraction pulmonary arteriography performed from a right atrial injection in a patient with Takayasu's arteritis demonstrating proximal occlusion of the right upper lobe artery and stenoses of the right lower lobe and left upper lobe segmental arteries. Stenoses, either segmental or tubular, focal or generalized, with decreased distal opacification can be found in multiple other entities, only a small fraction of which are true pulmonary vasculitides (scleroderma, systemic lupus erythematosus, idiopathic pulmonary fibrosis, sarcoidosis, radiation injury, bronchiectasis, chronic tuberculosis, pneumoconiosis, lung neoplasm, primary pulmonary hypertension, congenital peripheral pulmonary stenosis, and chronic pulmonary embolism). In many of these cases the history will elucidate the diagnosis, but the approach should also keep in mind possible treatable causes. (*Courtesy of* Himangshu Gupta.)

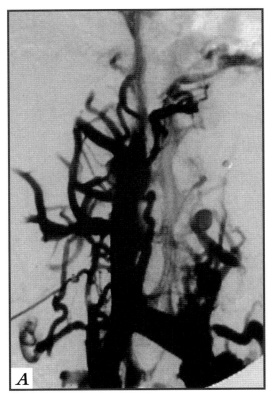

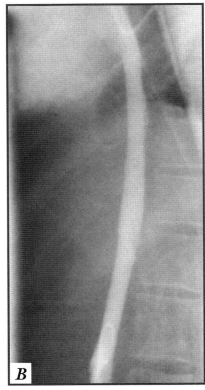

FIGURE 12-6. Digital subtraction angiography. This patient presented with abdominal pain and distension and swelling of the lower extremities. **A,** Frontal digital subtraction angiography inferior venocavogram demonstrating severe narrowing of the intrahepatic segment of the inferior vena cava (VC) with nonfilling of hepatic veins. No focal IVC web is seen. Collateral filling via the azygos system is indicative of increased pressures and partial obstruction. Other imaging studies showed hepatic vein involvement and ascites consistent with Budd-Chiari syndrome. **B,** Lateral view obtained after placement of a Wallstent (there was an initial trial of bolus lytic therapy) showing a widely patent IVC without opacification of collaterals. Filling via collaterals is a more reliable indicator of physiologic obstruction to venous flow than mean pressure gradients alone, as the latter are dependent on the fluid status of the patient, cardiac output, positioning, and degree of vascular tone, given the large capacitance of the venous system. However, mean pressure gradients between 6 and 9 mm Hg probably may be considered significant, and greater than 9 mm Hg, definitely significant [14]. Percutaneous transluminal angioplasty (PTA) of veins suffers from poor long-term patency overall, except perhaps for PTA of congenital IVC membranes [15]; there is development of myointimal hyperplasia, which may be handled with repeat PTA, stent, or atherectomy. In addition, long-term anticoagulation may be required after placement of metallic stents. For these reasons, interventional treatment of nonmalignant stenoses (other than those related to hemodialysis) is best handled on a case-by-case basis.

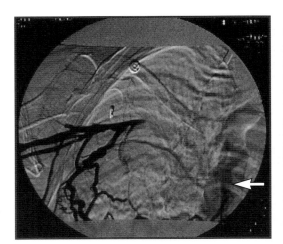

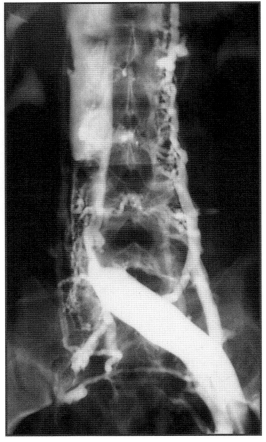

FIGURE 12-7. Subclavian venogram. Subclavian vein obstruction in a patient with a hypercoagulable state and a known long-term parenteral nutrition requirement. Magnetic resonance imaging had demonstrated occlusion of the superior vena cava (SVC), left and right brachiocephalic and left internal jugular veins. Diagnostic right arm venogram for access planning shows chronic right subclavian vein obstruction that was hard to probe with a guidewire, with large collateral flow via subscapular and intercostal veins to the azygos vein and distal SVC (*arrow*). Central venous stenosis and occlusion are becoming more common with the increased use of in-dwelling venous catheters for intravenous therapy and temporary hemodialysis. Other causes include extrinsic compression by neoplasm, extrinsic compression by other mass (such as bone, lymphadenopathy, or aneurysm), fibrosing mediastinitis, retroperitoneal fibrosis, postradiation or postsurgical fibrosis, luminal thrombus or tumor.

FIGURE 12-8. Inferior vena cavography. Inferior vena cava (IVC) occlusion in a posttonsillectomy patient who developed thrombophlebitis in the right greater saphenous vein, which was surgically ligated. The patient was placed on intravenous antibiotics. Examination performed for right leg swelling showed a large filling defect in the IVC, occlusion of the right common iliac vein, and flow through the ascending lumbar and paraspinal collaterals. Lower extremity deep venous thrombosis (DVT) is believed to account for 90% or more of pulmonary emboli. In addition, it is a source of significant late morbidity due to the postthrombotic syndrome, symptoms developing in 60% to 80% of patients after a single episode of proximal DVT [16]. Because complete recanalization is infrequent and return of normal valve function very infrequent on standard anticoagulant therapy, attempts are now being made to treat patients who have significant iliofemoral DVT with early lytic therapy or modern surgical thrombectomy techniques [17,18], with results showing greater success in complete lysis (approximately 65% of patients).

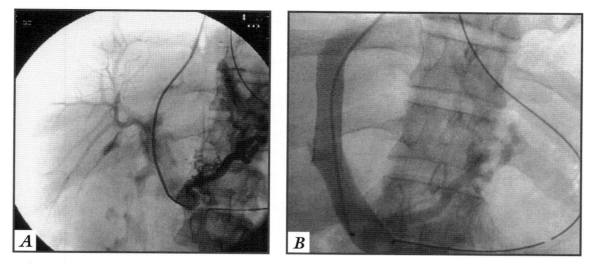

FIGURE 12-9. Portal venography. **A,** Portal venogram performed from a transjugular route demonstrating patency of portal vein branches, without filling defects, with hepatopetal flow, and with varices arising from the coronary vein. These studies are often performed, as here, during a transjugular intrahepatic portosystemic shunt procedure for patients with medically refractory esophageal or gastric variceal bleeding or medically unmanageable ascites, and for those with adequate liver reserve awaiting transplantation [19]. **B,** In this case, note the decreased variceal filling after transjugular portacaval shunt placement. Because of the patient's condition, embolization of the varices was also performed. Other indications for portal venography include the investigation of surgical shunts, congenital anomalies, and portal pressure measurements. For the evaluation of portal venous thrombosis and superior mesenteric and renal vein thrombosis, duplex sonography, computed tomography scanning, and magnetic resonance imaging have become the primary diagnostic methods [20].

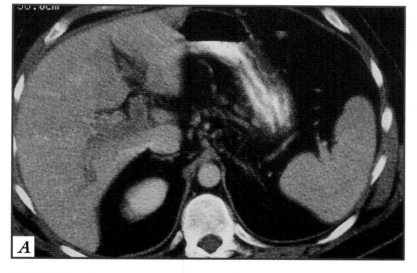

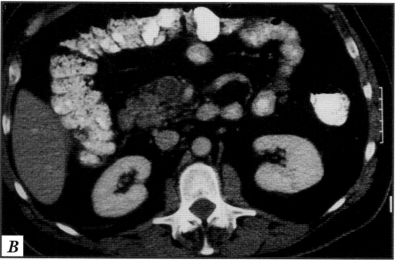

C. Presentation of Mesenteric Venous Thrombosis	
Pain (insidious)	81%
Gastrointestinal bleed	19%
Guaiac + stool	63%
Anorexia	44%
Previous deep vein thrombosis	44%
Pancreatic cancer	13%
Hepatitis	25%
Thrombocytosis	25%
Increased fibrinogen	13%
Decreased protein C/protein S	50%

FIGURE 12-10. Computed tomography. **A** and **B,** Computed tomography scan on an otherwise healthy 40-year-old patient who presented with the classic history of slowly progressive unrelenting nonpostprandial abdominal pain over 1 week. The pain was somewhat out of proportion to the physical examination; no peritoneal signs were present. There is segmental bowel wall thickening with filling defects noted in splanchnic and superior mesenteric veins, extending into the main branches of the portal vein. **C,** Presentation of mesenteric venous thrombosis. Mesenteric venous thrombosis is manifest by relatively subtle evidence of bowel congestion and stasis injury in association with suggestive comorbidity. (Legend *adapted from* Donaldson [21]; figure *from* Harward and coworkers [22]; with permission.)

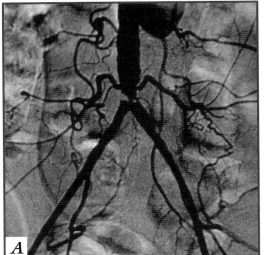

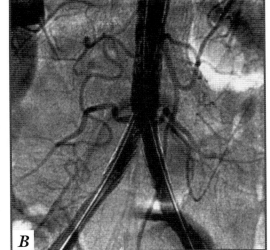

FIGURE 12-11. Pelvic arteriogram. **A,** Diagnostic study on a 41-year-old female patient, a long-time smoker, with fairly severe buttock claudication showing bilateral severe common iliac artery origin stenoses also involving the aortic bifurcation. **B,** Control study performed after the placement of distal aortic and bilateral common iliac stents. Iliac percutaneous transluminal angioplasty (PTA) has a technical success rate of 90% to 95% and a mean 5-year patency rate (pooled from several studies) of 69%; surgical therapy has a mean 5-year patency of 80% to 90% [23–25]. PTA patency rates are higher for the common iliac segment. For stenoses that are resistant to dilation, for common iliac origin stenoses, and for treatment of unstable dissection, stent placement is indicated, with a technical success rate of 95% to 98% and 5-year patency of 85% to 95%.

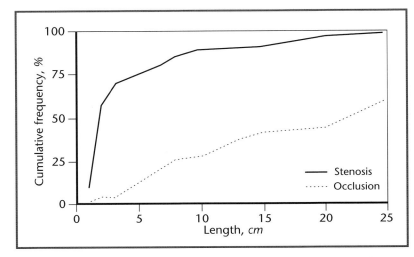

FIGURE 12-12. Cumulative relative frequency of stenoses and occlusions in the femoropopliteal system compared with their length. Among symptomatic patients, the frequency of significant lower extremity atherosclerotic disease involvement (from highest to lowest) is superficial femoral artery, iliac arteries, infrapopliteal arteries, popliteal artery, and common femoral artery. Multisegment disease is common with iliofemoral disease and femorotibial disease, each accounting for approximately one third of cases. There is a general tendency toward bilateral symmetry in segmental involvement, and diabetic patients demonstrate more diffuse as well as more infrapopliteal disease. (*Adapted from* Martin [26]; with permission.)

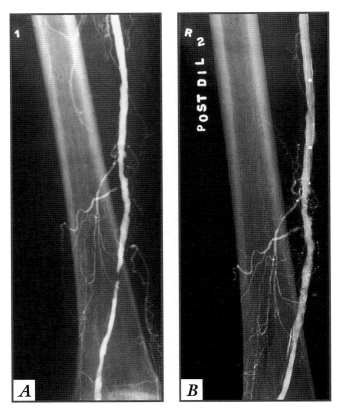

FIGURE 12-13. Superficial femoral artery (SFA) stenosis. **A,** This preliminary study shows an SFA stenosis at the adductor canal—the most common site for stenotic-occlusive disease in the SFA—in a diabetic man with ulcers and rest pain. **B,** After percutaneous transluminal angioplasty (PTA), there is significant improvement in the caliber of the artery; the characteristic collinear localized subintimal dissection of PTA is noted. No transverse flap is evident and, most importantly, no pullback pressure gradient was found.

(*Continued on next page*)

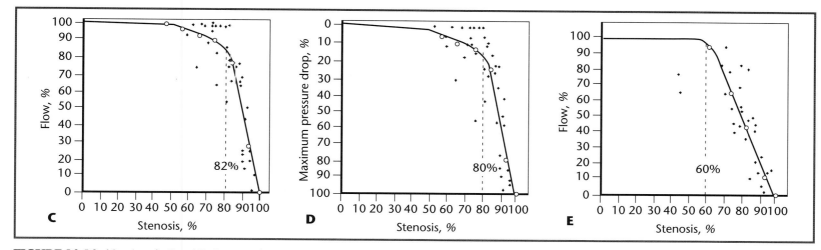

C

D

E

FIGURE 12-13. (*Continued*) **C** and **D**, Because the pressure drop and decrease in flow occur precipitously over a short range of lumen diameters, visual estimation of stenosis and its effects is not reliable, and pressure measurements are best obtained. Even with lesions that are angiographically not significant on two orthogonal views, pressure measurements may demonstrate signif-

icant gradient indicative of physiologically significant obstruction to flow. This is particularly true in the tortuous iliac arteries. **E**, Under conditions of increased flow (such as with exercise or with selective peripheral arterial vasodilation), the sharp drop occurs at lesser degrees of cross-sectional narrowing. (Parts *C* to *E* *adapted from* May and coworkers [27]; with permission.)

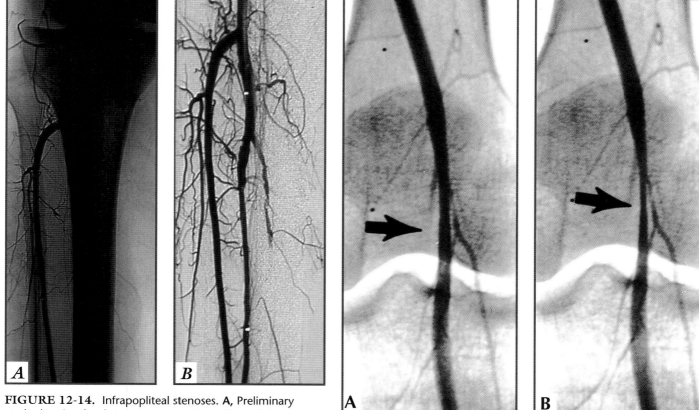

A

B

FIGURE 12-14. Infrapopliteal stenoses. **A**, Preliminary study showing focal stenoses in a patient with calf claudication that was limiting sports activity. **B**, Post–percutaneous transluminal angioplasty (PTA) study showing successful dilation of the stenoses. Although isolated focal limiting infrapopliteal disease is quite unusual, it can be limiting to an athletic patient. PTA in this region is fraught with greater risk of limb loss, particularly in patients with only a single runoff vessel. Long-term success depends on the presence of straight-line flow to the foot and the presence of stenosis (ideally a single short one) rather than occlusion; the need to use lytic therapy also is a poor prognostic factor [28].

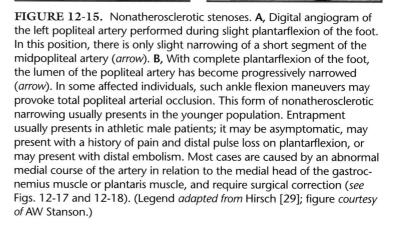

A

B

FIGURE 12-15. Nonatherosclerotic stenoses. **A**, Digital angiogram of the left popliteal artery performed during slight plantarflexion of the foot. In this position, there is only slight narrowing of a short segment of the midpopliteal artery (*arrow*). **B**, With complete plantarflexion of the foot, the lumen of the popliteal artery has become progressively narrowed (*arrow*). In some affected individuals, such ankle flexion maneuvers may provoke total popliteal arterial occlusion. This form of nonatherosclerotic narrowing usually presents in the younger population. Entrapment usually presents in athletic male patients; it may be asymptomatic, may present with a history of pain and distal pulse loss on plantarflexion, or may present with distal embolism. Most cases are caused by an abnormal medial course of the artery in relation to the medial head of the gastrocnemius muscle or plantaris muscle, and require surgical correction (*see* Figs. 12-17 and 12-18). (Legend *adapted from* Hirsch [29]; figure *courtesy of* AW Stanson.)

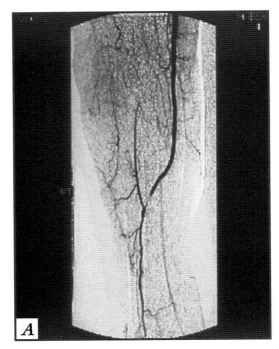

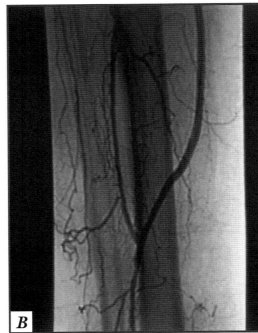

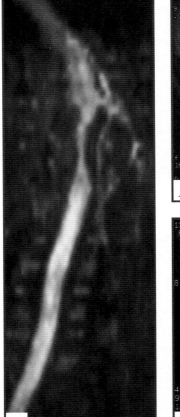

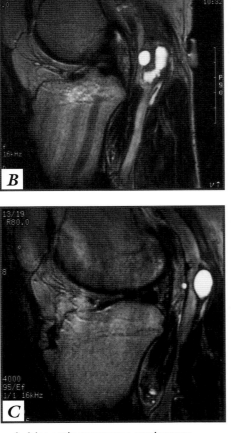

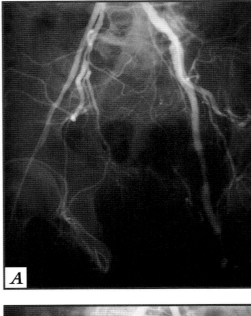

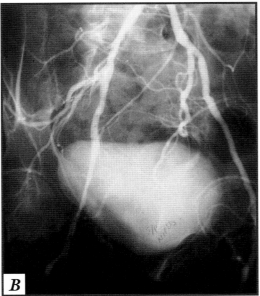

FIGURE 12-16. Bypass graft stenoses. Patient with an *in situ* saphenous vein femoroperoneal graft found to have a focus of stenosis during routine follow-up color-duplex ultrasound examination. Such routine surveillance is crucial in early identification of the failing graft, whose correction before failure can positively affect graft longevity [30]. **A,** Focal distal anastomotic stenosis (the usual site in approximately 80% of cases). **B,** Patency has been restored with percutaneous transluminal angioplasty (PTA). However, the long-term results of PTA have been relatively poor in the treatment of anastomotic graft stenoses, with 3-year patency rates approximately 15% to 40%.

FIGURE 12-18. Nonatherosclerotic stenoses. Apparent severe stenosis or occlusion of the right external iliac artery (**A**). Treatment with sublingual nifedipine was successful in relieving the spasm that had caused the femoral pulse originally present to disappear (**B**). No dissection relating to vessel access is evident. The lack of collaterals on the original study is suggestive of acute occlusion or spasm.

FIGURE 12-17. Popliteal artery. **A,** Magnetic resonance angiogram demonstrating a smooth eccentric narrowing of the midpopliteal artery. **B** and **C,** Magnetic resonance image showing the relationship of the cyst (with high T_2W signal) to the arterial wall and lumen. Adventitial cystic disease presents angiographically as a smooth, focal, spiral, or eccentric narrowing of the supratibial popliteal artery, often without poststenotic dilation. The popliteal artery is the most common site of disease, age of presentation (fourth or fifth decades) is earlier than is usually the case with atherosclerotic disease, and men are much more commonly affected. There may be a history of loss of pulse with knee flexion. Therapy is by surgical marsupialization. (*Adapted from* Miller and coworkers [31]; with permission.)

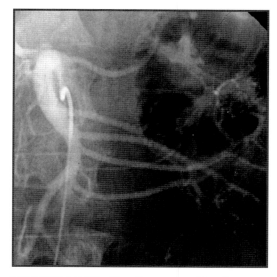

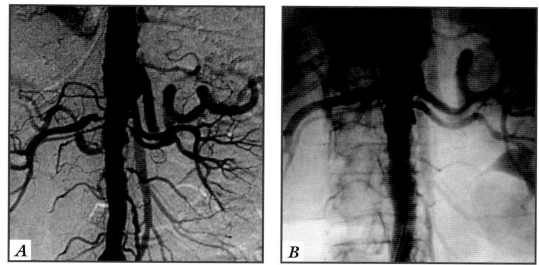

FIGURE 12-19. Standing waves. Standing waves are the regular indentations of the jejunal branch vessel lumen in this patient. They represent a transient nonpathologic physiologic finding that often resolve by the time of repeat injection (as in this case) or with use of a vasodilator. The appearance is more regular and shallow than is the finding in fibromuscular dysplasia (see Fig. 12-25).

FIGURE 12-20. Renal artery stenosis. An 83-year-old patient who underwent separate right coronary artery and left anterior descending coronary artery percutaneous transluminal coronary angioplasties for flash pulmonary edema 4 days and 2 days prior to the current study, necessitated by continued hypertension and apparent diastolic left ventricular dysfunction. A, Diagnostic study showing single right and two left renal arteries, all with severe ostial stenoses. B, After the placement of three Palmaz stents at the three ostia, there is wide patency of the three vessels; there is mild persistent stenosis of the inferior left renal artery due to the stent being placed slightly deep to the true renal ostium. The majority of renal artery stenosis is of atherosclerotic origin, with fibromuscular dysplasia being the second most common cause; other causes include vasculitis (Takayasu's arteritis), neurofibromatosis, radiation injury, and posttraumatic injury.

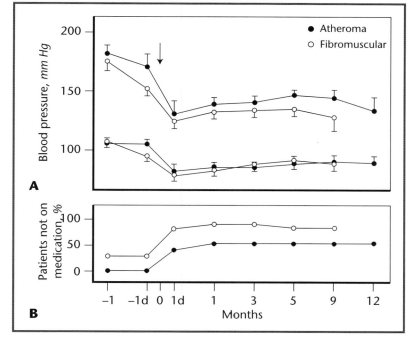

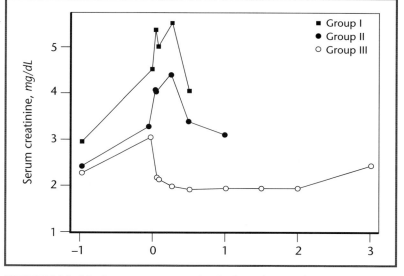

FIGURE 12-21. Percutaneous transluminal renal angioplasty (PTRA). Successful PTRA is usually followed by a rapid fall in blood pressure, and the blood pressure 24 hours after angioplasty usually predicts the long-term level (A). Data are for two groups of patients, 17 with atheromatous stenoses and 24 with fibromuscular dysplasia. B, Note that a greater proportion of fibromuscular patients remained off the antihypertensive medications following the procedure. Percutaneous transluminal angioplasty of atherosclerotic renal artery stenosis for hypertension has a primary 3- to 5-year patency rate of 70% and a secondary 3- to 5-year patency rate of 87%, with an approximately 80% initial technical success rate and an overall clinical success rate (cure or improvement of hypertension) of 75% [32,33]. Similar patency rates are seen with stent placement, but the initial technical success rate is higher (90%). (Legend adapted from Pickering [34]; figure from Sos and coworkers [35]; with permission.)

FIGURE 12-22. Percutaneous transluminal renal angioplasty (PTRA)—like surgery has the potential to improve renal function in patients with renovascular hypertension and azotemia. In this analysis, the effects of angioplasty were investigated in 55 consecutive patients [36]. The average age was 65 years, and all had atheromatous stenoses with a serum creatinine of at least 1.7 mg/dL. They were followed up for up to 4 years. The patients were divided retrospectively into three groups. In group I (47% of the total), there was a reduction of serum creatinine 3 months after the procedure, which in most cases was sustained after 3 years. In group II (35%), angioplasty was judged to be technically successful, but there was no improvement of renal function. In group III (18%), the stenosis could not be dilated. The follow-up periods for groups II and III were shorter because many either died or were started on dialysis. Note that all three groups showed a deterioration of renal function in the year preceding angioplasty. Those expected to benefit most from PTRA performed for renal insufficiency are those with bilateral renal artery stenosis with at least 8-cm kidney (ie, sufficient remaining parenchyma) but without intrarenal disease and serum creatinine less than 4 mg/dL. (Courtesy of Thomas G. Pickering.)

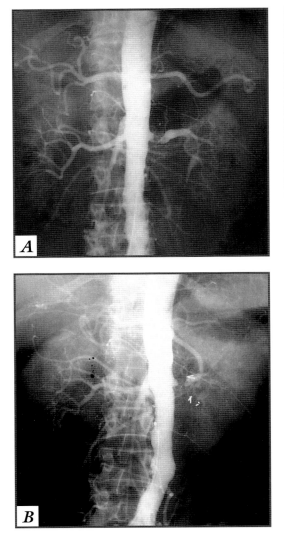

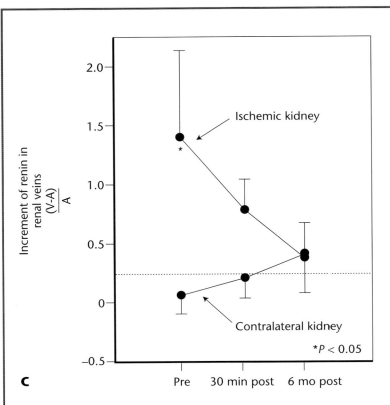

artery bypass patient should include celiac and pelvic arteriograms as well. **C,** Successful revascularization of the ischemic kidney results in a return of the renal vein renin pattern to normal: renin secretion decreases in the ischemic kidney and increases in the contralateral kidney. Measurements were made before, 30 minutes after, and 6 months after angioplasty. *Asterisk* indicates a significant difference between the values for the ischemic versus contralateral kidney. Renin values can differ widely between laboratories, and renin secretion is affected by a host of conditions, including upright position, salt loading, angiotensin-converting enzyme inhibitors, and β-blockers, and the test can result in a significant number of false-negative results. Therefore, the test is not widely used. (Part C *adapted from* Pickering and coworkers [32]; with permission.)

FIGURE 12-23. Left renal artery stenosis. **A,** Left renal artery stenosis in a 55-year-old patient with hypertension. Renin values were as follows: left renal vein peripheral to the adrenal and gonadal veins, 17.8%; right renal vein, 9.4%; inferior vena cava (IVC) superior to renal veins, 8.2%; IVC inferior to renal veins, 7.0. The normal range for this laboratory for a supine patient on a low-salt diet was 2.5 to 8.0 mg/mL/h. The ratio of affected to unaffected kidney was thus greater than 1.5. **B,** The patient underwent left splenorenal artery bypass with restenosis. Diagnostic arteriography for a potential renal

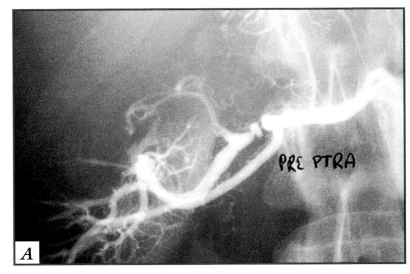

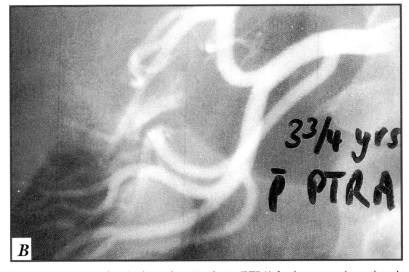

FIGURE 12-24. Renal arteriograms in a 40-year-old white woman with recent onset of hypertension. **A,** Medial fibroplasia of the middle portion of the right renal artery. **B,** Arteriogram taken 3.75 years after angioplasty when the patient was normotensive; there is no residual trace of stenoses.

Percutaneous transluminal renal angioplasty (PTRA) for hypertension related to fibromuscular dysplasia demonstrates approximately 95% initial success (50% cures, 45% improved), 85% primary and 93% secondary long-term patency with 10% recurrence rate. (*Courtesy of* Thomas G. Pickering.)

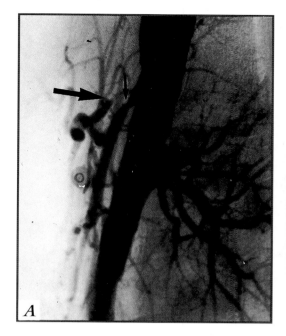

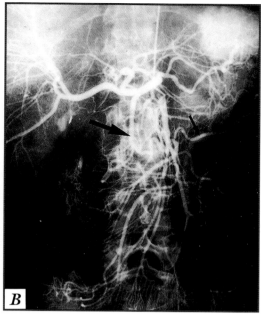

FIGURE 12-25. Mesenteric vascular insufficiency. **A,** Lateral aortogram of a patient with chronic abdominal pain and weight loss demonstrating subtotal occlusion of the celiac artery (*large arrow*), superior mesenteric artery (SMA), moderate stenosis, and inferior mesenteric artery occlusion. Atherosclerotic narrowing responds well to angioplasty, but compression syndrome related to median arcuate ligament compression requires surgery (diagnostic films obtained first on inspiration and then on expiration help to make this diagnosis).

B, Selective SMA injection showing a proximal SMA stenosis and celiac occlusion with reconstitution via retrograde flow through pancreaticoduodenal and gastroduodenal arteries (*large arrow*), and large left branch of the middle colic artery (*small arrow*). These collateral flows are a helpful physiologic indicator of obstruction to antegrade flow. (*Courtesy of* Clement Grassi.)

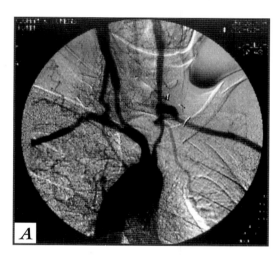

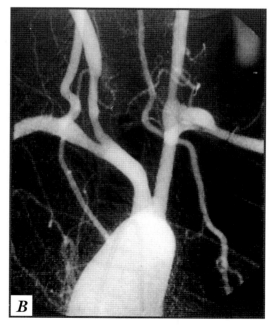

FIGURE 12-26. Carotid artery stenoses. **A,** Patient with a left carotid–subclavian artery bypass performed for subclavian steal syndrome who presented with recurrent arm claudication and a tubular stenosis of the left common carotid artery, most severe near the anastomosis. **B,** After failure of an initial angioplasty, two Palmaz stents were used to successfully restore wide patency to the common carotid artery, with resolution of symptoms. (*Courtesy of* Michael Meyerovitz.)

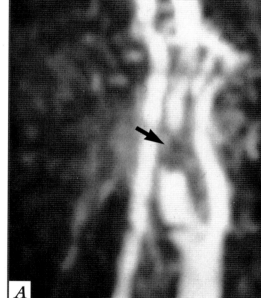

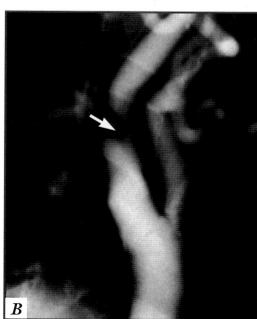

FIGURE 12-27.
A, Magnetic resonance (MR) angiogram of extracranial arteries, showing high-grade stenosis of the internal carotid artery (*arrow*). Recent advances in MR angiography technology have produced high-quality imaging of the neck and proximal intracranial vessels. The technique is noninvasive, and its accuracy equals that of duplex ultrasonography.

B, Conventional contrast angiogram of the carotid arteries from the same patient demonstrating a high-grade stenosis in the proximal carotid artery (*arrow*). Standard arteriography is still the preferred method, when MR angiography and ultrasound imaging have yielded ambiguous results regarding the status of extracranial carotid arteries, or when information regarding the status of the intracranial vasculature is required. Note the overestimation of the degree of stenosis on the MR angiogram (**A**), which has a low rate of false-negative results. (*Courtesy of* Frances E. Jensen and Mark A. Creager.)

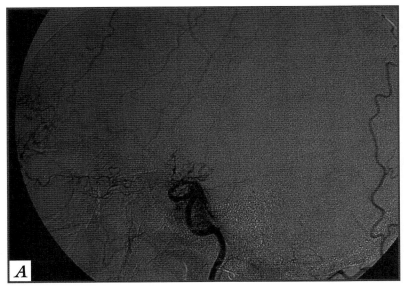

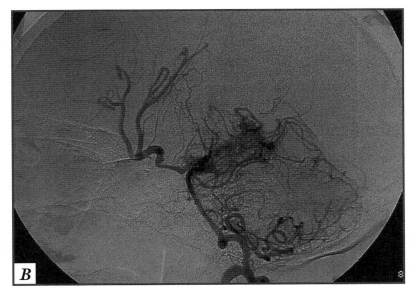

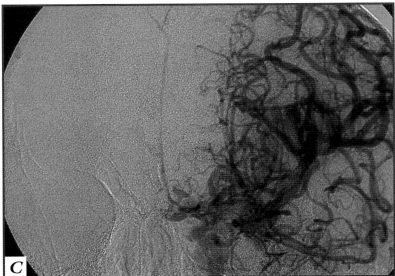

FIGURE 12-28. Cerebral arteriogram. Severe narrowing of the anterior cavernous carotid artery. **A,** Lateral view of cerebral angiogram demonstrating occlusion in the supraclinoid portion in a patient with sickle-cell disease and multiple systemic complications. **B,** Vertebral artery injection demonstrating somewhat enlarged thalamostriate and lenticulostriate arteries providing collateral flow (falling into the spectrum of Moyamoya disease). **C,** Frontal view of later phase of vertebral artery injection. Large leptomeningeal collaterals were demonstrable from other injections in this case. (*Courtesy of* Richard B. Schwartz.)

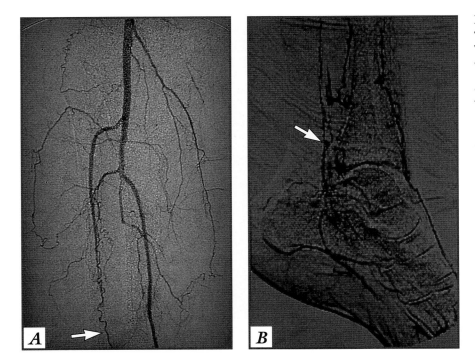

FIGURE 12-29. Buerger's disease. **A** and **B,** A 48-year-old woman who had stopped smoking 7 years previously when she was developing some rest pain symptoms. She began smoking again about 6 months before this study was performed for a nonhealing foot ulceration. The findings of abrupt proximal occlusions (only the left leg is shown), segmental filling of the vessels, and the corkscrew collaterals (*arrows*) coincide with the history to provide a diagnosis of thromboangiitis obliterans (Buerger's disease), although the disease is more commonly encountered in men. Definitive diagnosis is on the basis of histopathology (usually of amputated digits).

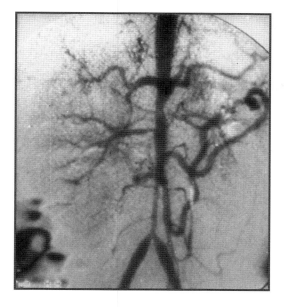

FIGURE 12-30. Takayasu's disease. Aortogram of a patient with Takayasu's disease demonstrating the characteristic smooth-walled, fairly abrupt, segmental narrowing of the infrarenal aorta. There is severe stenosis of the right renal artery and common iliac arteries, near occlusion of the left renal artery, and occlusion of the superior mesenteric artery, with large collateral flow from the inferior mesenteric artery through the arc of Riolan. Stenoses are the main manifestation (80%), and most cases involve the aorta; when the branches of the aorta are involved, the involvement is usually very proximal. Left subclavian and renal arteries are frequently involved, and carotid, coronary, and pulmonary arteries are sometimes involved, although arteriography may not show the full extent of disease. Stenosis combined with dilation and dilation alone are less common manifestations. (*Courtesy of* Himangshu Gupta.)

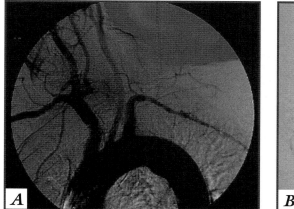

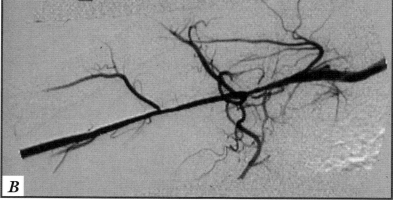

FIGURE 12-31. Stenoses of giant cell arteritis (temporal arteritis). **A** and **B**, These stenoses tend to be more distally placed (distal subclavian, axillary, brachial, external carotid branches, rarely intracranial branches), with more tapered narrowing than in Takayasu's arteritis. They also present in an older age group and predominantly in women, some of whom present with polymyalgia rheumatica. Involvement of the ophthalmic artery is a dreaded complication, and biopsy of the temporal artery can yield a diagnosis even when it is not frankly tender.

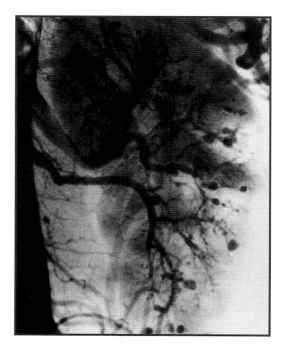

FIGURE 12-32. Renal arteriogram from a patient with polyarteritis nodosa. These renal microaneurysms are found in 75% of patients with this diagnosis. Also present are irregular stenoses of the intrarenal branches. Later, a nephrographic phase (not shown) demonstrated a subcapsular hematoma. (*From* Kandarpa and coworkers [37]; with permission.)

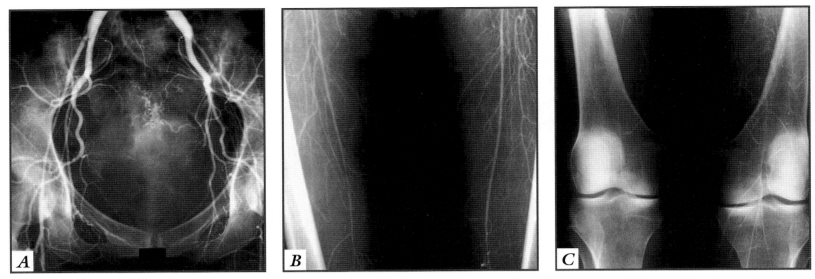

FIGURE 12-33. A to C, Ergotism. Ergotism refers to the toxic effects of ergot derivatives, most notably dihydroergotamine and methysergide. The bilaterally symmetric diffuse vasoconstriction most severe distally but also involving more proximal vessels in a hemodynamically stable patient would suggest the sort of vascular spasm seen in this condition; Raynaud's phenomenon would not be expected to extend so far proximally, but also results in diffuse bilateral narrowing of smaller vessels, and is responsive to warming. (*From* Husted and coworkers [38]; with permission.)

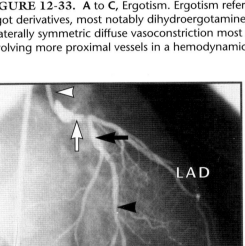
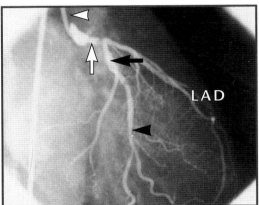

FIGURE 12-34. Left main coronary artery disease. Shown is a right anterior oblique angiogram of the left coronary artery of a patient with exertional angina that worsened over a period of several months. Angiography demonstrated tight stenosis (*white arrow*) in the distal left main coronary artery. The remainder of the coronary circulation was free of severe obstructive disease. The patient was treated with coronary artery bypass grafting with a left internal mammary artery graft to the anterior descending artery and a saphenous vein graft to the major circumflex (Cx) obtuse marginal branch. *White arrowhead* indicates the coronary catheter; *black arrow* indicates the Cx artery; *black arrowhead* indicates the obtuse marginal branch. LAD—left anterior descending coronary artery. (*Courtesy of* Eric R. Powers.)

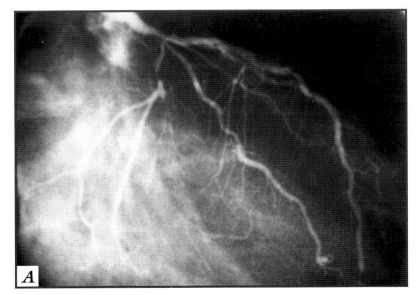

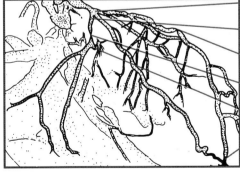

Moderate stenosis in the left main artery

Moderate stenosis in the proximal circumflex artery

Severe stenosis in the middle anterior descending artery

Severe stenosis in the proximal circumflex artery

Occlusion of a major circumflex branch

Moderate stenosis in the distal anterior descending artery

FIGURE 12-35. Multivessel coronary disease depicted by left (**A**) and right (**B**) coronary angiograms from a man with severe angina and abnormal left ventricular function, which was demonstrated by left ventriculography (not shown).

(*Continued on next page*)

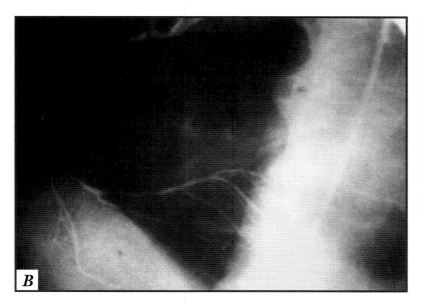

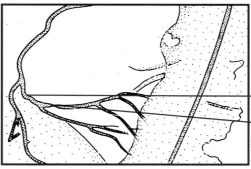

FIGURE 12-35. (*Continued*) Several areas of severe stenosis can be seen. Coronary artery bypass grafting was subsequently performed. (*Courtesy of* Eric R. Powers.)

Long lesion in the midportion of the right coronary artery

Discrete lesion in the distal portion of the right coronary artery

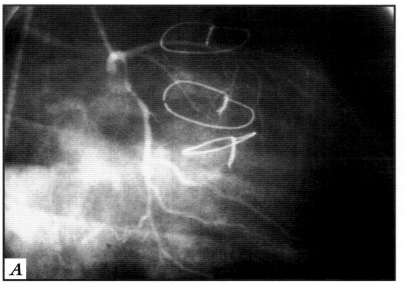

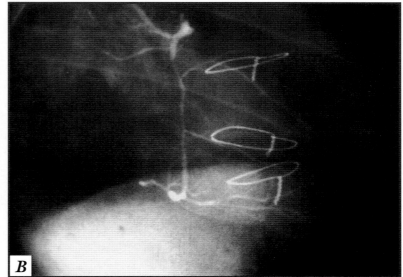

FIGURE 12-36. Transplant coronary disease. The coronary angiograms shown were obtained as part of a patient's routine annual evaluation 4 years after cardiac transplantation. Angiography performed 1 year before this study demonstrated mild coronary luminal narrowing. The study demon-

strates severe and diffuse narrowing of both left (**A**) and right (**B**) coronary arteries. This pattern of diffuse proximal and distal disease is common on posttransplant coronary disease. (*Courtesy of* Eric R. Powers.)

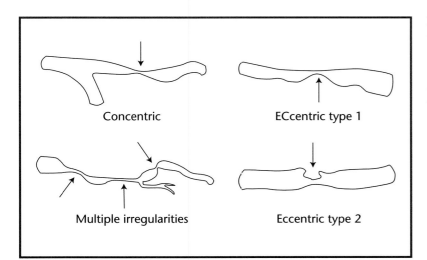

Concentric

ECcentric type 1

Multiple irregularities

Eccentric type 2

FIGURE 12-37. Types of stenoses. Severity of stenosis is only one feature of coronary lesions that has clinical significance; certain lesions are associated with unstable syndromes and subsequent myocardial infarction. The pathologic basis for clinical instability is believed to be ulceration of the plaque in many patients. In this illustration, stenoses are divided into four types based on angiographic appearance (*arrows* indicate stenoses) [39]. The angiographic appearance of the eccentric type 2 lesion is believed to be caused by plaque ulceration. (Legend *adapted from* Powers [40]; figure *adapted from* Ambrose and coworkers [39]; with permission.)

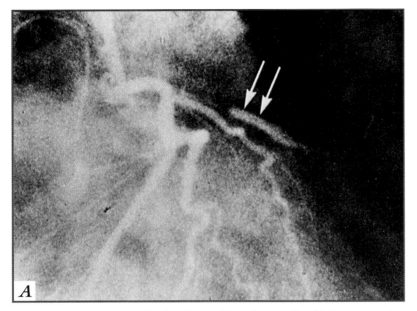

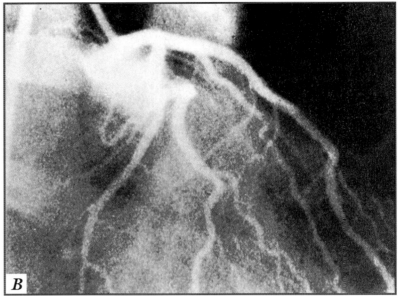

FIGURE 12-38. Prognosis of patients with variant angina. Variant angina is an unusual syndrome that is caused by coronary artery spasm. Coronary artery spasm of a patient who had typical variant (or Prinzmetal's) angina is illustrated. **A,** Spontaneous spasm of the anterior descending coronary artery occurred while the patient was in the cardiac catheterization laboratory. *Arrows* indicate a segment of the artery distal to the site of occlusion. **B,** Sublingual nitroglycerin was given, and angiography was repeated. A wide, patent artery without evidence of a fixed obstructing lesion is noted. In many patients with variant angina, coronary spasm can be precipitated by the intravenous administration of ergonovine. Coronary spasm causing the variant angina syndrome may occur at the site of fixed coronary stenosis or at a site without stenosis, as in this patient. The prognosis of patients with variant angina is influenced by the presence or lack of stenosis. In the study by Mark *et al.* [41], infarction-free survival probability at 3 years was 0.89 if significant fixed coronary stenosis was absent but only 0.46 if significant stenosis was present. (Legend *adapted from* Powers [38]; figure *from* Abrams [42]; with permission.)

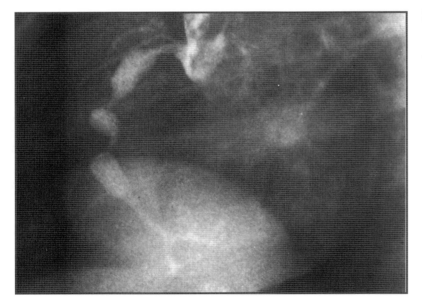

FIGURE 12-39. Kawasaki disease. Right coronary arteriogram from a 17-month-old girl who was diagnosed with Kawasaki disease at age 15 months. Two months after onset of disease, three aneurysms are present, with possible discrete stenoses between aneurysmal segments. (Legend *adapted from* Isselbacher and coworkers [43]; figure *from* Takahashi and coworkers [44]; with permission.)

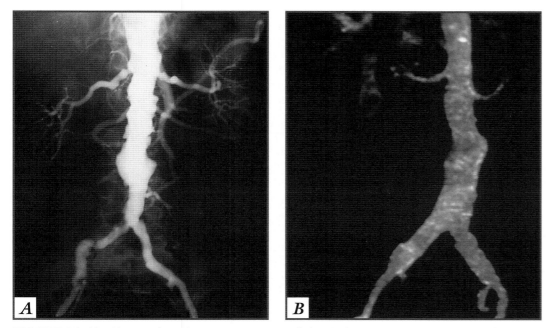

FIGURE 12-40. Abnormal aortic aneurysms. **A,** An abdominal aortic aneurysm is present, but because arteriography depends on opacification of the blood flow lumen (mural thrombus is often present in aneurysms), the true diameter of the aorta can be judged only by finding the faint line of calcification on either side of the lumen. For this reason, ultrasound, computed tomography (CT)

scan or CT angiography, and magnetic resonance (MR) scanor/MR angiography better evaluate the luminal diameter; the latter two also can give information regarding peri-aneurysmal leak or fibrosis, iliac extension or separate aneurysm, position of the neck of the aneurysm with respect to the renal arteries, number of renal arteries, inferior mesenteric artery patency, and condition of the celiac artery and superior mesenteric artery origins [45]. However, angiography may be necessary if there is known azotemia, brittle hypertension, bowel ischemia, or lower extremity ischemia.

B, Gadolinium-enhanced MR angiography of an aneurysm in another patient. Of aortic aneurysms, 80% are infrarenal, 12% are descending thoracic, and only 3% are thoracoabdominal. Of abdominal aneurysms, 75% are fusiform, 3% to 5% are inflammatory, and over 90% are infrarenal; approximately 20% to 25% of patients have concurrent significant iliofemoral occlusive disease. Rupture is related to size, with a smaller than 3.5-cm aneurysm having a negligible rate of rupture within 6 years, a 4- to 5-cm aneurysm having a 3% to 4% rate, and a larger than 5-cm aneurysm having a greater than 25% rupture rate.

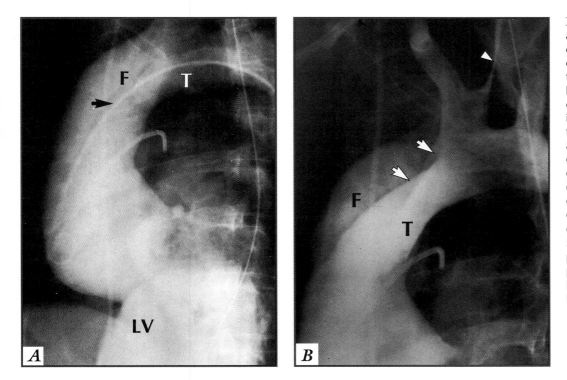

FIGURE 12-41. Left anterior oblique aortograms demonstrating a proximal aortic dissection and its associated cardiovascular complications. **A,** The aortic root is dilated. The true lumen (T) and false lumen (F) are separated by a faintly visible radiolucent line (following the contour of the pigtail catheter), which is the intimal flap (*arrow*). The abundance of contrast in the left ventricle (LV) is indicative of significant aortic insufficiency. **B,** The true lumen is better opacified than is the false lumen, and two planes of the intimal flap can now be distinguished (*arrows*). Additionally, the branch vessels are opacified and the marked narrowing of the right carotid artery (*arrowhead*) suggests that it is compromised by the dissection. (Legend *adapted from* Isselbacher and coworkers [43]. Figure for part A *from* Cigarroa and coworkers [46]; with permission. Figure for part B *courtesy of* Eric M. Isselbacher, Joaquin E. Cigarroa, and Kim A. Eagle.)

Diagnostic Information Sought in Patients with Suspected Aortic Dissection

Presence or absence of aortic dissection
Involvement of the ascending aorta
Extent of dissection
Sites of entry and re-entry
Thrombus in the false lumen
Branch vessel involvement by dissection
Aortic insufficiency
Pericardial effusion
Coronary artery involvement by intimal flap

FIGURE 12-42. Diagnostic information sought in patients with suspected aortic dissection. Although ideally one would prefer to define all of these anatomic characteristics in each case of aortic dissection, no single diagnostic study can provide all of this information. Instead, on a case-by-case basis one's clinical suspicion, together with consideration of available treatment options, should determine which diagnostic information is necessary for patient management. In fact, in some situations more than one diagnostic study may be required to define the salient features of an aortic dissection adequately [47]. (Legend *adapted from* Isselbacher and coworkers [43]; figure *adapted from* Cigarroa and coworkers [46]; with permission.)

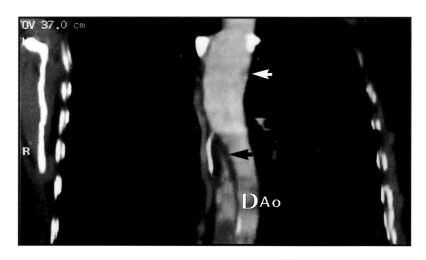

FIGURE 12-43. Computed tomography (CT) of aortic dissection. Newer techniques in CT scanning that produce superior images to those of conventional CT scanners have been introduced and are particularly useful in diagnosing aortic dissection. Shown is a CT scan generated using the traced-curve reformation technique, which has unfolded the aorta. This tomographic reformation in the coronal plane shows the aortic arch (*white arrow*) and an intimal flap (*black arrow*) in the descending aorta (DAo), which spirals as it progresses distally.

Whereas spiral CT now allows for extended coverage of craniocaudal anatomy in 30 to 40 seconds with high-contrast opacification of the aorta and great vessels, magnetic resonance imaging (MRI) scan allows fast multiplanar imaging. Whereas CT benefits from higher spatial resolution, MRI benefits from high-contrast resolution for detection of very small thrombosed channels or intramural hematoma, and cine MRI imaging may allow for detection of small flaps that are otherwise blurred due to their motion in the cardiac cycle, as in the case of dissecting aneurysm. (*Courtesy of* Eric M. Isselbacher, Joaquin E. Cigarroa, and Kim A. Eagle.)

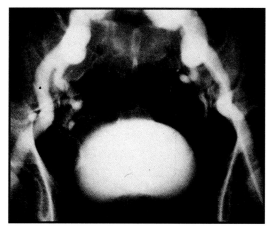

FIGURE 12-44. Abdominal angiogram demonstrating bilateral iliac aneurysms. Of iliac aneurysms, 75% are continuations of abdominal aortic aneurysm, with the common iliac artery being the most common site, followed by the internal iliac artery, and the external iliac artery. Isolated iliac aneurysms may be silent until they present with a mass effect on neighboring structures (bowel, iliac vein, ureter, or bladder) due to their large size; they may thus be associated with a high risk of rupture. (Legend *adapted from* Creager and Halperin [48]; figure *from* Creager and coworkers [49].)

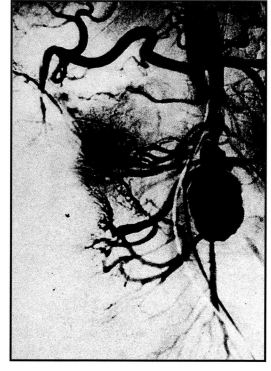

FIGURE 12-45. Mycotic aneurysm of the superior mesenteric artery that was subsequently excised; arterial reconstruction was achieved using autologous saphenous vein grafts. *Staphylococcus aureus* and *Salmonella* organisms are the most common bacterial isolates. (Legend *adapted from* Creager and Halperin [48]; figure *from* Whittemore and Mannick [50]; with permission.)

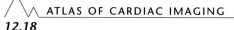

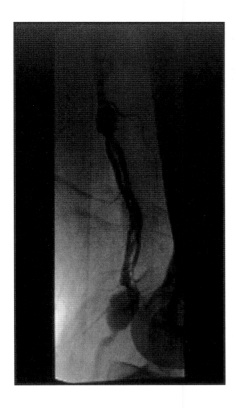

FIGURE 12-46. Popliteal aneurysm. These aneurysms constitute the most common aneurysm of the periphery (70%), with a heavy predominance among male patients. Fifty percent are bilateral, and 50% of patients have associated iliofemoral or aortic aneurysm. They more often present with thromboembolic disease than with the claudication that this patient gave as his prime symptom, and may present with acute popliteal artery thrombotic occlusion. This study demonstrates multiple channels related to recanalization of thrombus.

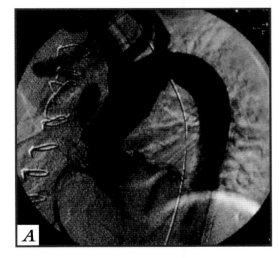

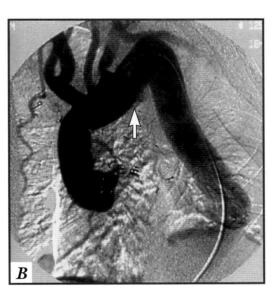

FIGURE 12-47. Aortic arch pseudoaneurysms. A and B, Two patients with surgically proven aortic arch pseudoaneurysms after aortic repairs. Both presented with fever, and whereas the patient in B also presented with hemoptysis, the patient in A demonstrated an episode of hypotension and slightly bloody right pleural effusion. Whereas the finding in A shows a clear extraluminal collection, that in B shows only a slight haziness and irregularity focally at the margin and contour convexity (arrow).

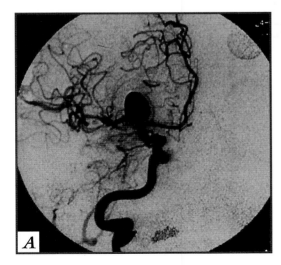

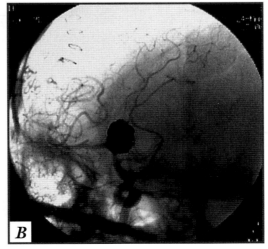

FIGURE 12-48. Subarachnoid hemorrhage (SAH). A and B, This patient presented with SAH, but at surgery the middle cerebral artery aneurysm proved to be too calcified at the wide neck to be reliably controlled, and embolization was performed with detachable Gianturco coils. A total of 75% of SAH cases are caused by berry aneurysm rupture; other causes include arteriovenous malformation, parenchymal hemorrhage with extension, and trauma. Forty percent of survivors have permanent neurologic sequelae. (Courtesy of F. Huang-Hellinger.)

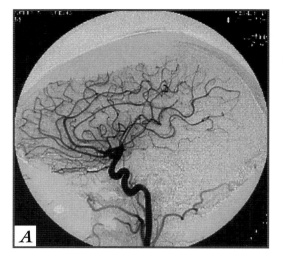

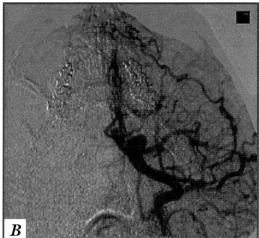

FIGURE 12-49. A and B, Aneurysm of the anterior communicating artery, whose relationships are best delineated on the submentovertex view (B). The supraclinoid internal carotid artery is the most common site, followed by the anterior communicating artery, followed by the middle cerebral artery; a small percentage involve the posterior circulation (posterior inferior cerebellar artery, basilar tip). There is a baseline 1% per year rate of rupture, greater for larger aneurysms; if the aneurysm has already bled, then there is a 3% to 4% per year rate (30% to 40% in the first month). (Courtesy of R. Klufas.)

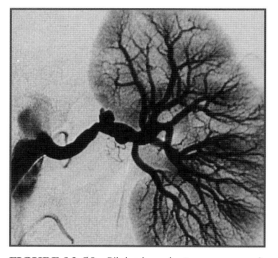

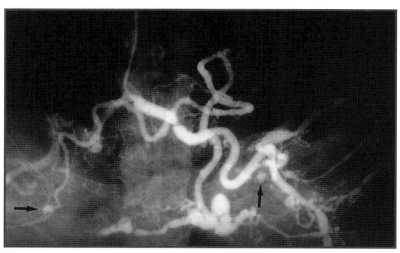

FIGURE 12-50. Bilobed renal artery aneurysm in a patient who was previously treated successfully with percutaneous transluminal renal angioplasty on the contralateral side for fibromuscular dysplasia–related renovascular hypertension, with resolution of hypertension. Aneurysms are seen with medial fibroplasia, the most common form of fibromuscular dysplasia, but are not often this large.

FIGURE 12-51. Patient with polyarteritis nodosa demonstrating hepatic and splenic microaneurysms as well as intrahepatic arterial narrowing. Although involvement of skin, muscle, and myocardium occurs, microaneurysms are rare in these locations. (See Fig. 12-32, which demonstrates the more common renal site for this disease.) Other causes of intrarenal aneurysm include atherosclerosis, traumatic pseudoaneurysm, and methamphetamine use. (From Chopra and Kandarpa [51]; with permission.)

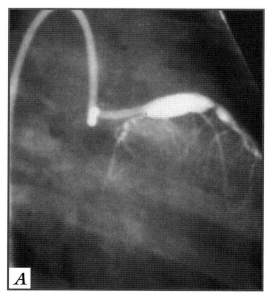

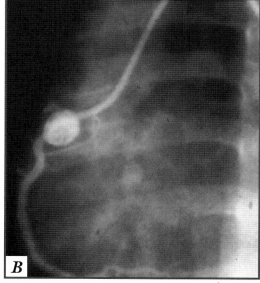

FIGURE 12-52. Coronary angiograms of patients demonstrating fusiform (A), saccular (B), (Continued on next page)

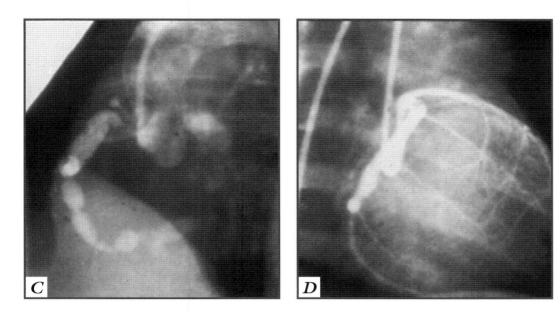

FIGURE 12-52. (*Continued*) and segmental (**C**) aneurysms and an ecstatic coronary artery (**D**). (*Courtesy of* Kathryn A. Taubert and Adnan S. Dajani.)

ARTERIAL EMBOLIC DISEASE

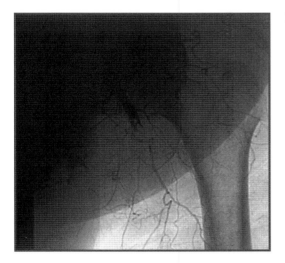

FIGURE 12-53. Common femoral artery embolus in a patient presenting with sudden-onset severe left leg pain, pulselessness, pallor with distal coolness, and paresthesia. Note the lack of collateral flow. Spasm can also contribute to the acute narrowing of the artery and convert a stenosis to an occlusion. In the lower extremity, emboli lodge in the following sites in descending order of frequency: femoral artery bifurcation, popliteal artery, iliac artery bifurcation, and aortic bifurcation. In the upper extremity, the brachial artery is the most common site, followed by axillary artery.

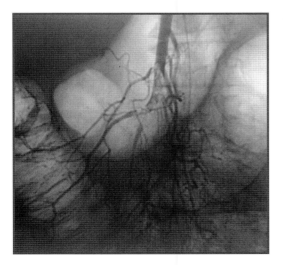

FIGURE 12-54. Superior mesenteric artery embolus in a patient who presented with abdominal pain that had grown quickly worse over the course of 1 day. The most common source of emboli is the heart, as in this patient with atrial fibrillation; other cardiac sources include mural thrombus and valvular vegetations. The next most common site is aneurysm or atheroma in a proximal artery.

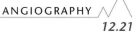

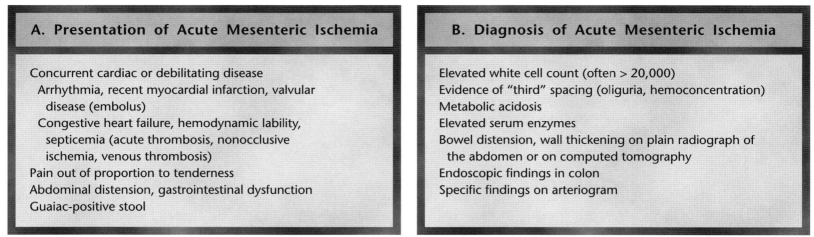

A. Presentation of Acute Mesenteric Ischemia

Concurrent cardiac or debilitating disease
  Arrhythmia, recent myocardial infarction, valvular
    disease (embolus)
  Congestive heart failure, hemodynamic lability,
    septicemia (acute thrombosis, nonocclusive
    ischemia, venous thrombosis)
Pain out of proportion to tenderness
Abdominal distension, gastrointestinal dysfunction
Guaiac-positive stool

B. Diagnosis of Acute Mesenteric Ischemia

Elevated white cell count (often > 20,000)
Evidence of "third" spacing (oliguria, hemoconcentration)
Metabolic acidosis
Elevated serum enzymes
Bowel distension, wall thickening on plain radiograph of
  the abdomen or on computed tomography
Endoscopic findings in colon
Specific findings on arteriogram

FIGURE 12-55. Acute mesenteric ischemia. **A,** Presentation of acute mesenteric ischemia. Acute mesenteric ischemia is manifest by the presence of suggestive causative comorbidity, severe visceral pain, and evidence of bowel dysfunction and early mucosal slough. **B,** Diagnosis of acute mesenteric ischemia. Diagnosis is confirmed by laboratory, endoscopic, and clinical evidence of diffuse inflammation and tissue injury together with arterial occlusion on arteriogram. (*Courtesy of* Magruder C. Donaldson.)

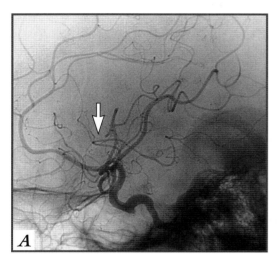

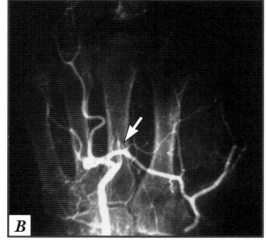

FIGURE 12-56. Appearance of microemboli in the small vasculature of **A,** the brain (operculofrontal artery obstruction; *arrow*) and **B,** the hand (common digital artery; *arrow*).

ARTERIAL HEMORRHAGIC DISEASE

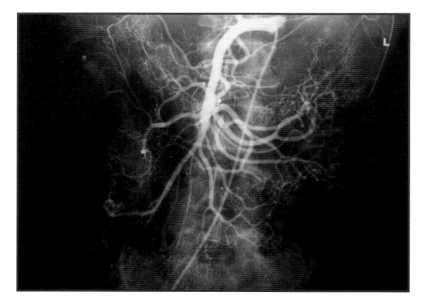

FIGURE 12-57. Bleeding diverticulum (note the luminal extravasation) in a patient who presented with melena. Seventy-five percent of lower gastrointestinal bleeding can be managed acutely with intravenous fluid and transfusion support, correction of coagulopathy, sedation, and bedrest, since the nature of the bleeding is self-contained or intermittent. Only those with brisk bleeding, extensive transfusion requirements, or cardiovascular instability require prompt arteriography. A radionuclide bleeding scan can help to confirm active bleeding and direct the angiographer to a particular site. Three quarters of the time, diverticular bleeding involves the ascending or transverse colon and can be controlled successfully in 90% of cases with intra-arterial vasopressin; embolization has also been used in patients intolerant of vasopressin or unable to cooperate with extended catheter therapy. Diagnostic arteriography for upper gastrointestinal bleeding has been replaced in most cases by endoscopy, sclerotherapy, endoscopic cautery, and medications (H_2^- and proton-pump antagonists, somatostatin).

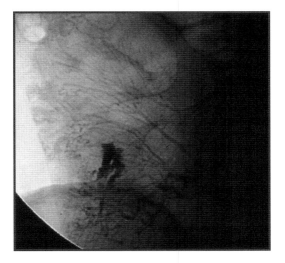

FIGURE 12-58. Cecal angiodysplasia. This represents another source of lower gastrointestinal bleeding: from dilated mucosal and submucosal veins in the cecum and ascending colon, which are not apparent endoscopically. Luminal extravasation is not commonly seen, but the early filling and persistent late opacification of veins in the region seen in this case are the hallmark; sometimes an abnormal tangle of feeding vessels at the bowel may be seen (as in this case).

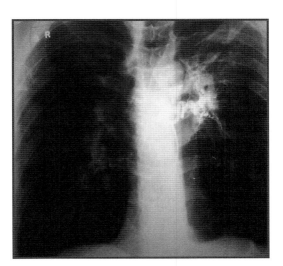

FIGURE 12-59. Enlarged tortuous bronchial arteries. In the adult with significant hemoptysis, chronic inflammatory causes of bronchial bleeding (bronchiectasis from any underlying process, including cystic fibrosis, bronchopulmonary aspergillosis, tuberculosis) are most common, but cavities (related to neoplasms, tuberculosis, sequestration, necrotizing pneumonias), and rarely, foreign bodies and arteriovenous malformation, can be causes. In infants, congenital heart disease with large bronchial collaterals (pulmonary atresia, tetralogy with a severe pulmonary stenosis component) can also be a cause. Visualization of extravasation is not the rule, and enlarged tortuous bronchial arteries (as in this case) or collaterals of other systemic arteries with a prominent blush may be the only finding, which is sufficient to warrant embolization in the appropriate clinical setting.

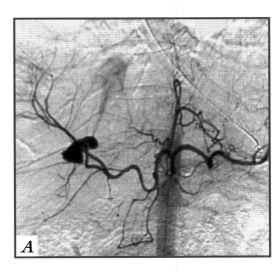
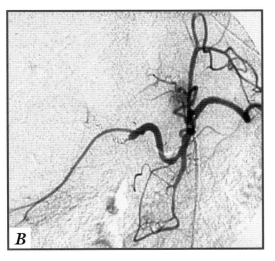

FIGURE 12-60. Trauma after motor vehicle accident. **A** and **B,** Hepatic pseudoaneurysm in a patient after motor vehicle accident, with rapidly falling hematocrit and liver laceration on computed tomography scanning. There is a laceration of a right hepatic artery branch with a leaking pseudoaneurysm; the artery was successfully embolized, which stabilized the patient's hemodynamic status. (*Courtesy of* Clement Grassi.)

 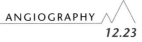

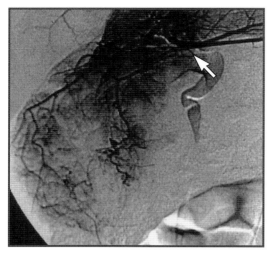

FIGURE 12-61. Hypervascularity, neovascularity, and draping of vessels supplying a cystic neoplasm of the pancreas. There is also a small area where vessel encasement is found (*arrow*). No arteriovenous shunting is seen.

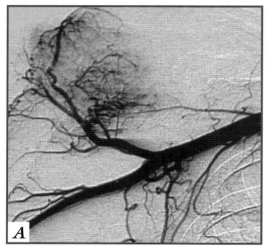

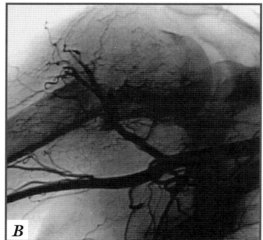

FIGURE 12-62. Right humeral metastatic lesion from renal cell carcinoma. Pre- (**A**) and postembolization (**B**) images. Embolization was performed to minimize blood loss at a rodding procedure planned to prevent pathologic fracture and control pain. (*Courtesy of* Clement Grassi.)

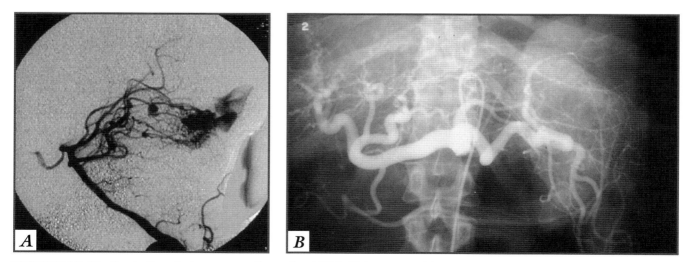

FIGURE 12-63. Cerebellar arteriovenous malformation (AVM). This 50-year-old patient had a history of prior subarachnoid hemorrhage. **A,** Although hypervascularity and arteriovenous shunting are present, there is no neovascularity in this cerebellar AVM, which represents a vascular malformation rather than neoplasm. The tangle of vessels represents the nidus. There is enlargement of the superior cerebellar artery supplying the region, and inflow aneurysms are also present. **B,** In this cirrhotic patient with portal hypertension, there is arterial enlargement due to increased hepatic arterial flow and corkscrewing of the intrahepatic arterial branches without hypervascularity or neovascularity (there is also splenomegaly). (*Courtesy of* F. Huang-Hellinger.)

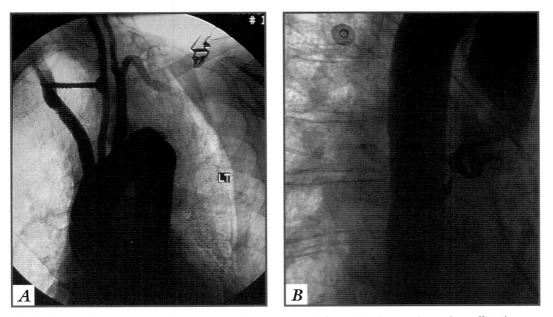

A

B

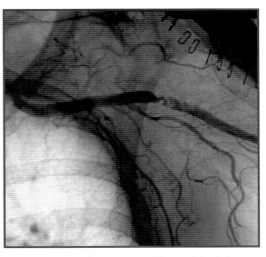

FIGURE 12-65. Extensive injury of the left axillary and brachial arteries from a motor vehicle accident. There is evidence of an intimal flap, mural hematoma or arterial contusion, spasm, and draping of vessels around surrounding hematoma. The artery remains patent, and no extravasation or pseudoaneurysm is found.

FIGURE 12-64. Arterial trauma. **A** and **B**, Traumatic aortic laceration in a patient who suffered a motor vehicle accident. Ninety-five percent of these injuries occur at the site of attachment of the ligamentum arteriosum, but other sites include the aortic root at the annulus, at the origin of the great vessels (usually brachiocephalic artery), and at the diaphragmatic hiatus. At least two orthogonal views of the arch, particularly the aortic isthmus, must be obtained. In this case there were two separate sites of injury—one a pseudoaneurysm at the isthmus and the other an unusual intimal flap of the descending thoracic aorta (not discernible on computed tomography scan), confirmed at surgery.

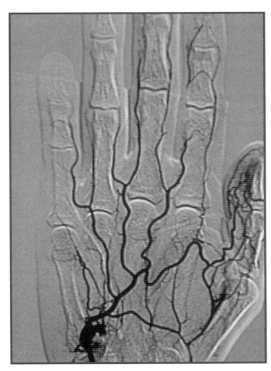

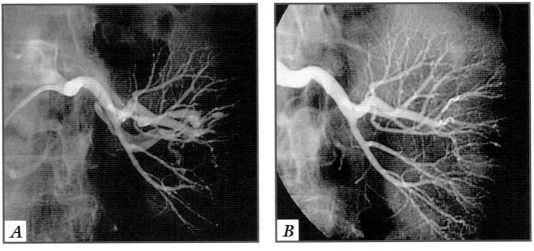

A

B

FIGURE 12-67. Iatrogenic arteriovenous (AV) fistula **A**, Iatrogenic AV fistula in a patient with Wegener's granulomatosis and azotemia presenting with gross hematuria after renal biopsy. **B**, Final arteriogram showing closure of the fistula via superselective platinum coil embolization; apart from the primary aim of closing the fistula, care had to be taken to preserve as much renal tissue as possible in this patient with renal insufficiency.

FIGURE 12-66. Hypothenar hammer syndrome. This syndrome is caused by repetitive nonpenetrating trauma to the ulnar nerve and artery opposite the hook of the hamate leading to ulnar artery aneurysm formation. Presentation is either due to a pulsatile mass or digital thromboembolism. A thenar hammer syndrome affecting the radial artery as it crosses the first metacarpal has also been reported.

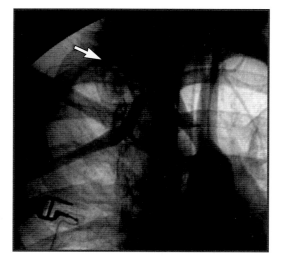

FIGURE 12-68.
Fusiform dilation of the axillary artery just lateral to the first thoracic rib in this patient who also has a cervical rib (*arrow*). This is a characteristic location, and appearance of arterial injury is associated with thoracic outlet syndrome (although neurologic and venous impingement are more common findings in this syndrome than is arterial impingement).

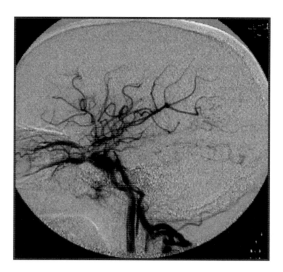

FIGURE 12-69.
Carotid-cavernous fistula. This patient suffered a motorcycle accident with head injury. Several weeks later he presented with visual disturbances including scotoma, eye pain, and exophthalmos. Cerebral angiogram demonstrates carotid-cavernous fistula that was later managed with detachable balloon embolization. (*Courtesy of* F. Huang-Hellinger.)

REFERENCES

1. Abrams HL: Historical notes. In *Abrams' Angiography*, edn 4. Edited by Baum S, Pentecost MJ. Boston: Little, Brown & Co; 1997:3–12.

2. Bettman MA: Radiographic contrast agents: history, chemistry, and variety. In *Abrams' Angiography*, edn 4. Edited by Baum S. Boston: Little, Brown & Co; 1997:13–21.

3. Dalen JE: When can treatment be withheld in patients with suspected pulmonary embolism? *Arch Intern Med* 1993, 153:1415–1418.

4. Worsley DF, Alavi A: Comprehensive analysis of the results of the PIOPED study. Prospective Investigation of Pulmonary Embolism Diagnosis Study.. *J Nucl Med* 1995, 36:2380–2387.

5. Stein PD, Athanasoulis C, Alavi A, *et al.*: Complications and validity of pulmonary angiography in acute pulmonary embolism. *Circulation* 1992, 85:462–468.

6. Wolfe MW, Skibo LK, Goldhaber SZ: Pulmonary embolic disease: diagnoses, pathophysiologic aspects and treatment with thrombolytic therapy. *Curr Prob Cardiol* 1993, vol:591–633.

7. Uflacker R, Strange C, Vujic I: Massive pulmonary embolism: preliminary results of treatment with the Amplatz thrombectomy device. *JVIR* 1996, 7:519–528.

8. Skibo L, Goldhaber SZ: Diagnosis of acute pulmonary embolism. In *Atlas of Heart Diseases: Cardiopulmonary Diseases and Cardiac Tumors*, vol 3. Edited by Braunwald E, Goldhaber SZ. Philadelphia: Current Medicine; 1995.

9. Sagel SS, Greenspan RH: Nonuniform pulmonary arterial perfusion. *Radiology* 1970, 99:541–548.

10. Remy-Jardin M, Remy J, Wattinne L, *et al.*: Central pulmonary thromboembolism: diagnosis with spiral volumetric CT with the single-breath-hold technique. Comparison with pulmonary angiography. *Radiology* 1992, 185:381–387.

11. Teigen CL, Maus TP, Sheedy PF II, *et al.*: Pulmonary embolism: diagnosis with electron beam CT. *Radiology* 1993, 188:839–845.

12. Oser RF, Zuckerman DA, Gutierrez FR, *et al.*: Anatomic distribution of pulmonary emboli at pulmonary angiography: implications for cross-sectional imaging. *Radiology* 1996, 199:31–35.

13. Remy-Jardin M, Remy J, Deschildre E, *et al.*: Diagnosis of pulmonary embolism with spiral CT: comparison with pulmonary angiography and scintigraphy. *Radiology* 1996, 200:699–702.

14. Mitchell SE: Inferior vena cava. In *Venous Interventional Radiology with Clinical Perspectives*. Edited by Savader SJ, Trerotola SO. New York: Thieme Verlag; 1996:285–297.

15. Park JH, Chung JW, Han JO, *et al.*: Interventional management of benign obstruction of the hepatic IVC. *JVIR* 1994, 5:403–409.

16. Lindner DJ, Edwards JM, Phinney ES, *et al.*: Long-term hemodynamic and clinical sequelae of lower extremity deep venous thrombosis. *J Vasc Surg* 1986, 4:436–442.

17. Comerota AJ, Aldridge SC, Cohen G, *et al.*: A strategy of aggressive regional therapy for acute iliofemoral venous thrombosis with contemporary venous thrombectomy or catheter-directed thrombolysis. *J Vasc Surg* 1994, 20:244–254.

18. Semba CP, Dake MD: Iliofemoral deep vein thrombosis: aggressive therapy with catheter-directed thrombolysis. *Radiology* 1994, 191:487–494.

19. LaBerge JM, Ring EJ, Gordon RL, *et al.*: Creation of transjugular intrahepatic portosystemic shunts with the Wallstent endoprosthesis: results in 100 patients. *Radiology* 1993, 187:413–423.

20. Matos C, Van Gansbeke D, Zaleman MM, *et al.*: Mesenteric venous thrombosis: early CT and US diagnosis and conservative management. *Gastrointestinal Radiol* 1986, 11:322–325.

21. Donaldson MC: Mesenteric vascular disease. In *Atlas of Heart Diseases: Vascular Disease*, vol 7. Edited by Braunwald E, Creager MA. Philadelphia: Current Medicine; 1995.

22. Harward TRS, Green D, Bergan JJ, *et al.*: Mesenteric venous thrombosis. *J Vasc Surg* 1989, 9:328–333.

23. Rholl KS: Percutaneous aortoiliac intervention in vascular disease. In *Abrams' Angiography*, vol 3. Edited by Baum S, Pentecost MJ. Boston: Little, Brown & Co; 1997:225–261.

24. Vorwerk D, Guenther RW, Schurmann K, *et al.*: Primary stent placement for chronic iliac artery occlusions: follow-up results in 103 patients. *Radiology* 1995, 194:745–749.

25. Long AL, Sapoval MR, Beyssen BM, *et al.*: Strecker stent implantation in iliac arteries: patency and predictive factors for long-term success. *Radiology* 1995, 194:739–744.

26. Martin EC: Transcatheter therapies in peripheral and noncoronary vascular diseases. *Circulation* 1991, 83(suppl 1):1–5.

27. May AG, DeWeese JA, Rob CG: Hemodynamic effects of arterial stenosis. *Surgery* 1963, 54:250.

28. Bull PG, Mendel IJ, Hold M, *et al.*: Distal popliteal and tibioperoneal transluminal angioplasty: long-term follow-up. *JVIR* 1992, 3:45–53.

29. Hirsch AT: Arterial occlusive diseases of the extremities. In *Atlas of Heart Diseases: Vascular Disease*, vol 7. Edited by Braunwald E, Creager MA. Philadelphia: Current Medicine; 1995.

30. Whittemore AD, Clowes AW, Couch NP, *et al.*: Secondary femoropopliteal reconstruction. *Ann Surg* 1981, 193:35–42.

31. Miller A, Salenius JP, Sacks BA, *et al.*: Noninvasive vascular imaging in the diagnosis and treatment of adventitial cystic disease of the popliteal artery. *J Vasc Surg* 1997, in press.

32. Pickering TG, Sos TA, Vaughn ED, *et al.*: Predictive value and changes of renin secretion in patients undergoing successful renal angioplasty. *Am J Med* 1984, 76:398–404.

33. Tegtmeyer CJ, Matsumoto AH, Johnson AM: Renal angioplasty. In *Abrams' Angiography*, vol 3. Edited by Baum S, Pentecost MJ. Boston: Little, Brown & Co; 1997:294–325.

34. Pickering TG: Renal vascular disease. In *Atlas of Heart Diseases: Vascular Disease*, vol 7. Edited by Braunwald E, Creager MA. Philadelphia: Current Medicine; 1995.

35. Sos TA, Pickering TG, Sniderman K, *et al.*: Percutaneous transluminal renal angioplasty in renovascular hypertension due to atheroma or fibromuscular dysplasia. *N Engl J Med* 1983, 309:274–279.

36. Pickering TG, Sos TA, Saddekni S: Renal angioplasty in patients with azotemia and renovascular hypertension. *J Hypertens* 1986, 4(suppl 6):S667–S669.

37. Kandarpa K, Chopra PS, Chakrabarti J, *et al.*:The vasculitides: current imaging and clinicopathologic correlations. *J Vasc Med Biol* 1991, 3:419–431.

38. Husted JW, Ring EJ, Hirsh LF: Intraarterial nitroprusside treatment for ergotism. *AJR Am J Roentgenol* 1978, 131:1090–1092.

39. Ambrose JA, Winters SL, Stern A, *et al.*: Angiographic morphology and the pathogenesis of unstable angina pectoris. *J Am Coll Cardiol* 1985, 5:609–616.

40. Powers ER: Coronary angiography. In *Atlas of Heart Diseases: Vascular Disease: Chronic Ischemic Heart Disease*, vol 5. Edited by Braunwald E, Beller GA. Philadelphia: Current Medicine; 1995.

41. Mark DB, Califf RM, Morris KG, *et al.*: Clinical characteristics and long-term survival of patients with variant angina. *Circulation* 1984, 69:880–888.

42. Abrams H: Angiography in coronary disease. In *Coronary Arteriography: A Practical Approach*. Edited by Abrams HL. Boston: Little, Brown & Co.; 1983:175–240.

43. Isselbacher EM, Cigarroa JE, Eagle KA: Aortic dissection. In *Atlas of Heart Diseases: Vascular Disease*, vol 7. Edited by Braunwald E, Creager MA. Philadelphia: Current Medicine; 1995.

44. Takahashi M, Schrieber RA, Wishner SH, *et al.*: Selective coronary arteriography in infants and children. *Circulation* 1983, 68:1021–1028.

45. Peterson MJ, Cambria RP, Kaufman JA, *et al.*: Magnetic resonance angiography in the preoperative evaluation of abdominal aortic aneurysms. *J Vasc Surg* 1995, 21:891–898.

46. Cigarroa JA, Isselbacher EM, DeSanctis RW, Eagle KA: Diagnostic imaging in the evaluation of suspected aortic dissection: old standards and new directions. *N Engl J Med* 1993, 328:35–43.

47. Sommer T, Fehske W, Holzknecht N, *et al.*: Aortic dissection: a comparative study of diagnosis with spiral CT, multiplanar transesophageal echocardiography and MR imaging. *Radiology* 1996, 199:347–352.

48. Creager MA, Halperin JL: Aortic and arterial aneurysms. In *Atlas of Heart Diseases: Vascular Disease*, vol 7. Edited by Braunwald E, Creager MA. Philadelphia: Current Medicine; 1995.

49. Creager MA, Halperin JL, Whittemore AD: Aneurysmal disease of the aorta and its branches. In *Vascular Medicine: A Textbook of Vascular Biology*. Edited by Loscalzo J, Creager MA, Dzau VJ. Boston: Little, Brown & Co.; 1992:903–930.

50. Whittemore AD, Mannick JA: Principles of vascular surgery. In *Vascular Medicine: A Textbook of Vascular Biology and Diseases*. Edited by Loscalzo J, Creager MA, Dzau VJ. Boston: Little, Brown & Co.; 1992:683–713.

51. Chopra PS, Kandarpa K: Arteritides: an angiographic perspective. *Applied Radiology* 1991:13.

Index